CLINICAL DECISION MAKING IN

Rehabilitatic

EFFICACY AND OUTCO

CLINICAL DECISION MAKING IN

Rehabilitation

E F F I C A C Y   A N D   O U T C O M E S

Edited by

John V. Basmajian, O.C., O.ONT., M.D., F.R.C.P.C.

Professor Emeritus of Medicine and Anatomy
Faculty of Health Sciences
McMaster University
Director Emeritus
Rehabilitation Centre
Chedoke-McMaster Hospital
Hamilton, Ontario, Canada

Sikhar N. Banerjee, M.B.B.S., F.R.C.P.C.

Professor
Department of Medicine
Dartmouth Medical School
Hanover, New Hampshire
Section Chief PM&R
Dartmouth-Hitchcock Medical Center
Lebanon, New Hampshire

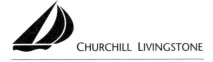 CHURCHILL LIVINGSTONE

New York, Edinburgh, London, Madrid, Melbourne, San Francisco, Tokyo

Library of Congress Cataloging-in-Publication Data

Clinical decision making in rehabilitation : efficacy and outcomes /
   edited by John V. Basmajian, Sikhar N. Banerjee.
         p.   cm.
      Includes bibliographical references and index.
      ISBN 0-443-08993-0
      1. Medical rehabilitation—Evaluation. I. Basmajian, John V. ,
   Date–   .   II. Banerjee, Sikhar Nath.
      [DNLM: 1. Rehabilitation—methods. 2. Outcome Assessment (Health
   Care)   3. Decision Making.   WB 320 C6414 1996]
   RM930.C56   1996
   617′ .03—dc20
   DNLM/DLC
   for Library of Congress   96-2745
                                                                      CIP

Distributed in the United Kingdom by Churchill Livingstone, Robert Stevenson
House, 1–3 Baxter's Place, Leith Walk, Edinburgh EH1 3AF, and by associated
companies, branches, and representatives throughout the world.

Accurate indications, adverse reactions, and dosage schedules for drugs are provided in this book, but it is possible that they may change. The reader is urged
to review the package information data of the manufacturers of the medications
mentioned.

The Publishers have made every effort to trace the copyright holders for bor-
rowed material. If they have inadvertently overlooked any, they will be pleased
to make the necessary arrangements at the first opportunity.

Acquisitions Editor: *Carol Bader*
Assistant Editor: *Ann Ruzycka*
Production Editor: *Robert M. Carmenini*
Production Supervisor: *Laura Mosberg Cohen*
Desktop Coordinator: *Alice Terry*
Cover Design: *Jeannette Jacobs*

Printed in the United States of America

First published in 1996   7   6   5   4   3   2   1

Contributors

Sikhar N. Banerjee, M.B.B.S., F.R.C.P.C.

Professor, Department of Medicine, Dartmouth Medical School, Hanover, New Hampshire; Section Chief PM&R, Dartmouth-Hitchcock Medical Center, Lebanon, New Hampshire

John V. Basmajian, O.C., O.ONT., M.D., F.R.C.P.C., F.R.C.P.S.(Glasg.), F.A.C.A., F.S.B.M., F.A.B.M.R., F.A.F.R.M.-R.A.C.P.(Australia), Hon.Dip.(St. L.C.)

Professor Emeritus of Medicine and Anatomy, Faculty of Health Sciences, McMaster University; Director Emeritus, Rehabilitation Centre, Chedoke-McMaster Hospital, Hamilton, Ontario, Canada

Ralph Bloch, M.D., Ph.D., F.R.C.P.(C.)

Professor, Institut für Aus-, Weiter-, und Fortbildung IAWF, Universität Bern, Medizinische Fakultät, Bern, Switzerland

Scott E. Brown, M.D.

Medical Director of Outpatient Rehabilitative Services, Department of Rehabilitation Medicine, Sinai Hospital of Baltimore, Baltimore, Maryland

Joan Crook, Ph.D., R.N.

Professor, School of Nursing, McMaster University School of Nursing, Hamilton, Ontario, Canada

Barbara J. de Lateur, M.D., M.S.

Professor and Lawrence Cardinal Shehan Chair of Rehabilitation Medicine, Department of Physical Medicine and Rehabilitation, Johns Hopkins University School of Medicine; Director, The Johns Hopkins Hospital, Baltimore, Maryland

M. Alan J. Finlayson, Ph.D., C.Psych.

Professor, Department of Psychiatry, Faculty of Health Sciences, McMaster University, Hamilton, Ontario, Canada; Executive Director, Columbia Neuro-rehab Centre, Toronto, Ontario, Canada

Scott H. Garner, M.D., F.R.C.P.(C.)

Associate Clinical Professor, Department of Medicine, Faculty of Health Sciences, McMaster University; Consultant, Acquired Brain Injury Program, Chedoke-McMaster Hospital, Hamilton, Ontario, Canada

Carolyn Gowland, M.H.Sc., P.T.

Associate Professor, School of Rehabilitation Science, Faculty of Health Sciences, McMaster University, Hamilton, Ontario, Canada

Virginia Graziani, M.D.

Assistant Professor, Department of Rehabilitation Medicine, Jefferson Medical College of Thomas Jefferson University, Philadelphia, Pennsylvania

Lawrence E. Hart, M.B.B.Ch., M.Sc., F.R.C.P.(C.), F.A.C.P., F.A.C.R.

Associate Professor, Department of Medicine, Faculty of Health Sciences, McMaster University; Director and Head of Rheumatic Disease Unit, Chedoke Division, Chedoke-McMaster Hospitals, Hamilton, Ontario, Canada

Ralph J. Marino, M.D.

Assistant Professor, Department of Rehabilitation Medicine, Jefferson Medical College of Thomas Jefferson University, Philadelphia, Pennsylvania

Robert S. McKelvie, M.Sc.(Physiology), M.D., F.R.C.P.C.

Career Scientist of the Ontario Ministry of Health; Associate Professor, Department of Medicine, Division of Cardiology, Faculty of Health Sciences, McMaster University; Medical Director of the Medical Diagnostic Unit, Hamilton Civic Hospitals, General Division, Hamilton, Ontario, Canada

David L. Sackett, F.R.S.C., M.D., F.R.C.P.(C.)

Professor of Clinical Epidemiology, Director, Nuffield Department of Clinical Medicine, NHS R&D Centre for Evidence-Based Medicine, Oxford University, Oxford, England; Formerly of Faculty of Health Sciences, McMaster University, Hamilton, Ontario, Canada

Karen M. Smith, M.D., F.R.C.P.C., F.A.C.R.M., F.A.B.E.M.

Associate Professor, Department of Rehabilitation Medicine, Queen's University Faculty of Medicine; Director of Regional Spinal and Brain Injury Rehabilitation Programs, Kingston General Hospital, Department of Rehabilitation, Kingston, Ontario, Canada

David G. Stubbing, M.B., M.S., M.R.C.P.(U.K.), F.R.C.P.(C.)

Associate Professor, Department of Medicine, Faculty of Health Sciences, McMaster University; Director, Respiratory Rehabilitation Program, Chedoke-McMaster Hospital, Hamilton, Ontario, Canada

Eldon Tunks, M.D., F.R.C.P.(C.)

Professor, Department of Psychiatry, Faculty of Health Sciences, McMaster University; Director of Pain Clinic, Chedoke-McMaster Hospital, Hamilton, Ontario, Canada

Preface

Many factors led to the writing of *Clinical Decision Making in Rehabilitation: Efficacy and Outcomes* but two predominate: (1) pressure from "outside" because of escalating health costs and (2) health clinicians' deep dissatisfaction with the current lack of valid evidence for many of their management methods (both old and new). The thinking clinician is fully aware that many state-of-the-art procedures are built on quicksand. Even in the lifetime of fairly recent graduates many hallowed ideas have been tossed out to be replaced by new dogma. These too may undergo the same fate in one generation.

The saying goes that "the practice of medicine is an art as well as a science." The art of medicine developed over centuries as teachers of medicine passed on their knowledge to their students who acted as apprentices to their masters. In this century, the allied professions had no choice but to adopt the same approach. Specific treatment methods were developed through experience from individual patients and keen observation of treatment effects. The scientific basis for the current practice of medicine and of rehabilitation grew after World War II when introduction of newer drugs and technologies revolutionized the practice of medicine.

As more and more newer treatment methods were introduced, the need for scientific evidence regarding efficacy of treatment methods became more evident. The exponential growth of the rehabilitation therapies and technologies since 1950 has depended almost equally on valid evidence of efficacy and on unquestioning acceptance of charismatic teaching. Skeptics are ignored, but often they have little evidence to base their rejections of widely accepted methods.

With increasing constraints on health-care resources, it is essential that finite resources are used efficiently. Obviously, paying agencies will continue to insist that they will only pay for treatment proven to be efficacious on the basis of scientific evidence. All rehabilitation professionals need to be aware of scientific evidence based on available literature regarding efficacy of their treatment methods.

This book is devoted to the analysis of the evidence in the literature in order to establish the level of efficacy of commonly employed rehabilitation management methods. Nothing is treated as sacred in analyzing the available evidence but care is taken not to reject treatments that hold some promise and are under current or proposed investigation. We recall the recent history of vascular surgery of carotid arteries for stroke patients and internal "mammary" implants into the myocardium. In both cases, extensive investigation proved them ineffective. On the other hand, we can cite the successful adoption of self-catheterization by paraplegic patients, a technique opposed by many clinicians until the overwhelming research evidence came into play.

Unfortunately, research results for many accepted procedures are absent to some degree, ranging from total absence to spotty and scattered results. While such evidence is gathered, we must make clinical choices of therapies. Even doing nothing or stopping a treatment are choices which may do harm or good or nothing at all. Certainly every thoughtful clinician should choose this avenue of approach but then must keep a watch for results in individual patients and to the mixed results obtained with a series of similar patients. If fortune smiles, the clinician may find evidence in the literature supporting individual decisions—perhaps in this book.

As clinicians and scientists, the editors have been preparing unknowingly for two decades to write or edit such a book. One of us (SB) has become immersed in epidemiologic and statistical analyses of clinical efficacy while the other (JB) has conducted many controlled trials of pharmaceutical and physical agents. We recruited a team of contributors on the basis of their expert knowledge of the chapter topic and their willingness to accept our stringent orders to follow an explicit pathway of practical importance to our readers. Then we edited ruthlessly to ensure compliance.

The editors called for firm guidelines and definitions (wherever possible) from each author of first degree and second degree evidence for the decision-making process. We here will re-emphasize the strong point of Chapter 1, that is, decision making by a clinician must be made with whatever is available for guidance. More often than not, clear evidence does not exist, certainly not solid proof of the level of efficacy from double-blind research studies. The effective clinician makes the best choice under the circumstances, so serving the patient optimally.

John V. Basmajian,
O.C., O.ONT., M.D., F.R.C.P.C.

Sikhar N. Banerjee,
M.B.B.S., F.R.C.P.C.

Acknowledgments

With genuine pleasure and admiration, we thank our previously innocent authors who shed their innocence as they labored to fulfill our imposing demands. Sometimes boldly and, at other times, timorously they ventured into the mine field. Avoiding the air of dogma that they were sniffing out in the field, they have done all who have an interest in it a great service in the here and now. They have set precedents for the future that must not be ignored.

Contents

1. Levels of Evidence and Clinical Decision Making in Rehabilitation / **1**
David L. Sackett

2. Stroke / **5**
Carolyn Gowland and
John V. Basmajian

3. Spinal Cord Injury / **19**
Karen M. Smith, Ralph J. Marino,
and Virginia Graziani

4. Traumatic Brain Injury / **41**
Scott H. Garner and M. Alan J. Finlayson

5. Low Back Pain / **55**
Diagnostic Approach / **55**
Ralph Bloch

   Nonsurgical Treatment of Acute Low Back Pain / **68**
Sikhar N. Banerjee

6. Persistent Pain / **93**
Eldon Tunks and Joan Crook

7. Chronic Airflow Limitation / **119**
David G. Stubbing

8. Cardiac Rehabilitation / **141**
Robert S. McKelvie

9. Lower Extremity Amputations / **153**
Sikhar N. Banerjee

10. Muscle Disease / **171**
Exercise and Orthotics / **171**
Barbara J. de Lateur

    Pharmacologic Treatment / **187**
Scott E. Brown

11. Arthritis / **203**
Lawrence E. Hart

12. Many Challenges Remain / **223**
John V. Basmajian

Index / **229**

1

Levels of Evidence and Clinical Decision Making in Rehabilitation

David L. Sackett

What rules of evidence should apply when experts generate recommendations for the clinical management of patients? Should only the thoroughly validated results of randomized clinical trials be admissible to avoid or minimize the application of useless or harmful therapy? Or, to maximize the potential benefits to patients (including those possible from unproved remedies), should a synthesis of the experiences of seasoned clinicians form the basis for such recommendations? Ample precedent exists for the latter approach, even when attempts are made to replace it.[1] For the following reasons, however, the nonexperimental evidence that forms the recalled experiences of seasoned clinicians will tend to overestimate efficacy:

1. Clinicians are more likely to recognize and remember favorable treatment responses when their patients comply with treatments and keep follow-up appointments. There are five documented instances in which compliant patients in the placebo groups of randomized trials exhibited far more favorable outcomes (including survival) than their noncompliant companions.[2-6] Therefore, because high compliance is a marker for better outcomes, even when treatment is useless, our uncontrolled clinical experiences often cause us to conclude that compliant patients must have been receiving efficacious therapy.
2. Unusual patterns of symptoms (e.g., transient ischemic attacks) or signs (e.g., high blood pres-

sure levels) and extreme laboratory test results, when they are reassessed even a short time later, tend to return toward the more usual, normal result.[7] Because of this universal tendency of "regression toward the mean," any therapy that is initiated (regardless of efficacy in the interim) will appear efficacious.
3. Routine clinical practice is never "blind," and both patients and their clinicians know when active treatment is underway. As a result, both the placebo effect (which has shown, for example, that angina pectoris can be relieved by mock internal mammary ligation[8]) and the desire of patients and clinicians for success can cause both parties to overestimate efficacy.

For these reasons, the "consensus" approach based on uncontrolled clinical experience risks precipitating the widespread application of treatments that are useless or even harmful. These same treatments are much less likely to be judged efficacious in double-blind, randomized trials than in an uncontrolled series of unblinded, "open" comparisons with contemporaneous or historical series of patients; hence the maxim: Therapeutic reports with controls tend to have no enthusiasm, and reports with enthusiasm tend to have no controls.

The foregoing discussion is not a mandate for discarding the large body of uncontrolled observations by clinicians who have used various treatments in an effort to assist the rehabilitation of their patients.

In many instances, randomized controlled trials have never been (and, arguably, never could be) carried out, and the only information base for generating some of the recommendations comes from uncontrolled clinical observations.

Nevertheless, it is important to base firm recommendations (and especially those involving risk to patients) on the results of rigorously controlled investigations and to be much more circumspect when counsel is based only on the results of uncontrolled clinical observations. The editors and authors of this book adopted this approach, which in turn led to the definition and adoption of both Levels of Evidence and Grades of Recommendations.

LEVELS OF EVIDENCE

The editors have suggested that the authors of this book, when summarizing what was known about the rehabilitation of a given clinical entity, should specify the level of evidence that was being used in each case according to the following classification.

Level I

Level I evidence consists of randomized trials with low false-positive (α) and/or low false-negative (β) errors (high power). A low false-positive (α) error applies to a "positive" trial that demonstrated a statistically significant benefit from experimental treatment. For example, Bracken et al.[9] randomized patients with acute spinal cord injuries to receive methylprednisolone, naloxone, or placebo. Patients randomized to methylprednisolone developed statistically significantly better motor power and sensation after 6 months compared with patients randomized to placebo.

A low false-negative (β) error (high power) applies to a "negative" trial that demonstrated either no effect of therapy or no difference between therapies, but was large enough to exclude the possibility of a clinically important benefit of active treatment over placebo, or of one active treatment over another (i.e., had very narrow 95 percent confidence limits that excluded any clinically important difference between treatment groups).

Level II

Level II evidence consists of randomized trials with high false-positive (α) and/or high false-negative (β) errors (low power). A "high false-positive (α) error" refers to a trial with an interesting positive trend that is not statistically significant. For example, in the aforementioned spinal cord injury trial,[9] some of the results among patients treated with naloxone appeared promising, but were not statistically significant.

A "high false-negative (β) error (low power)" applies to a "negative" trial that concluded therapy was not efficacious or that two treatments had similar efficacy. Because the trial involved small numbers of patients, however, the possibility of a clinically important benefit or difference between agents could not be excluded (i.e., wide 95 percent confidence limits on the contrast between treatment groups).

The advent of meta-analysis has had a major impact on levels of evidence. It allows two or more high-quality, homogeneous but small (and therefore Level II) trials to be converted into a single Level I overview.

Subgroup Analyses in Randomized Trials: A Special Note

Writers and readers of trial reports may be tempted to conclude that the efficacy of rehabilitative maneuvers differs in clinically important ways between subgroups of patients as defined by the etiology or severity of their conditions, the time between the onset of their symptoms and the administration of rehabilitative maneuvers, or other baseline features. Such subgroup analysis, especially when it is carried out in exploratory data "dredging," often leads to false-positive conclusions (that subgroups differ in their responsiveness to treatment when they do not). For this reason, decisions on whether apparent differences in subgroup responses are real should require positive answers to questions such as the following seven suggested by Oxman and Guyatt.[10]

1. Is the magnitude of the difference in subgroup responses clinically important (so that it would

lead to different treatment recommendations for each subgroup)?

2. Was the difference in subgroup responses statistically significant?

3. Did a hypothesis that the subgroups ought to differ precede rather than follow the analysis? This is a key point. For example, in the spinal cord injury trial,[9] methylprednisolone was effective only when started within 8 hours of the injury; thereafter it was ineffective. This conclusion is credible because it was based on a hypothesis stated before the trial was undertaken; it also satisfies several of the other guides listed here.

4. Was this subgroup analysis one of a small number of subgroup analyses performed in the study (1 in 20 of which should be significant by chance alone)?

5. Was the difference in subgroup responses suggested by comparisons within a study (as opposed to between two studies)?

6. Was the difference in subgroup responses consistent across two or more studies?

7. Is there indirect (e.g., biologic) evidence to support the hypothesized difference in subgroup responsiveness?

Level III

Level III evidence consists of nonrandomized concurrent cohort comparisons between contemporaneous patients who did and did not receive a rehabilitative maneuver. In Level III, the outcomes of patients who received and complied with a rehabilitative maneuver would be compared with those of contemporaneous patients who did not receive these same treatments (e.g., because of refusal, noncompliance, contraindication, local practice, nonavailability, or oversight). The biases described previously usually apply here. For example, the demonstration that stroke patients treated in a special stroke unit (when beds were available) fared better than contemporaneous patients treated on general medical wards (when the stroke unit was full) leaves substantial room for concern that subtle prognostic factors in patients presenting with stroke may have unconsciously influenced the vigor with which stroke unit beds were emptied to make room for them.[11]

Level IV

Level IV evidence consists of nonrandomized historical cohort comparisons between current patients who did receive a rehabilitation maneuver and former patients (from the same institution or from the literature) who did not. In this case, the outcomes of patients who received the maneuver (as a result of a local treatment policy) are compared with those of patients treated in an earlier era or at another institution (when and where different treatment policies prevailed). To the biases presented earlier, we must add those that result from inappropriate comparisons over time and space.

Level V

In the Level V approach—case series without controls—, the reader is simply informed about the fate of a group of patients. This series may contain extremely useful information about clinical course and prognosis, but can only hint at efficacy. For example, remarkably few complications were observed among a group of patients who had practiced long-term intermittent urethral self-catheterization, but the study sample composed only 9 percent of patients using this maneuver at hospital discharge, and there were no control subjects.[12]

THE GRADING OF RECOMMENDATIONS

Finally, the authors of this book were encouraged by the editors to classify their ultimate recommendations on the use of rehabilitation maneuvers into three grades, depending on the level of evidence used to generate them. The three grades of recommendations are (Table 1-1):

Grade A: Supported by at least one, and preferably more, Level I randomized trial(s).

Grade B: Supported by at least one Level II randomized trial.

Grade C: Supported only by Level III, IV, or V evidence.

Table 1-1. The Relation Between Levels of Evidence and Grades of Recommendations

Level of Evidence	Grade of Recommendation
Level I: Large randomized trials with clear-cut results (and low risk of error)	Grade A
Level II: Small randomized trials with uncertain results (and moderate to high risk of error).	Grade B
Level III: Nonrandomized, contemporaneous controls	Grade C
Level IV: Nonrandomized, historical controls	Grade C
Level V: No controls; case series only	Grade C

It is hoped that advances in our understanding of both these treatments and the mechanisms of the disorders in which they are applied will be matched by more Level I evidence in the future; such advances will be reflected in an ever-greater proportion of Grade A recommendations.

REFERENCES

1. National Institutes of Health Consensus Development Conferences: 1:1, 1977–1978
2. Coronary Drug Project Research Group: Influence of adherence treatment and response of cholesterol on mortality in the Coronary Drug Project. N Engl J Med 303:1038, 1980
3. Asher WL, Harper HW: Effect of human chorionic gonadotropin on weight loss, hunger, and felling of well-being. Am J Clin Nutr 26:211, 1973
4. Hogarty GE, Goldberg E: Drug and sociotherapy in the aftercare of schizophrenic patients. Arch Gen Psychiatry 28:54, 1973
5. Fuller R, Roth H, Long S: Compliance with disulfram treatment of alcoholism. J Chronic Dis 36:161, 1983
6. Pizzo PA, Robichaud KJ, Edwards BK et al: Oral antibiotic prophylaxis in patients with cancer: a double-blind randomized placebo-controlled trial. J Pediatr 102:125, 1983
7. Sackett DL, Haynes RB, Guyatt GH, Tugwell P: Clinical Epidemiology: A Basic Science for Clinical Medicine. 2nd Ed., Little, Brown, Boston, 1991
8. Cobb LA, Thomas GI, Dillard DH et al: An evaluation of internal-mammary-artery ligation by a double-blind technique. N Engl J Med 260:1115, 1959
9. Bracken MB, Shepard MJ, Collins WF et al: A randomized, controlled trial of methylprednisolone or naloxone in the treatment of acute spinal cord injury. N Engl J Med 322:1405, 1990
10. Oxman AD, Guyatt GH: A consumer's guide to subgroup analysis. Ann Intern Med 116:78, 1992
11. Strand T, Asplund K, Eriksson S et al: Stroke unit care—who benefits? Stroke 17:377, 1986
12. Kuhn W, Rist M, Zaech GA: Intermittent urethral self-catheterisation: long-term results. Paraplegia 29:222, 1991

2

Stroke

Carolyn Gowland
John V. Basmajian

The rehabilitation literature is full of gloomy statistics about stroke; they require no reiteration here. In this chapter we venture to the somewhat brighter side of the picture—the strides made in improving the outcomes for survivors—those who only a generation ago faded into the shadows of society and beyond. We are at the beginning of a crusade to find new ways and to improve old ways for stroke management. Much more must be done, but this chapter offers more optimism than pessimism, although both are woven into its fabric.

We must acknowledge the enormous help provided by an excellent publication by the Agency for Health Care Policy and Research of the US Department of Health and Human Services in preparing this chapter. Their "Clinical Practice Guideline No. 16: Poststroke Rehabilitation" (Guideline 16)[1] strongly indicates the importance of the rehabilitation team, including the patient, family, and other caregivers. We will draw on the guideline throughout this chapter.

Over the years, the Chedoke-McMaster Stroke Team evolved a clinical decision-making paradigm for use in stroke rehabilitation. This paradigm was first published as the clinical management process for the "Assessment and Treatment of Physical Impairments Leading to Disability after Brain Injury" in 1994.[2] This process is similar to that recommended in the newly released Guideline 16 noted previously.

CLIENT-CENTERED AND EVIDENCE-BASED PRACTICE

The principles underlying client-centered practice arose from the consumer rights movement of the 1970s. Consumers or clients, in response to receiving services they often deemed ineffective and overpriced, are now demanding services that in their view meet their *needs* and are of *value*. To make intelligent choices, clients, which in stroke rehabilitation includes not only the patient but the family and caregivers, need appropriate information and should be, as much as possible, actively involved in decision making at every step in the process. It must be stressed that both clients and others paying for services are willing to pay for or endure only those aspects of rehabilitation care they deem valuable or that will have a significant effect on things of value. Examples of these services include (1) the ability to independently toilet—probably the single most motivating need; (2) improved "function," which according to most patients with stroke means walking, speaking, and arm function; (3) improved ability to carry out self-care activities; (4) improved "quality of life," which often equates with ability to cope, sense of empowerment and control, satisfactory adjustment to disability, satisfaction with life and with the health care received, and the ability to access services. Family and caregivers tend to voice the degree of burden, independence in self-care, cognition, and behavior as primary considerations.[1] Guideline 16 additionally notes important examples of attributes of value such as survival, normalized health patterns (such as nutrition, continence, and sleep), freedom from pain and emotional distress, independence in complex daily functions and social roles, and successful family function.

As important as client-centered practice is to rehabilitation, it has a limitation: it focuses only on the needs of clients, not on their ability to have these needs met, that is, to *benefit* from the services provided. Evidence-based practice, on the other hand, focuses on what can be changed, that is, on the ability of the client to *benefit* from the services and interventions provided. The development and use of evidence in the process of clinical decision making are fundamental to the provision of cost-effective rehabilitation care. The most classic example of this concept in stroke deals with the function of the arm and hand. Clearly no one would contest a patient's need for a functional arm. However, evidence-based practice provides essential information about the likelihood of rehabilitation being able to address this need. In the majority of patients with a completed stroke resulting in paralysis of the hand, function is not a realistic goal and cannot be achieved. Hence the ability to adjust to and cope with such a loss, which is often achievable with humane advice and practical help, is often overlooked as the primary goal that would be most beneficial.

Information about the ability of clients to benefit from services, along with the choice of intervention, should be determined from the best available scientific evidence regarding effectiveness and cost-effectiveness.[3] This information comes from three sources: valid theory, evidence in the research literature, and demonstration in the clinical setting.

First, rehabilitation should be based on valid theories and sound theoretical models.[4] As a result of the development and testing of scientific theories, the body of knowledge focusing on the underlying mechanisms of impairments, disabilities, and handicaps will be advanced and applied to the development of new and appropriate intervention strategies. However, therapy derived only by induction from a valid theory may not be effective, and demonstrating the validity of the theoretical rationale does not provide adequate evidence of effectiveness.

The second information source, and currently the most valid, is direct evidence of effectiveness arising from clinical effectiveness studies.[3]

A, B, and C Levels of Evidence

The scheme for appraising the level of evidence that was originally developed by Sackett[5] was modified for the Guideline 16.[1] For stroke rehabilitation, the levels of evidence are defined as follows:

A Level: Supported by the results of two or more randomized controlled trials (RCTs) that have good internal validity, and also specifically address the question of interest in group of patients comparable to the one to which the recommendation applies (external validity).
B Level: Supported by a single RCT meeting the criteria given above for A-level evidence, by RCTs that only indirectly address the questions of interest, or by two or more nonrandomized clinical trials (case control or cohort studies) in which the experimental and control groups are demonstrably similar or multivariate analyses have effectively controlled for group differences.
C Level: Supported by a single non-RCT meeting the criteria for B-level evidence, by studies using historical controls, or by studies using quasiexperimental designs such as pretreatment and posttreatment comparisons.

The literature often fails to provide adequate information about effective therapy for systematic or specific use. In those cases, a third source of information is usually relied on—direct evidence of effectiveness gained in the clinical setting. To select treatment interventions, clinicians often must extrapolate what might be effective from their experience with other patients and from what is reported in books and articles by experts in the field. When thoughtful consensus is obtained, this form of evidence becomes more powerful. The power of clinical evidence is increasing even more as we derive it from the use of standardized measures and databases, combining these data with those of other facilities and compiling results to provide information.

In Guideline 16, evidence on effectiveness from the literature is used in conjunction with expert consensus. This approach is both appropriate and popular, but will be enhanced by the provision of sound evidence from the clinical setting. Guideline 16 addresses this needed change by recommending that "Rehabilitation programs should maintain up-to-date information on staffing patterns, services offered, and quality indicators and outcomes and should make this information widely available to health care providers, medical facilities, and the public. Health care providers and hospitals who refer patients to rehabilitation programs should be knowledgeable about the capabilities of programs in their communities."[1]

WHO CLASSIFICATION OF IMPAIRMENT, DISABILITY AND HANDICAP: A BASIS FOR DECISION MAKING

The task of managing the rehabilitation of stroke victims cannot be undertaken without a mechanism for classifying patient problems. The World Health Organization's (WHO) International Classification of Impairment, Disability and Handicap (ICIDH),[6] provides a useful framework for such a purpose. The key terms in this classification are defined as follows:

Impairment: Any loss or abnormality of psychological, physiologic or anatomic structure or function.
Disability: Any restriction or lack of ability to perform an activity in a manner or within the range considered normal. Disability represents a departure from the norm in terms of performance of the individual, as opposed to that of an organ or mechanism.
Handicap: A disadvantage for a given individual, resulting from an impairment or a disability, that limits or prevents the fulfillment of a role that is normal for that individual (depending on age, sex, and social and cultural factors).

Generally speaking, patients are motivated by their degree of handicap. When mild impairments or disabilities do not interfere with an individual's ability to carry out normal roles, there may be no perceived need for services. Patients who can fulfill all of their expected roles in life, that is, patients with no handicap, even in the presence of an impairment or disability, may not be motivated to comply with therapeutic regimens. The major reason for seeking help relates to some breakdown in ability to perform one's roles. When the degree of handicap is great, the most effective approach to addressing the problems may be at the level of impairment or disability. For example, improving the balance of a patient can have a considerable impact on the ability to walk and even the ability to carry out social roles.

MEASUREMENT

The Purposes of Measures

Generally speaking, there are three main purposes to assess health status: (1) to discriminate (diagnose or classify) among patients, (2) to predict future status, and (3) to evaluate outcome or the effectiveness of interventions.[7] In stroke rehabilitation, as elsewhere in health care, properly constructed, valid, and reliable measures are needed for all these purposes.

Discriminant Measures

Feinstein et al.[8] noted that reliable and valid assessments that incorporate classification of individuals into homogeneous subgroups foster logical prediction, treatment, and evaluation decisions. In the call for action of the National Symposium on Methodological Issues in Stroke Outcome Research, Basmajian[9] reinforced the need to discriminate among individuals with stroke. Such measures are particularly important in this condition where the clinical characteristics, severity of involvement, and natural history vary widely. Within any single class, the patients should have common problems, prognoses, and treatment goals.

Predictive Measures

Initial assessments should provide information about significant prognostic variables so that you are able to predict high-risk subgroups, subgroups suitable for specialized care, the amount of change, and the expected outcome. Prediction plays a more important role when reliable predictive equations are available. When impairment is predicted to be permanent, goals should concentrate on the minimization of disability and handicap. Prediction also plays an important role in the identification of high risk subgroupings of patients within our case loads. The identification of who is at high risk for severe shoulder pain, for example, is an essential piece of information when deciding how to allocate precious resources. A major part of the unique body of knowledge and specialized practice relates to the remediation of impairment. The clinical evaluation system can aid in determining when remediation is realistic.

Evaluative Measures

The measurement of outcomes is rapidly becoming a standard of rehabilitation practice. An assessment used to determine whether change has *taken place over time* should be capable of detecting important clinical change (i.e., change which is of value to the clients when such change exists, and "no change" states when the patient remains stable). This property is referred to as responsiveness. The extent to which the instrument can responsively detect meaningful change is an important consideration when evaluating the effectiveness of therapeutic interventions or programs. Typically, outcome measures should have this property.

Predicting Risk-Adjusted Outcomes

The usefulness of outcome information can be enhanced when the actual outcomes can be compared to expected outcomes. This comparison is possible when an accurate outcome prediction is made at the outset. In addition, the ability to estimate expected outcomes at the time of admission can substantially enhance program and discharge planning. In stroke, outcomes are known to be predictable but highly variable among individuals. This variability among patients is due to many factors, not least of which is the severity of the stroke, and hence the degree of impairment and disability. The proposed solution to dealing with this variability when interpreting the true impact of services is to develop and use *risk-adjusted outcomes* as a routine

part of program management. To achieve this goal, predictive equations composed of weighted risk or prognostic indicators can often be used to explain a significant amount of the variance in outcomes.[10] These predictions can be used to adjust for expected change when planning interventions and evaluating outcomes.

Standardized Measures with Appropriate Psychometric Properties

Standards for the use of measures in rehabilitation have been developed by the Advisory Group on Measurement Standards of the American Congress of Rehabilitation Medicine.[11] Assessments using standardized measures should be performed by professionals appropriately trained and experienced in their use.

The Quick Reference Guide for Clinicians in Guideline 16 lists preferred standard instruments for patient assessment in stroke. The source of the instrument, the approximate time to administer it, and its strengths and weaknesses are listed. Since the preparation of the guideline, the Chedoke-McMaster Stroke Assessment has been published.[10] This measure has been developed and validated with consideration of all the concepts on measurement. For example, the validation studies include determination of what was valued in rehabilitation by clients after the patient had been home for 6 to 24 months. It also provides equations for predicting and risk-adjusting outcomes.

CLINICAL DATA SET FOR STROKE REHABILITATION

The purpose of a clinical database is to enhance clinical decision making, both as it relates to individual clients and for various aspects of program evaluation. The Uniform Data Set for Medical Rehabilitation (UDS$_{MR}$) is an example of a data set contained within a database. The UDS$_{MR}$ was developed as a minimum data set that would include only common and useful client functional attributes. It is intended to be discipline-free and acceptable to clinicians, administrators, and researchers in rehabilitation. The UDS$_{MR}$ includes the Functional Independence Measure (Adult FIM), a valid and reliable measure of client function and burden on caregiver.[12]

A data set is "nothing more than a collection of information, including client demographics and the scores from standardized measures."[13] A database can be defined as simply "data from a data set organized for rapid search and retrieval (as by a computer)."[13] For clinicians not familiar with databases or data sets, it is important to distinguish between a database and a measure. A database is merely a system for collecting data; unlike a measure, it need not be standardized and issues of validity and reliability are not relevant. The data fields that make up the set may be altered as needed.

Patient information relating to the *clinical decision-making paradigm* that considers the delivery of patient care from first encounter to last follow-up is measured. During initial stages in the rehabilitation process, data are needed to manage the patient's problems. This information includes various factors that mediate the disabilities and handicaps. The purpose of the initial data set is to document the patient's problems. Thus, data on the various factors that mediate disabilities and handicaps should be considered. Included should be initial data on physical impairments; client demographics; outcome determinants; cognitive, communication, and behavioral status; and relating disabilities and handicaps. In conjunction with subsequent assessments, the initial assessment provides for the evaluation of change. Cost-effective practice dictates that the time spent on gathering findings is unjustified unless the information is needed for goal setting, selection of treatment, or the evaluation of outcome.

Contents of the Data Set

Table 2-1 lists common problems to consider when developing a stroke data set.

REHABILITATION IN THE ACUTE SETTING

Based on expert consensus, Guideline 16 has several recommendations that relate to rehabilitation management in the acute setting. First, it recommends that whenever possible, patients with acute

Table 2-1. Stroke Rehabilitation Data Set

Disorder
  Medical history
  Medical status
  Neurologic status
  Prognostically important comorbidity such as coronary disease, diabetes, mental deterioration, personality disorder
  Prognostically important complications and comorbidity secondary to stroke such as depression, dysphagia and aspiration, sleep disturbance, falls, skin breakdown, hemianopsia, deep vein thrombosis, urinary tract infection, contractures
Impairments
  Sensorimotor: postural control and balance, voluntary movements (including gait), sensation, tone/spasticity, range of motion, strength, coordination, involuntary movements
  Shoulder and central (thalamic) pain
  Speech and language
  Swallowing
  Cognition and emotion
  Perception
  Depression
Disabilities
  Functional independence in self-care, bowel and bladder care, mobility including gross motor function, walking and other forms of locomotion, communication, behavior
  Personal attributes such as ability to cope, sense of empowerment and control, adjustment to disability, satisfaction (with life and health care), ability to make informed decisions, ability to access services
Activities of daily living including automobile driving
  Arm and hand function
  Fitness
  Burden on caregivers
Handicaps
  Occupational
  Recreational
  Family (including sexual)
  Societal
Discharge Planning
  Living environment
  Available financial resources
  Available social and community supports
  Available family and caregiver support
  Vocational potential

strokes should receive coordinated diagnostic, acute management, preventive, and rehabilitative services.[1] Second, patients who survive the acute stroke and their families should be thoroughly instructed in the effects and prognosis of the stroke, potential complications, and the needs and rationales for treatments.[1] Third, discharge planning should begin at the time of admission. Goals are to determine the need for rehabilitation, arrange the best possible living environment, and ensure continuity of care after discharge.[1]

CHOOSING A REHABILITATION SETTING

Both Guideline 16 and the Cochrane Database of Systematic Reviews have conducted a literature review to determine the relative benefit of specialized stroke units over general medical care.[1,14] Of the 19 studies that were reviewed, the majority were randomized clinical trials.[15–33] The overall conclusion from these reviews is that "stroke patients managed within specialist stroke units are more likely to be alive and living at home a year after the stroke than those managed in general medical wards. Stroke unit care does not apparently increase the time spent in hospital. Based on strong consensus, Guideline 16 recommends that screening for possible admission to a rehabilitation unit should be performed as soon as the patient's neurologic and medical condition permits. "Patients who are medically unstable are generally not suitable for any type of rehabilitation program."[1]

Guideline 16 further examined the evidence on the benefits of early activation of stroke patients.[1] Although none of the studies reviewed[19,34,35] were randomized trials, they concluded that "patients with an acute stroke should be mobilized as soon after admission as is medically feasible." They further recommend that patients should be encouraged to perform self-care activities as soon as medically feasible.

Not all patients require the intensive services of a specialized stroke unit. Alternative forms of rehabilitation, including rehabilitation in nursing facilities, outpatient and day-hospital rehabilitation, and home rehabilitation, are becoming more common. Increasingly, authors,[36] have reported improved survival and greater likelihood of returning home with appropriate multidisciplinary team care given as soon as the acute phase is drawing to an end. Based on summarizing the results of seven studies,[27,37–42] five of which were randomized trials, Guideline 16 recommends that "admission to an interdisciplinary rehabilitation program should generally be limited to patients with disabilities in two or more of the following areas of function: mobility, performance of the basic activities of daily living, bowel or bladder control, cognition, emotional functioning, pain management, swallowing, and communication."[1] Recent publications by Gladman et al.[43] found that when home services included the rehabilitation team, they were often preferred by younger patients while the frail elderly benefited more from day hospital attendance.

STEPS IN THE CLINICAL DECISION-MAKING PROCESS

This section describes the nine steps in the clinical decision-making process (Fig. 2-1) we have developed for use in rehabilitation regardless of the setting.

Step 1: Gather Initial Data

The primary purpose of the initial assessment is to provide the baseline data needed to define the nature and severity of problems in terms that will aid in the selection of relevant interventions. Additionally, this assessment must provide the data needed to predict outcomes, to plan treatments, and to evaluate functional outcomes. Well-standardized measures of impairment, disability, and handicap should be selected by rehabilitation professionals trained in their administration. The ability to distinguish between classes of patients is important for identifying appropriate treatments. The content of the initial assessment is outlined in the stroke rehabilitation data set listed previously in the section on measurement. The exact content and the specific measures are determined by the setting and overall objectives of the program within that setting.

Based on a consensus of expert opinion, Guideline 16 recommends that the rehabilitation team should complete a baseline assessment for most patients within 3 working days after admission to an intense rehabilitation program in an inpatient rehabilitation facility or nursing facility, within 1 week of admission to a low-intensity nursing facility program, or within three visits for an outpatient or home rehabilitation program. Initial evaluation by a physician and a nurse, including medical and neurologic examinations completed within 24 hours of admission or, in the case of outpatient and home programs, on the first visit. All information should be fully documented in the patient's record. Discharge planning should begin at the time of the admission, be carried out by the multiple members of the rehabilitation team, and should intimately involve the patient and family.

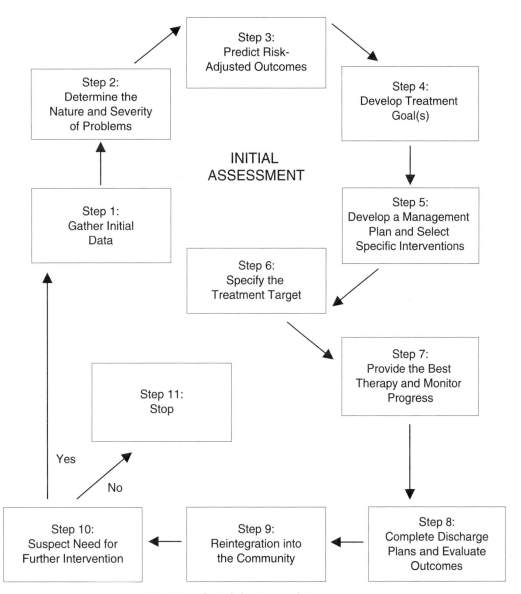

Fig. 2-1. Clinical decision-making process.

Step 2: Determine the Nature and Severity of the Problems

From the data gathered in the initial assessment, the nature and severity of a patient's impairment problems are identified. The importance of these impairments and their interactions with each other, particularly cognition, communication, and behavior, are then considered along with the patient's disabilities, handicaps, resources, and potential for change.

Step 3: Predict Risk-Adjusted Outcomes

Knowledge of the patient's prognostically significant signs, symptoms, characteristics, and behaviors can help predict probable outcome. These determinants of outcome can be grouped into three categories: those independent of the episode or disorder (e.g., age, premorbid fitness, personal preferences, and motivation), those related to the disease itself (e.g., type and extent of brain damage), and those that reflect the pattern of recovery (e.g., stage of recovery and duration of motor paralysis).

Using known statistically significant prognostic indicators the following should be predicted:

1. Status at the completion of the rehabilitation program
2. Who is at high risk for specific complications (e.g., moderate to severe shoulder pain)
3. Who will require specialized care (e.g., functional training of the upper limb)

When available, such as with the Chedoke-McMaster Stroke Assessment,[10] equations for predicting risk-adjusted outcomes for individual patients can be used. Such equations result from systematic literature review, followed by the gathering of clinical data, which is then subjected to regression analysis to identify equations with the highest possible statistical significance and predictive validity.[44] Using such equations, a clinician can estimate probable outcomes. These predicted outcomes, in conjunction with clinical judgment, provide the basis for selecting an appropriate therapeutic program or intervention and for evaluating the effectiveness of interventions and programs.

A note of warning when using predictive equations: These tools *provide information only for enhancing clinical judgment* and should not be the only consideration when goal setting. We recommend that treatment goals aim to surpass, not just meet, predicted values. However, prognosis must be considered when selecting treatment goals, planning preventative strategies, and advising the family. The provision of weeks of intensive therapy aimed at the cure of likely permanent impairments not only is an inefficient use of clinician time, but also could prevent the patient from learning compensatory strategies to help make a satisfactory adjustment to permanent impairment.

Step 4: Develop Treatment Goals

Sackett, et al.[13] remind us that the successful accomplishment of three tasks leads to the rational treatment of any patient: (1) identify the goals of treatment, (2) select the specific treatment, and (3)

Table 2-2. The Eight Ultimate Goals of Treatment

Remediate
  1. Remediate the underlying disorder or impairments
  2. Relieve current symptoms
  3. Remediate disabilities
Prevent
  4. Prevent recurrent strokes
  5. Prevent secondary disorders, impairments, and disability
Compensate and Adapt
  6. Train patients to compensate for disabilities and handicaps
  7. Adapt the environment and train caregivers in the management of permanent disabilities and handicaps
  8. Optimize patient and family adjustment to permanent disability and handicap

specify the treatment target. Within the impairment, disability and handicap classification, the perspective of goal setting is shifted from the medical model, which emphasizes curing the underlying disorder, to a multifaceted rehabilitation model, which considers prevention, remediation, restoration, adaptation, and adjustment. Although the ultimate goal is optimal function and adjustment,[4] treatment aimed at minimizing or curing the underlying impairments is the first priority of rehabilitation; postural control and voluntary movement obviously are needed before walking or hand function are possible. Modifying the work of Sackett et al.[3] provides us with eight ultimate goals of treatment (Table 2-2).

Guideline 16 recommends that both short- and long-term goals need to be realistic in terms of current levels of disability and the potential for recovery. Goals should be mutually agreed to by the patient, family, and rehabilitation team. They should be documented in the medical record in explicit, measurable terms.[1]

Step 5: Develop a Management Plan and Select Specific Interventions

The principles of both client-centered and evidence-based practice described earlier drive both the planning of the program and the selection of the specific interventions. Evidence for and against the effectiveness of various interventions has been mounting for many years and can be expected to increase substantially. In some cases, interventions are now supported by Level A, B, or C type evidence. Interpretation of the results from many of these studies, however, is suspect because of the all too common problems of conducting randomized trials using small sample sizes, patient samples with substantial heterogeneity (particularly in degree of severity) and ill-defined or too global outcomes. The rehabilitation management plan should indicate the specific treatments planned and their sequence, intensity, frequency, and expected duration.

Table 2-3 summarizes the effectiveness literature for various interventions and patient problems and indicates the level of evidence in support of its effectiveness. Table 2-4 summarizes the consensus opinions of the experts who deliberated over best practices in Guideline 16.

Step 6: Specify the Treatment Target

Having selected the best treatment, consider the treatment target, or what is to be expected as a reasonable outcome. The target guides the clinician in knowing when to stop treatment, change its inten-

Table 2-4. Consensus in Support of Addressing Specific Problems

Remediate
  Sensorimotor impairments
  Bladder and bowel incontinence
  Sleep disturbances
  Self-care activities
  Speech and language impairments
  Mild to moderate cognitive and perceptual impairments
Prevent
  Recurrent strokes
  Aspiration
  Seizures
  Shoulder pain
  Deep vein thromboses
  Skin breakdown
  Falls
Compensate or Adapt
  Compensate for disabilities in self-care and other important tasks and activities
  Provide adaptive devices, equipment (including wheelchairs) and orthoses for use to optimize independence and reduce burden on caregivers when remediation and compensation efforts fail

Table 2-3. Levels of Evidence in Support of the Effectiveness of Interventions

Level A
  Improvement in function of the leg when EMG biofeedback is used in conjunction with TENS[45,46]
  No improvement in function of the arm when EMG biofeedback is compared to other forms of therapy[47,48]
  Improvement in balance with physical therapy[49–52]
  No universal differences in functional outcomes when comparing different types of physical therapy[53–59]
  Improved arm function in selected patients with "forced use"[60,61]
  No improvement in family functioning with education[62–65]
Level B
  Improvement in foot drop with EMG biofeedback[57,66–70]
  Improvement in balance and function with acupuncture[71,72]
  No improvement in arm function with inflatable pressure splints[73]
  Improvement in spasticity with active antagonist strengthening[74]
  Improvement in test performance without functional change from cognitive and perceptual training[75–78]
  No improvement in dysphagia with use of intensive therapy intervention[79]
  Improvement in family functioning with counseling in conjunction with education[80]
  Improvement in family's ability to provide support with training and education[80]
Level C
  Improvement in shoulder pain with a prevention program[81]
  Improvement in communication and language in patients with aphasia when provided with speech therapy[82–89]
  Improvement in depression with drug management[90,91]

Abbreviations: EMG, electromyographic; TENS, transcutaneous electrical nerve stimulation.

sity, or switch to some other treatment.[3] When an individual achieves a target, review the goals, reconsider the treatment being given, and either discontinue treatment or specify a new treatment target.

Step 7: Provide the Best Therapy and Monitor Progress

While treatment is being provided with as much technical skill as possible, assessment and treatment interact in a constant iterative way, and progress should be objectively assessed on an ongoing basis. The complexity of the relationships among various impairments (e.g., physical, cognitive, communicative, and behavioral) requires that rehabilitation of one impairment or disability not occur in isolation. Members of the health care team must work together in a cooperative effort to optimize the patient's rehabilitation potential. If patient problems are not responding to care as predicted, treatment goals and the treatment plan should be reexamined.

Step 8: Complete Discharge Plans and Evaluate Outcomes

Guideline 16 recommends that discharge from a rehabilitation program should occur when reasonable treatment goals have been achieved. Absence of progress on two successive evaluations before the achievement of the rehabilitation goals should lead to reconsideration of the treatment regimen or the appropriateness of the current setting. Once discharge is imminent, discharge assessment should be carried out. The objective of this assessment is to measure the outcome of the rehabilitation process. This assessment should focus on both the extent to which disabilities and handicaps were minimized and the clinically important changes that were achieved. The use of generally agreed on standardized outcome measures is essential.

Step 9: Reintegration into the Community

Surveillance after discharge should stop only for those who do not have residual problems or reach the status of the healthy disabled (i.e., are free from handicap). Those with chronic impairment or disability leading to persistent handicap should continue to be monitored. Both medical and rehabilitation services will be required and support and assistance should be available for patients, family, and caregivers. Guideline 16 recommends that "clinicians need to be sensitive to potential adverse effects of caregiving on family functioning and the health of the caregiver. They should work with the patient and caregivers to avoid negative effects, promote problem solving, and facilitate reintegration of the patient into valued family and social roles."[1] In our experience with patients who have moderate to severe residual deficits, more than 50 percent of caregivers report providing in excess of 10 hours a day in direct caregiving. This burden can be overwhelming unless addressed. Information on community resources should be provided to the families and caregivers of stroke survivors, and assistance in obtaining needed services should be offered.

Guideline 16 recommends that "the stroke survivor's progress should be evaluated within 1 month after return to a community residence and at regular intervals during at least the first year, consistent with the person's condition and the preferences of the stroke survivor and family. Monitoring of physical, cognitive, and emotional functioning and integration into family and social roles is especially important."[1]

"Continued rehabilitation services should be considered to help the stroke survivor sustain the gains from the rehabilitation program and to build on patient and family strengths and interests as that patient becomes reintegrated into the home and community. Services should be phased out as measurable benefit diminishes."[1] Specific needs such as those relating to sexuality, automobile driving, or return to work should be reconsidered once the patient has returned to the community.

CONCLUSION

It is our hope that this chapter accurately reflects (1) the current state of problems that have been addressed by clinicians and clinical researchers to date, (2) the most useful solutions that have evolved and have been published, and (3) the serious gaps that persist in our knowledge and practice.

The last decade has produced a rich harvest of clinical scientific results that are beginning to influence the decision-making processes. However, the new methods require further validation, testing, and improvement if we are to achieve optimal effectiveness in the rehabilitation of the disabilities and handicaps that follow strokes.

REFERENCES

1. Agency for Health Care Policy and Research US Department of Health and Human Services: Post-Stroke Rehabilitation, Clinical Practice Guideline No. 16. Rockville, MD, 1995
2. Gowland C, Gambarotto C: Assessment and treatment of physical impairments leading to disability. In Finlayson A, Garner S, (eds): Brain Injury Rehabilitation: Clinical Considerations. Williams & Wilkins, Baltimore, 1993
3. Sackett DL, Haynes RB, Guyatt GH, Tugwell P: Clinical Epidemiology. A Basic Science for Clinical Medicine. 2nd Ed. Little, Brown, Toronto, 1991
4. Harris SR: Efficacy of physical therapy in promoting family functioning and functional independence for children with cerebral palsy. Pediatr Phys Ther 2:160, 1990
5. Sackett DL: Rules of evidence and clinical recommendations on the use of antithrombotic agents. Chest, suppl. 89:2s, 1986

6. World Health Organization (WHO): International classification of impairments, disabilities and handicaps. A manual of classification relating to the consequences of disease. World Health Organization, Geneva, 1980

7. Kirshner B, Guyatt G: A methodological framework for assessing health indices. J Chronic Dis 38:27, 1985

8. Feinstein AR, Josephy BR, Wells CK: Scientific and clinical problems in indexes of functional disability. Ann Intern Med 105:413, 1986

9. Basmajian JV: The call for action. Stroke, suppl. 21:II, 1990

10. Gowland C, VanHullenaar S, Torresin W et al: Chedoke-McMaster Stroke Assessment: Development, Validation and Administration Manual. Chedoke-McMaster Hospitals and McMaster University, Hamilton, Ontario, 1995

11. Johnston MV, Keith RA, Hinderer SR: Measurement standards for interdisciplinary medical rehabilitation. Arch Phys Med Rehabil 73:s3, 1992

12. State University of New York at Buffalo School of Biomedical Sciences The Centre for Functional Assessment Research: Guide for the Uniform Data Set for Medical Rehabilitation (Adult FIM) Version 4.0. 1993.

13. Strub RL, Black FW: The Mental Status Examination in Neurology. FA Davis, Philadelphia, 1977

14. Cochrane: Database of Systematic Reviews. BMJ, BMA House, Tavestock Square, London, 1995

15. Stevens RS, Ambler NR, Warren MD: A randomized controlled trial of a stroke rehabilitation ward. Age Ageing 13:65, 1984

16. Smith ME, Garraway WM, Smith DL, Akhtar AJ: Therapy impact on functional outcome in a controlled trial of stroke rehabilitation, Arch Phys Med Rehabil 63:21, 1982

17. Strand T, Asplund K, Eriksson S et al: A non-intensive stroke unit reduces functional disability and the need for long-term hospitalization. Stroke 16:29, 1985

18. Garraway WM, Akhtar AJ, Hockey L, Prescott RJ: Management of acute stroke in the elderly: follow-up of a controlled trial. BMJ 281:827, 1980

19. Hamrin E: II. Early activation in stroke: does it make a difference? Scand J Rehabil Med 14:101, 1982

20. Wood-Dauphinee S, Shapiro S, Bass E et al: A randomized trial of team care following stroke. Stroke 15:864, 1984

21. Hamrin E: III. One year after stroke: a follow-up of an experimental study. Scand J Rehabil Med 14:111, 1982

22. Garraway WM, Akhtar AJ, Prescott RJ, Hockey L: Management of acute stroke in the elderly: preliminary results of a controlled trial. BMJ 1040, 1980

23. Feldman DJ, Lee PR, Unterecker J et al: A comparison of functionally orientated medical care and formal rehabilitation in the management of patients with hemiplegia due to cerebrovascular disease. J Chronic Dis 15:197, 1962

24. Garraway WM, Akhtar AJ, Smith DL, Smith ME: The triage of stroke rehabilitation. J Epidemiol Community Health 35:39, 1981

25. Indredavik B, Bakke F, Solberg R et al: Benefit of a stroke unit: a randomized controlled trial. Stroke 22:1026, 1991

26. Kalra L, Dale P, Crome P: Improving stroke rehabilitation. Stroke 24:1462, 1993

27. Sivenius J, Pyorala K, Heinonen OP et al: The significance of intensity of rehabilitation of stroke—a controlled trial. Stroke 16:928, 1985

28. Peacock PB, Riley CHP, Lampton TD et al: The Birmingham stroke, epidemiology and rehabilitation study. In Stewart GT (ed): Trends in Epidemiology Charles C Thomas, Springfield, Ill, 1972

29. Stevens RS, Ambler NR: The Dover Stroke Rehabilitation Unit: A randomised controlled trial of stroke management. In Rose FC (ed): Advances in Stroke Therapy. Raven Press, New York, 1982

30. Gordon EE, Kohn KH: Evaluation of rehabilitation methods in the hemiplegic patient. J Chron Dis 19:3, 1995

31. Aitken PD, Rodgers H, French JM et al: General medical or geriatric unit care for acute stroke? A controlled trial. Age Aging, suppl. 2, 22:4, 1993

32. Kalra L, Dale P, Crome P: Do stroke units benefit elderly stroke patients? Age Aging, suppl. 1, 23:5, 1994

33. Strand T, Asplund K, Eriksson S et al: Stroke unit care—who benefits? Comparisons with general medical care in relation to prognostic indicators on admission. Stroke 17:377, 1986

34. Asberg KH: Orthostatic tolerance training of stroke patients in general medical wards. An experimental study. Scand J Rehabil Med 21:179, 1989

35. Hayes SH, Carroll SR: Early intervention care in the acute stroke patient. Arch Phys Med Rehabil 67:319, 1986

36. Stonnington HH, Browne JA: Team approach to management. In Branstater ME, Basmajian JV (eds): Williams & Wilkins, Baltimore, 1987

37. Young JB, Forster A: The Bradford community stroke trial: results at six months. BMJ 304:1085, 1992

38. Wade DT, Collen FM, Robb GF, Warlow CP: Physiotherapy intervention late after stroke and mobility. BMJ 304:609, 1992

39. Wade DT, Langton-Hewer R, Skilbeck CE et al: Controlled trial of a home-care service for acute stroke patients. Lancet 1:323, 1985

40. Tucker MA, Davison JG, Ogle SJ: Day hospital rehabilitation—effectiveness and cost in the elderly: a randomised controlled trial, BMJ 289:1209, 1984

41. Smith DS, Goldenberg E, Ashburn A et al: Remedial therapy after stroke: a randomised controlled trial. BMJ 282:517, 1981

42. Feigenson JS, Gitlow HS, Greenberg SD: The disability oriented rehabilitation unit: a major factor influencing stroke outcome. Stroke 10:5, 1979

43. Gladman JRF, Lincoln NB, Barer DH: A randomised controlled trial of domiciliary and hospital-based rehabilitation for stroke patients after discharge from hospital. J Neurology Neurosurg Psychiatry 56:960, 1993

44. Gowland C: Predicting physical outcomes in stroke: Implications for clinical decision making. Cambridge, MA. Paper presented at the Sixth Annual Stroke Rehabilitation Conference, 1994.

45. Cozean CD, Pease WS, Hubbell SL: Biofeedback and functional electric stimulation in stroke rehabilitation. Arch Phys Med Rehabil 69:401, 1988

46. Winchester P, Montgomery J, Bowman B, Hislop H: Effects of feedback stimulation training and cyclical electrical stimulation on knee extension in hemiparetic patients, Phys Ther 63:1096, 1983

47. Moreland J, Thomson MA: Efficacy of electromyographic biofeedback compared with conventional physical therapy for upper-extremity function in patients following stroke: a research overview and meta-analysis. Phys Ther 74:534, 1994

48. de Weerdt WJG, Harrison MA: The efficacy of electromyographic feedback for stroke patients: a critical review of the main literature. Physiotherapy 72:108, 1986

49. Tangeman PT, Banaitis DA, Williams AK: Rehabilitation of chronic stroke patients: changes in functional performance. Arch Phys Med Rehabil 71:876, 1990

50. Winstein CJ, Gardner ER, McNeal DR et al: Standing balance training: effect on balance and locomotion in hemiparetic adults. Arch Phys Med Rehabil 70:755, 1989

51. Shumway-Cook A, Anson D, Haller S: Postural sway feedback: its effect on reestablishing stance stability in hemiplegic patients. Arch Phys Med Rehabil 69:395, 1988

52. Hocherman S, Dickstein R, Pillar T: Platform training and postural stability in hemiplegia. Arch Phys Med Rehabil 65:588, 1984

53. Sunderland A, Tinson DJ, Bradley EL et al: Enhanced physical therapy for arm function after stroke: a one year follow-up study. J Neurol Neurosurg Psychiatry 57:856, 1994

54. Sunderland A, Tinson DJ, Bradley EL et al: Enhanced physical therapy improves recovery of arm function after stroke. A randomised controlled trial. J Neurol Neurosurg Psychiatry 55:530, 1992

55. Jongbloed L, Stacey S, Brighton C: Stroke rehabilitation: sensorimotor integrative treatment versus functional treatment. Am J Occup Ther 43:391, 1989

56. Dickstein R, Hocherman S, Pillar T, Shaham R: Stroke rehabilitation: three exercise therapy approaches. Phys Ther 66:1233, 1986

57. Lord JP, Hall K: Neuromuscular reeducation versus traditional programs for stroke rehabilitation. Arch Phys Med Rehabil 67:88, 1986

58. Logigian MK, Samuels MA, Falconer J: Clinical exercise trial for stroke patients. Arch Phys Med Rehabil 64:364, 1983

59. Stern PH, McDowell F, Miller JM, Robinson M: Effects of facilitation exercise techniques in stroke rehabilitation. Arch Phys Med Rehabil 51:526, 1970

60. Taub E, Miller NE, Novack TA et al: Technique to improve chronic motor deficit after stroke. Arch Phys Med Rehabil 74:347, 1993

61. Wolf SL, Lecraw DE, Barton LA, Jann BB: Forced use of hemiplegic upper extremities to reverse the effect of learned nonuse among chronic stroke and head injured patients. Exp Neurol 104:125, 1989

62. Friedland JF, McColl M: Social support intervention after stroke: results of a randomized trial. Arch Phys Med Rehabil 73:573, 1992

63. Jongbloed L, Morgan D: An investigation of involvement in leisure activities after a stroke. Am J Occup Ther 45:420, 1991

64. Pain HSB, McLellan DL: The use of individualized booklets after stroke. Clin Rehabil 4:265, 1990

65. Towle D, Lincoln NB, Mayfield LM: Service provision and functional independence in depressed stroke patients and the effect of social work intervention on these. J Neurol Neurosurg Psychiatry. 52:519, 1989

66. Mandel AR, Nymark JR, Balmer SJ et al: Electromyographic versus rhythmic positional biofeedback in computerized gait retraining with stroke patients. Arch Phys Med Rehabil 71:649, 1990

67. Mulder T, Hulstijn W, Van Der Meer J: EMG feedback and the restoration of motor control. Am J Phys Med 65:173, 1986

68. Burnside IG, Tobias HS, Bursill D: Electromyographic feedback in the remobilization of stroke patients: a controlled trial. Arch Phys Med Rehabil 63:217, 1982

69. Shiavi RG, Champion SA, Freeman FR, Bugel HJ: Efficacy of myofeedback therapy in regaining control of lower extremity musculature following stroke. Am J Phys Med 58:185, 1979

70. Basmajian JV, Kukulka CG, Narayan MG, Takebe K: Biofeedback treatment of foot-drop after stroke com-

pared with standard rehabilitation technique: effects on voluntary control and strength. Arch Phys Med Rehabil 56:231, 1975

71. Johansson K, Lindgren I, Widner H et al: Can sensory stimulation improve the functional outcome in stroke patients? Neurology 43:2189, 1993

72. Magnusson M, Johansson K, Johansson BB: Sensory stimulation promotes normalization of postural control after stroke. Stroke 25:1176, 1994

73. Poole JL, Whitney SL, Hangeland N, Backer C: The effectiveness of inflatable pressure splints on motor function in stroke patients. Occup Ther J Res 10:360, 1990

74. Wolf SL, Catlin PA, Blanton S et al: Overcoming limitations in elbow movement in the presence of antagonist hyperactivity. Phys Ther 74:826, 1994

75. Carter LT, Howard BE, O'Neil WA: Effectiveness of cognitive skill remediation in acute stroke patients. Am J Occup Ther 37:320, 1983

76. Carter LT, Caruso JL, Languirand MA, Berard MA: Cognitive skill remediation in stroke and non-stroke elderly. Clin Neuropsychiatry II:109, 1980

77. Weinberg J, Diller L, Gordon WA et al: Training sensory awareness and spatial organization in people with right brain damage. Arch Phys Med Rehabil 60:479, 1979

78. Weinberg J, Diller L, Gordon WA et al: Visual scanning training effect on reading-related tasks in acquired right brain damage. Arch Phys Med Rehabil 58:479, 1977

79. DePippo KL, Holas MA, Reding MJ et al: Dysphagia therapy following stroke: a controlled trial. Neurology 44:1655, 1994

80. Evans RL, Matlock AL, Bishop DS et al: Family intervention after stroke: does counseling or education help? Stroke 19:1243, 1988

81. Braus DF, Krauss JK, Strobel J: The shoulder-hand syndrome after stroke: a prospective clinical trial. Ann Neurol 36:728, 1994

82. Poeck K, Huber W, Willmes K: Outcome of intensive language treatment in aphasia. J Speech Hear Disord 54:471, 1989

83. Hartman J, Landau WM: Comparison of formal language therapy with supportive counseling for aphasia due to acute vascular accident. Arch Neurol 44:646, 1987

84. Wertz RT, Weiss DG, Aten JL et al: Comparison of clinic, home, and deferred language treatment for aphasia. A Veterans Administration Cooperative Study. Arch Neurol 43:653, 1986

85. Lincoln NB, McGuirk E, Mulley GP et al: Effectiveness of speech therapy for aphasic stroke patients. A randomised controlled trial. Lancet 2:1197, 1984

86. Shewan CM, Kertesz A: Effects of speech and language treatment on recovery from aphasia. Brain Lang 23:272, 1984

87. Wertz RT, Collins MJ, Weiss D et al: Veterans Administration cooperative study on aphasia: a comparison of individual and group treatment. J Speech Hear Res 24:580, 1981

88. Basso AT, Capitani E, Vignolo LA: Influence of rehabilitation on language skills in aphasic patients. A controlled study. Arch Neurol 36:190, 1979

89. Butfield E, Zangwell O: Re-education in aphasia: a review of 70 cases. J Neurol Neurosurg Psychiatry 9:75, 1946

90. Reding MJ, Orto LA, Winter SW et al: Antidepressant therapy after stroke: a double-blind trial. Arch Neurol 43:763, 1986

91. Lipsey JR, Robinson RG, Pearlson GD et al: Nortriptyline treatment of post-stroke depression: a double-blind study. Lancet 1:297, 1984

3
Spinal Cord Injury

Karen M. Smith
Ralph J. Marino
Virginia Graziani

In the management of spinal cord-injured patients (SCI), several management decisions must be made that cover the spectrum from the initial to long-term management, all aimed at reducing morbidity and mortality, enhancing quality of life, and minimizing handicap. It is not possible to review all of these areas in one chapter; discussion is limited to those areas that are controversial or are being actively researched. Most of the discussion pertains to traumatic SCI, except where specified.

As in the preceding chapters, studies will be evaluated according to the five levels of evidence, with summary statements made on the intervention of interest. The summary statement includes a grade of recommendation.

SURGICAL INTERVENTION IN ACUTE TRAUMATIC SPINAL CORD INJURY

Decompression to Improve Neurologic Outcome

Evidence from animal studies suggests that decompression of the spinal cord may enhance neurologic recovery. Several studies have shown that functional recovery decreases with increasing time of compression.[1-3] Delamarter et al.[2] applied 50 percent constriction to dog spinal cord for periods up to 1 week. Recovery was seen only in those decompressed within 1 hour. Recovery is also inversely related to the compressive force.[1]

It is difficult to translate these results in animals to human SCI. The amount of force imparted to the spinal cord cannot be measured in humans. It is not known whether recumbency, with or without traction, is sufficient to decompress the cord. It may not be necessary to completely reconstitute the spinal canal area at the time of surgery. Johnson et al.[4] followed 17 patients with thoracolumbar stabilization without decompression. Mean spinal canal area postoperatively was 71 percent of normal, and improved to 86 percent on follow-up. Similar findings were noted by Levine et al.[5] However, Willen et al.,[6] in a study of the natural history of burst fractures at T12 and L1, found that bone fragments occupying more than 50 percent of the canal were not resorbed.

The usual course of recovery after SCI should be kept in mind when evaluating recovery after nonrandomized surgical interventions. Many recent studies have examined recovery after traumatic SCI. Reports by Waters et al.[7-10] indicate that recovery is most marked in the first 6 months postinjury, tapers off in the second 6 months, and changes little from 12 to 24 months. These studies are based on the American Spinal Injury Association (ASIA) standards (ASIA 1992) and rely on serial manual muscle testing of certain muscles. More sensitive measures of strength, such as myometry, may demonstrate continued improvements beyond 1 year.[11,12] In the zone of injury, individual muscles may improve up to 24-months postinjury.[13] In complete quadriplegia, the chance of functional recovery decreases with distance below the level of injury. Graziani et al.[14]

found a 70 percent one-year recovery to at least three-fifths strength in the myotome just below the level of injury. This rate decreased to 12 percent for the myotome two levels below the injury level and zero percent three levels below. Muscles at the level of injury with some initial strength recover more readily than those with zero strength; greater than 90 percent versus 43 percent, respectively, reach at least three-fifths strength by 1 year.[10,15,16]

Information from the National SCI database indicates that only 6.7 percent of those admitted with a complete (Frankel A) SCI convert to incomplete by discharge. Of these, only one fourth regain functional strength. In contrast, 37.4 percent of those who are sensory incomplete (Frankel B) improve; half of those who improve reach functional levels.[17] Those with preserved pin sensation have a better prognosis than those with only touch preserved.[18] Over half (53.6 percent) of those with Frankel C injuries improve to functional levels.[17] Those who are younger (less than 50 years old) have a significantly better chance of recovery than older individuals.[19] It is also important to note that changes in motor scores are common during the first few days after injury. Blaustein et al.[20] compared 24- and 72-hour motor scores in 26 motor complete cervical SCI patients. Although average score did not change, individual scores changed in 21 subjects, with improvement or deterioration of up to 8 points, approximately equal to a one motor level change in strength.

There are no randomized studies in humans on the effect of spinal cord decompression on neurologic recovery. What is available consists of cohort studies with concurrent or historical controls, or case series without controls. A report by Kiwerski[21] of outcomes of 1761 patients with cervical SCI from 1965 to 1991 illustrates some of the pitfalls of trying to compare treatments in nonrandomized groups. Kiwerski recognized that his surgical and nonsurgical groups were not similar, and did not perform formal comparisons. The conservative group of 798 patients had a 20 percent mortality compared to an 8.6 percent mortality in the surgical group. For those with complete injuries the mortality rate was 36 percent in the conservative group and 19 percent in the surgical group. Hospital length of stay (LOS) for survivors was reported as 27 weeks and 17 weeks for the conservative and surgical groups, respectively.

However, the LOS data are skewed, and median times are 9 to 12 weeks for both groups, suggesting perhaps that surgery is withheld from those with life-threatening injuries or those who develop serious complications, making it difficult to compare the interventions in case series.

Although surgery may be performed for many reasons, the question of concern here is whether decompression of the spinal cord, either by closed methods or by surgery, can improve recovery after traumatic SCI. There are case reports of significant recovery within hours after rapid realignment of cervical fracture dislocation.[22] Although skull traction for acute cervical spine fractures is not without risks,[23] Cotler et al.[24] demonstrated that reduction could be accomplished safely within hours in skilled hands with close monitoring. None of the 24 patients in their series deteriorated, despite traction weights up to 140 lb, and several had marked recovery in the first week postinjury.

Weinshel et al.[25] reviewed the type of surgery, either decompression and fusion versus fusion alone, with neurologic recovery in cervical SCI. They reported that 41 of 74 of those decompressed gained function in the next nerve root as opposed to only 6 of 16 in the fusion group ($P < .05$). Because the type of surgery was left to the discretion of the surgeon in this retrospective study, and no effort was made to evaluate compression of neural elements in the fusion group, this comparison may not be valid. There was not a significant difference between the groups with regard to recovery of cord function. Bose et al.[26] reported a series of 28 patients with cervical central cord injury, half of whom had surgical intervention. The surgical group was operated on at an average of 20 days after injury. This group had a greater average motor score improvement at discharge than the conservative group. However, the surgical group had a longer average LOS and, therefore, a longer time to recover than the nonoperative group.

Krengel et al.[27] looked at early decompression in incomplete thoracic paraplegia. Lower extremity recovery was better than that of historical controls. A comparison of decompression and fusion in thoracolumbar fractures found a 68 percent recovery of the neurologic deficit in those decompressed compared to a 44 percent recovery in those only fused.[28] Finally, Hu et al.[29] examined the effect of decompression on recovery from incomplete paraplegia after lumbar fracture. The average improvement in ASIA motor score for those decompressed was 10 points. Those who had fusion without decompression gained an average of 4.2 points ($P < .05$). This difference reached statistical significance, but may not be clinically significant.

Foreign Body Removal

The value of surgery to remove retained fragments in penetrating injuries has been evaluated with mixed results. Yashon et al.[30] did not find neurologic improvement in patients who underwent surgery for fragment removal. Simpson et al.[31] reviewed 160 cases of penetrating trauma, 37 of whom had surgery for various reasons. Only 2 of 11 who had fragment removal improved. Furthermore, the surgical group had significantly more complications than the nonoperative group. Both studies were nonrandomized, concurrent cohort comparisons.

On the other hand, a prospective nonrandomized study by Waters and Adkins[32] found no difference in complications between those with and those without the bullet removed. Neurologic outcomes were similar for those with injuries between T1 and T11. The 13 subjects with T12 to L4 injuries who had bullet removal had a significantly greater recovery on the ASIA motor index score than the seven who did not. Besides the lack of randomization in this study, there are several other possible sources of bias and confounding. Of the original 90 subjects, only 66 were available for 1 year follow-up. The rationale for grouping those with injuries from T12 to L4 is poorly justified. This area includes the conus and the cauda equina, areas that may have different patterns of recovery. A study of burst fractures in the thoracolumbar junction revealed fewer complete lesions and more patients with pain at the L1 level than at the T12 level.[6] Therefore, the results of this study by Waters should be viewed as suggestive but tentative in support of bullet removal in patients with cauda equina injuries.

Summary

Evidence supporting surgical decompression following traumatic SCI to improve neurologic outcome comes from Level III, IV, or V studies resulting in a Grade C recommendation for acute surgical decompression following SCI. Similarly, the Grade C recommendation for fragment removal in selected cases (i.e., below T12) comes from review of one Level III study. This finding is countered by two Level III studies suggesting no benefit from fragment removal in general SCI. This finding is confounded by two Level III studies suggesting no benefit from fragment removal in general SCI.

Early Versus Late Surgery

Even among those who advocate surgery to improve neurologic recovery in SCI, there is controversy about the timing of surgery. Those against early surgery say that it does not improve outcome[33] and that it increases the risk of deterioration.[34] Those who support early surgery state that it allows early mobilization, avoids the complications of prolonged bedrest,[35] and provides the best environment for neurologic recovery.[36]

Marshall et al.[34] voiced caution on early surgery based on the results of a multicentered prospective descriptive study of 283 patients with traumatic SCI. Of the 134 patients who underwent surgery, four deteriorated. All four had surgery within 5 days of injury. Heiden et al.[37] thought that patients operated on within 1 week of injury had a higher rate of pulmonary complications than those operated on later. They did not find improved recovery in their surgical groups of patients with cervical injuries. There was a 1.5 to 5 percent incidence of increased neurologic deficit in operated patients, but the timing of surgery (less than or greater than 48 hours) was not described. Anderson and Bohlman[38] have recommended late anterior decompression to improve motor function in cervical spine injuries. They reported 51 patients with motor complete quadriplegia who received a decompressive procedure between 1 month and 8 years after injury. Improvement in at least one new motor root occurred in 49 percent of patients. They felt that the neurologic improvement was a result of the surgery. Because the median time of surgery was 6 months after injury, however, their means of identifying neurologic plateau, an indication for surgery, may have been insensitive. Katoh and El Masri[39] reviewed a series of 53 patients with complete cervical SCI treated conservatively. Of the 40 patients followed for at least 12 months, 19 (47.5 percent) recovered motor power in local muscles that were initially paralyzed.

On the other hand, Aebi et al.[40] reviewed 100 patients with cervical spinal injuries. One-third of their patients improved neurologically. Seventy-five percent of those who improved had fractures that were reduced manually or surgically within 6 hours of injury. Levi et al.[35] presented a retrospective case series of 103 patients with cervical SCI treated with anterior decompression. There was no difference in neurologic outcomes between the patients operated on within 24 hours and those operated on later than 24 hours after injury.

Summary

The literature on surgery after SCI presents a mixed bag of Levels III and V studies with conflicting results. A review of the indications of surgery by Donovan[41] concluded that surgery to improve neurologic outcome could not be recommended at this time, based on the available evidence, but this evidence is not strong enough to proscribe surgery. In select patients, where there is salvageable cord, early decompression has the theoretical potential to significantly improve outcome. This surgery is not without risks, and patients occasionally deteriorate regardless of the type of treatment given. To obtain any resolution on this issue of the benefits of early versus late decompression and fusion following acute SCI, further research is needed.

Heterotrophic ossification is discussed in chapter 4 on page 47.

PHARMACOLOGIC TREATMENT OF ACUTE SPINAL CORD INJURY

Experimental studies on acutely injured spinal cords have revealed a sequence of events from near normal appearance of the cord to petechial hemorrhage to central necrosis, which develops over the hours to days after injury. This information has led to the search for interventions that can abort this cascade of events and limit the extent of injury. This search has been bolstered by the finding that functional recovery may occur with salvage of only 10 percent of spinal axons.[42] Evidence suggests that free radical formation and subsequent lipid peroxidation of cell membranes is responsible for the secondary injury observed after SCI.[43,44] There are several recent reviews of basic and clinical research in the pharmacologic treatment of SCI.[45–48] We focus here on results of interventions in humans.

The second National Acute Spinal Cord Injury Study (NASCIS) was the first clinical trial to demonstrate that a treatment, methylprednisolone (MP), given after injury could improve neurologic recovery.[49] A randomized, placebo-controlled, double-blind trial, it evaluated the effects of high-dose MP and naloxone on recovery after traumatic SCI. Although the first NASCIS study did not demonstrate any benefit for MP,[50] animal studies indicated that the dose used may have been too low.[51] The second NASCIS trial used a 30 mg/kg bolus followed by an infusion of 5.4 mg/kg per hour for the next 23 hours. There was a statistically greater improvement in motor and sensory function at 6 months for those treated with MP than for those given placebo. There was no functional outcome measure in the study, however, leaving open the question of whether the average 5 point gain in motor score for the MP group was clinically significant.

Further analysis of data from NASCIS 2 indicated that the main effect of MP on neurologic recovery was below the injury level, with relatively small improvement at the injury level.[52] This analysis also suggested that treatment with MP greater than 8 hours after injury resulted in decreased neurologic recovery. Of concern is the finding that the placebo group treated greater than 8 hours after injury gained a similar percentage of lost motor function (33.9 percent) as the MP group treated within eight hours (34.3 percent). A third NASCIS trial, now underway, is using the Functional Independence Measure to assess functional recovery and may answer some of the concerns of the second study.

Another class of drugs that has been studied in human spinal cord injury is the gangliosides. The GM_1 ganglioside has been shown to accelerate motor neuron sprouting in vitro[53] and to improve recovery in spinal cord-injured cats.[54] In 1991, Geisler et al.[55] reported results of a randomized, controlled trial of GM_1 ganglioside in SCI. The GM_1-treated subjects had significantly greater recovery based on improvement in Frankel grades and improvement in ASIA motor scores, than did the control group. Subsequent analyses of the data indicated that the bulk of the recovery occurred in muscles of the lower extremities, consistent with enhanced survival of the white matter tracts.[56] The mean time of administration of the GM_1 study drug was 48 hours after injury, indicating that the mechanism of action is different from that of MP, which must be given within 8 hours of injury. Consequently, a new study is underway to evaluate the effects of GM_1 versus placebo after MP, to see whether there are interactions or synergies between the two drugs.[57] As with the MP trial, this study did not include a functional evaluation and was unable to demonstrate that the improvement seen was clinically significant.

A final class of drugs that has shown promise in acute SCI is the 21-aminosteroids. These potent inhibitors of lipid peroxidation are free of the glucocorticoid effects of steroids.[58] In addition to their vitamin E sparing properties, 21-aminosteroids react with hydroxyl radicals to create a metabolite with potent antilipid peroxidation properties of its own.[59] In a spinal cord compression injury model, tirilazad, one of the 21-aminosteroids, given 30 minutes after injury improved neurologic recovery of cats.[60] The third NASCIS trial is evaluating the effect of a 48-hour treatment with tirilazad after a bolus of MP to an infusion of MP for 23 or 48 hours after the bolus.[52]

Summary

There are a few Level I trials on drug interventions in acute SCI. The initial reports await confirmation and demonstration of clinical rather than only statistical benefit. For patients with closed injuries and no contraindication to steroids, MP should be administered in a 30 mg/kg bolus followed by an infusion of 5.4 mg/kg per hour for 23 hours, provided that the bolus can be given within 8 hours of injury.

NEUROGENIC BLADDER MANAGEMENT

Many issues relate to the management of neurogenic bladder, only a small number of which can be dealt with in this chapter. The management decisions that need to be dealt with include the following:

1. Method of bladder emptying in acute and chronic phases
2. Diagnosis of urinary tract infection (UTI)
3. Prophylaxis of UTI
4. Treatment of UTI
5. Management of complications (e.g., stones, diverticuli, reflux)
6. Sexuality and fertility issues

This section describes the management decisions concerning issues 1, 3, and 4. The goal of management in these three issues is the same: reducing morbidity and mortality resulting from genitourinary problems. There is no consensus on the diagnosis of UTI after SCI. Many authors have attempted maneuvers to increase accuracy of localization, but none are reliable, other than perhaps ureteral catheterization or needle puncture, which is too invasive for routine clinical use.[61,62]

Bladder Emptying

There are 124 references relevant to the MeSH headings Spinal Cord Injuries and Catheterization from 1966 to 1994. Of these, supplemented with one author's (KMS) personal files and review of references, 28 articles were thought relevant to the long-term management of neurogenic bladder to facilitate bladder emptying. As noted earlier, the literature on surgery after SCI presents a mixed bag of Level III and V studies, with conflicting results in general.

A review of the indications of surgery by Donovan[41] concluded that surgery to improve neurologic controls could not be recommended at this time based on the available evidence. Nor is evidence strong enough against surgery. In select patients, where there is salvageable cord, early decompression has the theoretical potential to improve bladder emptying. Twelve articles were case series that described the complications experienced by patients using one type of management.[63–74] The remaining 15 articles compared various types of management including intermittent catheterization (sometimes subclassified as being done by self or others), suprapubic or indwelling catheter drainage, triggered voiding, or postsphincterotomy condom drainage.

These studies used a variety of methodologies for the cohort studies, including use of a historical cohort group, concurrent cohort group, prospective or retrospective recruitment, division based on initial management or long-term management, and varying lengths of follow-up, from 1 to 20 years. This variety makes synthesis of the evidence difficult if not impossible without a full meta-analysis. To complicate the process even further, the studies have produced conflicting results. Seven have concluded that the use of indwelling catheters increased infections or complications,[75–81] six have shown decreased or at least no difference in infections or complications with indwelling urethral or suprapubic tube management,[82–87] and two found "triggered" voiding to be superior to both indwelling or intermittent catheterization.[88,89]

Eight of the studies compared the various methods of bladder management and reported an average follow-up of 30 months or more postinjury, with the majority of studies following patients for 5 to more than 30 years.

Four of these studies concluded that indwelling catheter management was associated with increased complications.[77–79,81] Timoney and Shaw[77] describe follow-up on 14 patients who started and remained on intermittent catheterization, and compared these findings to the experience of 14 patients managed on long-term indwelling catheterization. Follow-up was 49 months on average. The initial population was 52 women. Long-term management included a variety of other techniques and complications experienced by the whole group, but they were not clearly outlined. Complications are described in the indwelling and intermittent catheter groups included reflux and upper tract changes. Statistical analysis was not performed, but trends in the complications that developed were not apparent.

Hall et al.[78] reviewed 898 SCI patients followed for 2 or more years through their clinic and found bladder stones in 261 and kidney stones in 198. A higher percentage of patients in both stone-forming groups used indwelling catheters (62.5 percent and 56.6 percent, respectively). No statistical analysis was performed on these data, and we do not know if the groups were otherwise similar at baseline.

McGuire and Savastano[79] retrospectively reviewed the charts of 35 female patients followed through their clinic for an average of 7 years. They found that complications of intravenous pyelogram (IVP) changes, autonomic dysreflexia, stones, erosion of the urethra, urine leakage, and UTI to be more prevalent with indwelling catheter management versus intermittent catheterization. They do not give much information to determine whether the groups were similar at baseline, but the higher level injuries seemed to be overrepresented in the indwelling catheter group.

Barkin et al.[81] followed 101 patients initially managed by intermittent catheterization and compared them with 101 matched controls not managed by intermittent catheterization during the acute management immediately after injury. Only 17 patients remained on intermittent catheterization at the end of the 25 month follow-up. There was increased febrile infection and two UTI septic deaths in the control population, as well as stones and urethral strictures and erosions. The controls, however, were matched on the basis of age, sex, duration, and completeness and level of lesion. They were not matched on urodynamic profiles or associated injuries, which may have influenced the outcomes of interest.

In the next group of studies of interest, the authors firmly disagreed with the preceding findings concluding that indwelling catheter management is not associated with any increased risk of complications. Dewire et al.[82] retrospectively reviewed 57 consecutive quadriplegic patients, none of whom were lost to follow-up over 10 years, with some being followed for 20 years. The patients were well described and similar at baseline except the catheter group was slightly older and injured in falls (39 versus 31 years at injury). The patients were not described according to their urodynamic profiles. These authors found no statistically significant difference in complication rates, but they would need to have had four times the sample size to detect a 25 percent difference. There was a trend to increased numbers of stones, pyelonephritis, erosions, and strictures in the indwelling group. Also disturbing is a ratio of 3:1 deaths in the catheter to noncatheter groups as a result of urosepsis or renal failure.

Chao et al.[86] followed 73 veterans with SCI for an average of more than 30 years postinjury. Thirty-two used an indwelling catheter, and 41 used other forms of management. The complication rates were small but comparable between groups, except perhaps for a trend to increased scarring and bladder stones in the catheterized group. The creatinine clearance was comparable between the two groups.

Jackson and DeVivo[87] examined the rates of complications between a group of 108 women and 434 men following SCI. The majority of women managed their bladder by indwelling catheter, whereas few men used indwelling catheters. Only the men who used ilioconduit was the association with deterioration in effective renal plasma flow significant. These patients were followed for up to 16 years, but the numbers followed for this length of time were small (63) and may have missed an important difference for infrequent complications.

Viera et al.[88] found that in 99 SCI patients followed for an average of 30 months, patients with a retrained bladder had statistically significant less abnormal renal clearance values than those managed with intermittent catheterization. The indwelling catheter group was too small for statistical analysis.

The basic underlying problem in trying to reach a consensus is that the cohort study design may not be able to control for an underlying bias that is influencing the outcome. That is, is there an underlying reason why an individual chooses indwelling catheter management that may be causing increased or decreased risk of complications? This point is made in the final study where the urodynamic finding of detrusor hyperreflexia was more closely related to evidence of upper urinary tract damage than was the method of bladder management, intermittent or indwelling catheterization, or voiding.[90]

Thus, the issue of ideal bladder management following SCI is not resolved. It is not clear whether long-term complications and renal damage are linked to any particular method. To resolve this dilemma, a randomized controlled trial may be needed, but such a study is probably not practical because of the length of time needed for follow-up (10 to 20 years). Thus, a prospective concurrent cohort study with well-matched controls may provide the answer to guide clinical decisions. In the interim, bladder management decisions are sometimes now made with respect to the method that best fits with the individual patient's social, vocational, functional, and financial resources and goals.

Treatment of UTI

Two issues deserve the bulk of attention in terms of the management of UTI following SCI:

1. Efficacy of antibiotics in prophylaxis of UTI
2. Treatment of symptomatic versus asymptomatic bacteriuria

Efficacy of Prophylaxis

From 1966 to 1994, there were 89 articles corresponding to the MeSH headings of the Prophylaxis of UTI following SCI. Of these, 14 were potentially relevant. On review of the articles, only eight dealt with the prophylaxis of UTI using oral antibiotics. The six remaining articles studied the efficacy of using various antiseptics for instillation into the bladder. These maneuvers are perhaps too laborious and impractical for long-term outpatient bladder management. Therefore, the eight articles dealing with oral treatment are reviewed here.[91–98]

Three studies were Level I trials with random assignment of patients and two of these used placebos.[91–93] Biering-Sorensen et al.[91] found that ciprofloxacin prophylaxis significantly reduced the number of UTI. Gribble and Puterman[92] found that septra prophylaxis reached statistical and clinical significance in reducing the number of symptomatic UTI and the number of laboratory UTI (i.e., positive urine cultures). Banovac et al.[93] found a statistically significant reduction in the percentage of positive urine cultures in patients treated with methenamine. The first two papers, however, note that the incidence of complications—rash, pseudomembranous colitis, drug fever, and the emergence of resistant organisms—is high in the treated group and may limit the long-term usefulness of this therapy. Two controlled randomized trials did not show any statistically significant difference between treatment and control groups.[94,95] However, the number of patients per group is such that a 25 percent risk reduction would be missed in the experimental group.

The remaining randomized trial showed a trend with reduction in the clinical infection rate.[96] This study population, however, may have been too small to detect a difference, thus providing perhaps Level II evidence of the efficacy of prophylactic antibiotics.

The two remaining cohort studies showed a reduction in laboratory infection, also termed *bacteriuria* or *positive urine culture*, in treated groups.[97,98]

The Grade A recommendation that prophylactic antibiotics—septra, ciprofloxacin and methenamine—can reduce the incidence of bacteriuria and symptomatic UTI following SCI comes from three Level I trials, one Level II trial, and two Level III trials. However, this proven efficacy must be balanced by the clinician against the side effects and development of resistant organisms noted by most authors.

Treatment of Asymptomatic Bacteriuria

Two review articles[61,62] illustrate the differing opinions on the treatment of asymptomatic bacteriuria. Asymptomatic bacteriuria is defined as significant growth on urine culture in the absence of clinical signs or symptoms. In 1992, a consensus group[62] advocated no treatment, whereas Stover et al.[61] earlier thought this recommendation was controversial. Series that have routinely cultured SCI patient's urine have found bacteriuria rates of 77, 50.6 and 78 percent.[99–101] Also, the bacterial flora change frequently unrelated to antibiotic usage.

Only four studies directly addressed the treatment of bacteriuria following SCI.[94,96,101,102] Lewis et al.[101] described 52 patients followed for an average of 3 months. Bacteriuria was not treated. Symptomatic infections responded to antibiotics within 2 days on average. The authors thought that this response supported the treatment of only symptomatic infections.

Sotolongo and Koleilat[102] followed 56 patients for 5 years with yearly cultures, serum creatinine, and upper tract imaging; none were treated for asymptomatic bacteriuria. In 1990, they reported no deterioration in the tests, but interestingly, the results were retracted without explanation, in 1992.[103]

The last two studies were nested studies within trials of prophylactic antibacterials.[94,96] Patients were randomized to those receiving and those not receiving antibiotics for asymptomatic bacteriuria. There was no difference in the development of further clinical or laboratory evidence of UTI. The groups were small and the results did not reach statistical significance. This could mean finding either that this interesting positive trend was not significant because of the small numbers or that we missed the beneficial effect of treating asymptomatic bacteriuria because of the small numbers.

In summary, one Level 5 study and two Level 2 studies result in a Grade B recommendation that asymptomatic bacteriuria may not need to be treated with antibiotics. Further study is warranted in this area, preferably a randomized controlled trial with long-term outcomes to determine whether there is any detrimental effect on renal function if bacteriuria is not treated.

FUNCTIONAL ELECTRICAL STIMULATION

Electrical neuromuscular stimulation techniques have been used for many applications in the SCI patient. These applications can be categorized into the treatment of consequences, prevention of secondary complications, and the restoration of functional movement of the extremities as described by Yarkony et al.[104] Therapeutic electrical stimulation as used primarily in research protocols is directed at facilitating neural regeneration.

Some of the applications in the treatment of consequences and prevention of secondary complications include stimulation for diaphragmatic pacing control of neurogenic bladder and bowel, enhancing ejaculation, reduction of pain, prevention of venous thrombosis, prevention and treatment of decubitus ulcers, spasticity, treatment of deconditioning as a result of lack of exercise, treatment for muscle atrophy, and prevention of pulmonary infection as a result of limited ability to cough.[104]

Lower Extremity Stimulation

Functional electrical stimulation (FES) is defined here as electrical stimulation directed at the restoration of functional movement of the extremities. Using this definition, the medline database was searched using the MeSH headings Spinal Cord Injuries and Electric Stimulation Therapy, for the time period 1966 to 1994, and including all languages. The findings were supplemented by one author's (KMS) personal files and review of the reference lists of potentially relevant articles. In all, 175 citations were found 10 of which were relevant to the clinical use of FES in facilitating standing or ambulation. The bulk of articles are technical studies refining the parameters of stimulation for gait or examining the physiology of muscles following stimulation.

After more detailed review of the 10 relevant articles, two reported before-after studies evaluating physiologic and functional effects of FES systems and eight were case series.[105–114] The physiologic parameters evaluated included muscle biopsy, measures of the metabolic cost of stimulation, fitness evaluations, and gait analysis. Functional outcomes have included objective assessments of the speed and distance walked and subjective qualitative gait assessments. These effects are almost universally positive, but there is a high attrition rate in those that decide to carry on with long-term stimulation for ambulation.[110] This outcome may be a reflection of the energy requirements of FES ambulation, the speed of ambulation afforded, and the complexity of currently available systems. In other words, attrition may be more a reflection of the effectiveness than of the efficacy of the procedure.

Thus, support for the various FES systems in facilitating ambulation are based on Levels IV and V evidence. Thus, a Grade C recommendation was made concerning the use of FES as it applies to the treatment of gait disturbances following SCI. However, as Rattay and Mayr[111] point out, only 10 percent of the original SCI population may be considered appropriate for this technology. Kralj et al.[110] estimates only 5 percent of the population is appropriate.

One may argue as to whether a randomized trial is needed if FES is used to make a previously non-ambulatory population ambulatory, as may be the case in a complete paraplegic, for example. However, the full "costs" of the technology need to be examined including equipment, therapy, and the indirect costs of, for example, the time spent away from vocational pursuits. The utility of FES should probably be balanced with, for example, the utility of work toward improving recovery following SCI. Also, the scope of outcomes used in research should probably be expanded to include a measure of quality of life. Thus, any beneficial effects of FES systems would be observed using physiologic, functional, handicap, and quality of life measures.

Upper Extremity Stimulation

FES systems for the upper extremity have not been widely published. Betz et al.[115] described surgical transposition of a muscle and subsequent triggered stimulation with the concurrent use of an orthosis in a C4 quadriplegic patient, who learned to feed himself using this system.

Nathan and Ohry[116] described two individuals with C4 complete quadriplegia who used a voice-activated FES system that triggered preprogramed sequences of muscle stimulation that provided the individuals with grasp to allow writing, eating, and drinking. This system was used in conjunction with residual shoulder girdle movements and mechanical splinting.

Gorman and Peckham[117] and Peckham and Creasey[118] reviewed the current research into FES systems for the upper extremity and evaluated 10 patients. When these 10 quadriplegics were evaluated with 10 functional upper extremity activities, 89 percent completed the activities with the neuroprosthesis, whereas only 49 percent could complete them without. They also note that 27 percent of patients that have the appropriate level of quadriplegia from SCI were subsequently excluded because of nerve root denervation. These same data were also published by Wijman et al.[119]

Thus, we have a Grade C recommendation supporting the use of FES in the upper extremity to improve function in select quadriplegics.

SPASTICITY

Drug Treatment of Spasticity

Spasticity occurs in more than 75 percent of SCI patients and is manifested clinically by increased resistance to passive stretch, flexor and/or extensor spasms, hyperactive deep tendon reflexes (DTR), and clonus.[120,121] The decision to treat spasticity should be based on whether the spasticity is causing pain or interfering with function or nursing care. Physical modalities are the first line of treatment for spasticity. If these measures are unsuccessful, then pharmacologic agents or surgical management may be used. Many of the studies that have evaluated the effectiveness of pharmacologic agents for "spinal spasticity" utilize subjects with several different diagnoses, including traumatic SCI, myelopathy due to spondylosis, multiple sclerosis (MS), and idiopathic or hereditary spastic paraparesis. Few of these studies present specific data on those with traumatic SCI; in those that do, the numbers are often too small to reach any statistically significant conclusions (Table 3-1).

Diazepam

Diazepam is the oldest antispasticity medication that is still widely used.[122] It is a centrally acting benzodiazepine that appears to potentiate the presynaptic inhibitory effects of γ-aminobutyric acid (GABA).[123] In a double-blind cross-over study[124] of 21 subjects, four of whom had spinal lesions, diazepam resulted in a significant reduction in resistance to passive stretch and spasms when compared to placebo. There was no significant change in muscle strength. The results are not stratified according to diagnosis; therefore it is not certain whether the spinal lesion subjects responded similarly to the entire group. In another double-blind cross-over study[125] of 19 subjects, however, diazepam, 6 and 15 mg/day, had no statistically significant effect on the time it took for the lower limb to drop from 180 to 90 degrees of knee flexion and no effect on the range of motion when compared to placebo. Grip strength was significantly diminished and the time it took to walk a maze was increased. Only four of the 19 subjects had spinal cord lesions, all the result of cervical spondylosis. When the data on these four patients were analyzed individually there was a difference in trend when compared with the entire group.[125]

Diazepam 45 mg/day, was superior to placebo and to amytal in a double-blind cross-over study[126] involving 22 subjects with traumatic SCI when evaluated by a physician, nurse, and therapist not involved in the subject's treatment. Neither the subject nor the treating physical therapist, however, noted any statistically significant difference between the treatments. The response to treatment was graded by each evaluator as worse, no effect, better,

or much better; but the authors do not describe the methods of evaluation.[126]

The effectiveness of diazepam in complete and incomplete spinal lesion has been studied. In an open label trial of 14 subjects,[127] diazepam given intravenously resulted in a statistically significant decrease in the excitability of the monosynaptic reflex arc in patients with MS, incomplete traumatic SCI, and transverse myelitis, but not in patients with complete traumatic SCI. The authors postulate that diazepam, therefore, may exert its effect primarily at a supraspinal level. Only neurophysiologic measures of spasticity were evaluated in this study, and no clinical correlation was provided.[127] In another open trial[128] aimed at comparing responses in complete and incomplete spinal lesions, 10 subjects were evaluated before and after intravenous diazepam. The evaluation consisted of "observations of movements and reactions" and evaluation of the general appearance and duration of motor unit activity noted on surface EMG following a physical stimulus to the lower extremity. In both complete and incomplete SCI the drug could be effective or ineffective against spasticity but no statistical analysis was provided.[128]

In summary, two double-blind cross-over studies have demonstrated a statistically significant improvement in spasticity in SCI subjects taking diazepam; however, in one study, there were only four SCI subjects,[124] and in the other the outcome measures were subjective and benefit was not seen by all observers.[126] Another study demonstrated no change in the speed of knee flexion with diazepam, but a trend was noted in the SCI subgroup. However, no clinical correlation was given.[125] The trials perhaps qualify for two Level II trials[124,125] and one Level I trial,[126] giving a Grade A recommendation that diazepam may be considered for the treatment of spasticity following SCI, although improvement is not uniform across studies.

Baclofen

Baclofen is a centrally acting antispasticity medication that is commonly used in SCI. It is an analog of the inhibitory neurotransmitter GABA and appears to act in the spinal cord on polysynaptic inhibitory pathways.[123] A double-blind cross-over study of

Table 3-1. Drug Treatment of Spasticity

Author	Population			Intervention			Outcome		
	Size	Randomized	SCI	Blind	Drug	Standardized and Objective Measures	Results	Level of Evidence	Grade of Recommendation
Wilson & McKechnie (1966)[124]	21	Crossover	4	Yes	Diazepam Placebo	No	Decreased resistance to stretch	Level II	Grade B
Cocchiarella et al. (1967)[125]	19	Crossover	4	Yes	Diazepam Placebo	Yes	No change in limb drop but a trend in SCI patients	Level II	Grade B
Corbett et al. (1972)[126]	22	Crossover	22	Yes	Diazepam Placebo	No	Three observers felt spasms improved, patient and treating PT felt no difference	Level I	Grade A
Jones et al. (1970)[129]	6	Crossover	6	Yes	Baclofen Placebo	Some objective Some subjective	Less resistance to passive range and less excitable stretch	Level II	Grade B
Basmajian & Yucel (1974)[130]	11	Crossover	3	Yes	Baclofen Placebo	Some objective Some subjective	EMG, spasms, DTR, clonus, pain, and function all improved No statistics	Level II	Grade B
Duncan et al. (1976)[131]	22	Crossover	11	Yes	Baclofen Placebo	Some objective Some subjective	Decreased spasm and resistance to stretch DTR, gait and clonus No statistics	Level II	Grade B
Hinderer et al. (1990)[132]	5	Crossover	5	Yes	Baclofen Placebo	Yes	No change Passive ankle movement No change	Negative	
Basmajian & Super (1973)[134]	23	Crossover	5	Yes	Dantrolene Sodium Placebo	Some yes	EMG response, spasm, clonus, DTR, strength all improved	Level II	Grade B
Monster (1974)[135]	147	Crossover	60	Yes	Dantrolene Sodium Placebo	Some yes	Subjective rating of ADL and clonus better, statistics not described	Cannot tell	
Weiser et al. (1978)[136]	35	Crossover	0	Yes	Dantrolene Sodium Placebo	Some yes	Tone, clonus, gait, and spasms improved in 8 that completed study	Level II	Grade B
Luisto et al. (1982)[137]	14	Crossover	8	Yes	Dantrolene Sodium Placebo	Some yes	PROM, clonus, DTR, improved	Level II	Grade B
Maynard (1986)[139]	12	No open label	12	No	Clonidine	No	No change in ADL Reported spasms better in 7 but CVA and seizure side effect	Level V	Grade C
Donovan et al. (1988)[140]	55	No	55	No	Clonidine	No	56 percent had decreased tone	Level V	Grade C
Nance et al. (1989)[141]	6	Yes	6	Yes	Clonidine Placebo	Yes	EMG yes No change in DTR or clonus	Level I	Grade A
Mathias et al. (1989)[143]	10	No	10	No	Tizanidine	Yes	Ashworth Scale improved	Level V	Grade C

Abbreviations: ADL, activities of daily living; DTR, deep tendon reflexes; PROM, passive range of motion; CVA, cerebrovascular accident; EMG, electromyography; PT, physical therapist.

29

baclofen versus placebo in six SCI subjects demonstrated improved resistance to passive range of motion (PROM) in all of the subjects and fewer spasms in four of the subjects taking 60 to 75 mg baclofen compared to placebo. All six subjects had less excitability of quadriceps stretch reflex demonstrated by reduced surface EMG activity while on baclofen. There was no difference in response to baclofen between the complete and incomplete subjects. This study utilized a small number of subjects and the authors did not note whether any of the improvements were statistically significant. Additionally, there was no comment on any impact the treatments had on function.[129]

A double-blind cross-over trial of baclofen versus placebo was conducted on 11 patients, three of whom had SCI.[130] Evaluation included EMG response to tendon tap and voluntary contraction, frequency of spasms, deep tendon reflexes (DTRs), clonus, subjective impressions regarding pain, motor status and presence of spasms, and weekly assessment of routine activity. The investigator felt that the response of the three SCI subjects was "much superior" while taking baclofen. There were no statistics performed on these results and the number of SCI subjects was small.[130]

Baclofen resulted in a significantly decreased number of spasms and resistance to passive range of motion when compared to placebo in a double-blind cross-over design study of 22 subjects, 11 of whom had spinal cord lesions other than MS.[131] No consistent change in DTRs or clonus was noted, and there was no change in muscle strength. Seven patients presented with a "spastic gait," which did not improve while on baclofen. The specific gait evaluation performed was not described. This study did not stratify the results according to neurologic disease, therefore, it is not possible to determine how the SCI subjects responded as a group.[131]

In a multiple baseline, double-blind study[132] of five traumatic SCI subjects, baclofen, 40 and 80 mg/day, did not result in any significant reduction of viscous or elastic stiffness measurements generated by passive sinusoidal ankle motion when compared to placebo. No other clinical or functional response to treatment was reported. The authors note that this study involved only patients who had previously been on baclofen but had discontinued treatment for unknown reasons. Therefore, this sample may represent a selection bias of subjects who do not respond to baclofen.[132]

In summary, two double-blind crossover studies have demonstrated the effectiveness of baclofen in reducing spasms, spasticity, and EMG activity with passive stretch and improving function in SCI subjects, although the numbers of subjects in each study was small.[129,130] Another demonstrated no change in spastic gait but reduced spasms and resistance to passive stretch.[131] The final study demonstrated that baclofen did not produce any decreased stiffness during passive ankle movement but this was a small study with a potentially biased population.[132] Thus, possibly three qualify for Level II trials that result in a Grade B recommendation that baclofen be considered for treatment of spasticity in SCI, but it may not produce improvement in all aspects of the clinical spectrum of problems seen with increased spasticity.

Dantrolene Sodium

Dantrolene sodium (Dantrium) diminishes spasticity by acting directly on skeletal muscle by depressing the release of calcium ions from the sarcoplasmic reticulum.[133] In a double-blind crossover study of dantrolene sodium in 23 subjects, five of whom were SCI, four subjects withdrew because of side effects (one while on placebo), and the results of treatment in four other cases were not decisive enough to draw conclusions. It is not clear how many of the remaining 15 subjects were SCI, but all had a statistically significant improvement while on dantrolene sodium compared to placebo. Evaluation was based on electrophysiologic studies, observation, and ratings of spasticity, strength, clonus, and tendon jerks. Almost all patients reported some weakness, which was severe enough to cause three patients to withdraw from the study.[134] A double-blind crossover study of a much larger group of 147 subjects included approximately 60 SCI subjects.[135] The overall clinical responses, as measured by a physician, improved in 83 percent, activities of daily living (ADL) assessment improved in 43 percent, and clonus was reduced in 90 percent of the entire patient population while on dantrolene sodium. Changes resulting from datrolene sodium were more qualitative than quantitative. Results of the statistical analyses were not provided.[135]

In a study specifically designed to evaluate the effectiveness of dantrolene sodium in chronic spinal cord disease,[136] the subject population consisted of nine with MS, eleven with spondylotic myelopathy, eight with hereditary spastic paraplegia, four with syringomyelia, and three miscellaneous subjects. In this double-blind crossover study, improvement on dantrolene was found to be statistically significant for tone in the limbs, knee and ankle clonus, flexor spasms, and gait. Eight patients who completed the trial had muscle weakness, which adversely affected their stance and gait while on dantrolene sodium but which improved when the dose was lowered.[136]

Fourteen subjects completed another double-blind crossover study of dantrolene sodium, eight of whom were SCI.[137] There was a statistically significant decrease in resistance to passive stretch, clonus, and hyperreflexia without significant reduction of muscle strength. No significant improvement was noted in ADLs. Response to treatment was not stratified by diagnostic group, however, the authors note that patients with SCI seemed to tolerate dantrolene better than the other patients.[137]

Hepatic injury may occur with the use of dantrolene sodium. Chan[138] reviewed 122 cases of hepatic injury from dantrolene sodium that was reported to the manufacturer through 1987.[138] Forty-seven subjects had asymptomatic transaminase elevations, 12 had additional mild hyperbilirubinemia, 36 had jaundice, and 27 patients died. There was an over-representation of women over 35 years and patients with MS in the fatal group compared to the entire group, although this finding was not statistically significant. Mean dantrolene dose was 582 mg/day in the fatal group, compared to 263 mg/day in the non-fatal group.

In summary, dantrolene sodium reduced resistance to passive stretch, spasms, and clonus in four double-blind crossover studies. In two studies, the number of subjects was small but the results still reached statistical significance, although not performed separately on SCI patients. In one study with a larger number of subjects, no statistical analysis of the results was provided. Dantrolene sodium caused significant weakness, which may impair function. Hepatic toxicity, including death, is

a concern and physicians should monitor liver function studies of those taking the drug. Thus there are three, possibly four, Level II trials that support a Grade B recommendation for considering dantrolene sodium in the treatment of spasticity following SCI. This recommendation has to be balanced with the reported side effects of weakness, hepatic toxicity, and death.

Clonidine

Clonidine is a centrally acting α_2-agonist that exerts antispasticity effects.[139] An open clinical trial of clonidine in 12 SCI subjects demonstrated a reduction in spasticity by patient report and by observation of spasticity during functional activities and a reduction in muscle tone and spasm in seven of the subjects. Five of the responders discontinued treatment because of the following intolerable side effects: syncopal seizures in two responders, cerebrovascular accident in one responder, lethargy in three responders, and nausea and vomiting in one. The authors note that reduction in spasticity was clonidine dose-related and that little improvement was observed until a dose of at least 0.3 mg a day was reached. Three of the five nonresponders did not reach this dose before discontinuing because of side effects.[139] Another open clinical trial of 55 SCI subjects who had established spasticity unresponsive to baclofen demonstrated a decrease in hypertonicity in 56 percent of subjects treated with clonidine. The authors did not provide specifics regarding this evaluation. Seventeen of the nonresponders did not reach maximum dosage (0.1 mg four times a day) before discontinuing the drug because of side effects, disappointment with lack of response, and noncompliance.[140] In a single-blind study of six SCI subjects, treatment with clonidine resulted in a statistically significant reduction of the vibratory inhibition of the H reflex when compared to placebo. There was no significant change in measurement of the Achilles DTR or clonus. The authors reported no functional response to the treatment.[141]

In summary, clonidine is supported by one Level I and two Level V trials with stronger evidence of laboratory versus functional effect but also significant side effects, often at less than therapeutic doses. Therefore, this is a Grade A recommendation supporting the use of clonidine for the treatment of spasticity, but side effects may limit its usefulness.

Tizanidine

Tizanidine is an imidazole derivative that diminishes spasticity by depressing polysynaptic reflexes.[142] In an open trial involving 10 traumatic SCI subjects, there was a statistically significant reduction in spasticity, as measured by the Ashworth Scale, following a single oral dose of 8 mg and lasting 4 hours. There was no effect on voluntary muscle power.[143] Tizanidine is not approved for use in Canada or the United States.

Crossover Studies

Several studies have compared the effectiveness of various antispasticity medications. Two double-blind crossover studies compared baclofen and diazepam. Neither study found a statistically significant difference between the two drugs.[144,145] Another study found no difference in response between dantrolene sodium and diazepam.[146] A double-blind crossover trial comparing tizanidine with baclofen in 32 MS and four syringomyelia subjects found no statistically significant difference between the two drugs.[147]

Ten subjects, four with compressive myelopathy, were evaluated in a double-blind crossover study comparing the effects of tizanidine, baclofen, and placebo on spastic gait using polarized light goniometry. Only minimal subjective and objective changes in gait were noted with either drug when compared to placebo.[148]

Intrathecal Treatment of Spasticity

Baclofen

Baclofen is quite effective in reducing spasms and spasticity in SCI subjects when delivered intrathecally. In a double-blind crossover study, 10 SCI subjects underwent implantation of an intrathecal pump which was filled with either saline or baclofen. Evaluation included assessment of number of spasms, resistance to passive range of motion. EMG responses during passive and/or active movement, DTRs, and voluntary control of the lower extremities. There was a statistically significant improvement on each evaluation scale while on baclofen infusion as compared to saline.[149] Loubser et al.[150] compared intrathecal baclofen (ITB) and saline infusion in nine SCI subjects and found that baclofen produced a significantly greater decrease in resistance to passive range of motion and reflex score when compared to saline. Eight subjects demonstrated improved mobility and self-care. One ambulatory motor incomplete subject developed muscle weakness while on ITB and his ambulatory function decreased.[150] Penn[151] reported a series of 62 subjects, 30 with SCI, treated with ITB and followed for up to 84 months. The improvement noted in resistance to passive range of motion and number of spasms immediately after treatment was maintained through follow-up; however, subjects required gradually increasing dose over the first 2 years after which the required dose tended to stabilize.

Morphine Sulfate

Morphine sulfate administered intrathecally in open clinical trials has been effective in controlling spasticity in SCI subjects and those with other neurologic disorders.[152] In a series of 32 subjects, 25 had complete or good relief of their spasticity with a bolus injection. No quantitative measure of spasticity was provided. Twelve subjects underwent implantation of an intrathecal pump or reservoir and only one became drug tolerant.[152] No controlled studies have been performed on intrathecal morphine for treatment of spasticity.

In summary, considering intrathecal baclofen is a Grade A recommendation; the use of intrathecal morphine for the treatment of spasticity would be a Grade C recommendation.

Surgical Treatment of Spasticity

Surgical treatment of spasticity is usually reserved for cases in which less invasive treatments have failed. Surgical procedures include neurotomy, anterior and posterior rhizotomy, myelotomy, and spinal cord stimulation. No well-controlled studies provide evidence for the advantage of one procedure over another; however, many case series have been reported.

Anterior Rhizotomy

In 1947, a series of 28 SCI subjects treated with anterior rhizotomy from T11 through S1 and followed for

3 to 19 months postoperatively was described.[153] The authors report that the "severe, deforming spasms were relieved in all cases," but there was "non-disabling residual spasticity" in five cases. Functional gains, weight gain, and healing of decubitus ulcers were also reported. The authors do not comment on any complications except for one case of development of a completely flaccid bladder.[153] Other authors note that anterior rhizotomies produce marked muscle loss and should be performed only on subjects with complete motor paralysis.[154,155]

Myelotomy

Myelotomy is also generally reserved for those without residual motor function. In a series of 24 subjects, longitudinal myelotomy resulted in "satisfactory results" in 22 subjects.[154] The authors do not describe the patient population or the specific results of the procedure. In a retrospective review of seven SCI subjects treated with longitudinal myelotomy and followed from 4 to 26 months, only one subject had no recurrence of spasticity.[156] This same subject lost spontaneous bladder voiding function, and another subject had decreased penile sensation and loss of sexual function. These authors conclude that myelotomy is not successful in controlling spasticity in SCI.[156]

Neurectomy

For those with incomplete SCI, section of the obturator, sciatic, femoral, and tibial nerves has been reported to result in improvement in spasticity.[155,157] Dorsal rhizotomy also may be performed on incomplete SCI subjects, and results in reduction of spasticity and spasms without directly impairing voluntary movement or causing marked muscle atrophy.[155] Percutaneous radiofrequency rhizotomy (PRFR) has been studied prospectively in a series of 25 subjects,[158] two with SCI. Both SCI subjects had improvement in their tone and relief of their spasms through follow-up of 6 months in one subject and 18 months in the other subject. There were no complications and no patient had a change in bowel, bladder, or sexual function.[158]

A retrospective review[159] of one center's experience with neurosurgical management of spasticity in 118 subjects, over half with traumatic SCI, was reported in 1990. Techniques utilized on the SCI subjects were PRFR, sciatic neurectomy via percutaneous radiofrequency approach, open neurectomies of the sciatic and posterior tibial nerve branches combined with tenotomies of the hamstring and Achilles tendons, and longitudinal myelotomy. The authors do not stratify their results based on neurologic diagnosis; however, they note excellent improvement in resistance to passive range of motion was noted in 85 percent of those who underwent PRFR, 96 percent of those treated with sciatic neurectomy, and 100% who underwent neurectomy and tenotomy or myelotomy. Sixty-one percent of those undergoing PRFR had recurrent spasticity that required either repeat PRFR or other procedures. Forty-one percent of all subjects continued on oral antispasticity medication postoperatively.[159]

Spinal Cord Stimulation for Spasticity

There have been several reports of beneficial effects of spinal cord stimulation (SCS) on spasticity in SCI subjects. In a series of 59 subjects who had SCS on a trial basis for 7 days, the authors reported a marked or moderate clinical benefit in 37 subjects (63 percent). Fifteen of 30 subjects who had implantation with a permanent system responded to a follow-up questionnaire; six were continuing to use the SCS, two were waiting for repairs, three stopped using SCS because of lack of benefit, and four others stopped for miscellaneous reasons.[160] Neurophysiologic evaluation of reflex activity in 15 SCI subjects who reported beneficial clinical effects from SCS was performed. The data was analyzed by a single observer who was unacquainted with the clinical status of individual patients and not involved in the SCS trial. Changes occurred in 55 percent of the neurophysiologic responses during SCS, but with widely varying patterns of response.[161] A report of a series of 16 subjects with severe spasms secondary to myelopathy noted significant therapeutic benefit in 14 subjects, mainly less frequent and less severe spasms. Other beneficial effects in this series included improved bowel and bladder function in some subjects and increased voluntary motor control in one subject. Complications included infection, wire breakage, and skin breakdown over the insertion of the electrode.[162]

Other reports of SCS in SCI are not as positive. In one series of 15 SCI subjects tested percutaneously for a few days, only three demonstrated enough improvement to proceed to permanent implantation. Of these, one subject showed no change and the other two showed only very minimal changes.[163] In another series of seven SCI subjects, all had improvement in spasms and clonus, but five had technical problems and required additional surgery. Only four continued to use their system 12 to 30 months after implantation. The authors noted that the changes obtained by chronic SCS were moderate and that it is essential to educate and train the patient to utilize SCS with regular physical therapy in the first weeks after implantation. They also noted that results were poorer in subjects treated who had fewer physical therapy facilities available to them.[164]

There have been no controlled studies on SCS in SCI. Subjects usually can identify when the SCS is on and, therefore, blinding would be difficult to maintain. Additionally, factors such as postimplantation physical therapy have not been consistent and may have biased outcomes. Many technical difficulties and failures are reported, which often require repeat surgery.

In summary, with respect to more invasive treatments for spasticity, these procedures are supported only by case series or Level V studies. Thus, there is a Grade C recommendation that rhizotomy, myelotomy, neurotomy, and spinal cord stimulation be considered for the treatment of spasticity following SCI. These therapies are usually applicable to a subpopulation of SCI patients, and relief is often incomplete and may be temporary. Further prospective, matched cohort studies are warranted, at a minimum, but randomized controlled trials are preferable.

REFERENCES

1. Dolan EJ, Tator CH, Endrenyi L: The value of decompression for acute experimental spinal cord compression injury. J Neurosurg 53:749, 1980
2. Delamarter RB, Sherman JE, Carr JB: The pathophysiology of spinal cord damage and subsequent recovery following immediate or delayed decompression. J Am Paraplegia Soc 17:105, 1994
3. Rivlin AS, Tator CH: Effect of duration of acute spinal cord compression in a new acute cord injury model in the rat. Surg Neurol 10:30, 1978
4. Johnsson R, Herrlin K, Hagglund G, Stromqvist B: Spinal canal remodeling after thoracolumbar fractures with intraspinal bone fragments. 17 cases followed 1–4 years. J Ortho Scand 62:125, 1991
5. Levine M, Lin S, Balderston R, Cotler J: Fate of residual retropulsed bone fragments in surgically managed thoracolumbar burst fractures. J Am Paraplegia Soc 17:98, 1994
6. Willen J, Anderson J, Tomooka K, Singer K: The natural history of burst fractures at the thoracolumbar junction. J Spinal Disord 3:39, 1990
7. Waters RL, Adkins RH, Yakura JS, Sie I: Recovery following complete paraplegia. Arch Phys Med Rehabil 73:784, 1992
8. Waters RL, Adkins RH, Yakura JS, Sie I: Motor and sensory recovery following complete tetraplegia. Arch Phys Med Rehabil 74:242, 1993
9. Waters RL, Adkins RH, Yakura JS, Sie I: Motor and sensory recovery following incomplete paraplegia. Arch Phys Med Rehabil 75:67, 1994
10. Waters RL, Adkins RH, Yakura JS, Sie I: Motor and sensory recovery following incomplete tetraplegia. Arch Phys Med Rehabil 75:306, 1994
11. Schwartz S, Cohen ME, Herbison GJ, Shah A: Relationship between two measures of upper extremity strength: manual muscle test compared to handheld myometry. Arch Phys Med Rehabil 73:1063, 1992
12. Isaac Z, Herbison G, Cohen M, Ditunno J: Superiority of the use of a force transducer to the MMT in quantifying changes in strength post-SCI. J Am Paraplegia Soc 17:94, 1994
13. Ditunno JF, Stover SL, Freed MM, Ahn JH: Motor recovery of the upper extremity in traumatic quadriplegia: a multicenter study. Arch Phys Med Rehabil 73:431, 1992
14. Graziani V, Crozier KS, Herbison GJ et al: Strength recovery in the three levels of zone of partial preservation in motor complete quadriplegia after one year post-injury. J Am Paraplegia Soc 15:122, 1992
15. Mange KC, Marino RJ, Gregory PC et al: Course of motor recovery in the zone of partial preservation in spinal cord injury. Arch Phys Med Rehabil 73:437, 1992
16. Wu L, Marino RJ, Herbison GJ, Ditunno JF: Recovery of zero-grade muscles in the zone of partial preservation in motor complete quadriplegia. Arch Phys Med Rehabil 73:40, 1991
17. Stover SL, Fine PR (eds): Spinal Cord Injury: The Facts and Figures. The University of Alabama at Birmingham, Birmingham, 1986
18. Crozier KS, Graziani V, Ditunno JF, Herbison GJ: Spinal cord injury: prognosis for ambulation based on sensory examination in patients who are initially

motor complete. Arch Phys Med Rehabil 72:119, 1991

19. Penrod LE, Hedge SK, Ditunno JF: Age effect on prognosis for functional recovery in acute, traumatic central cord syndrome. Arch Phys Med Rehabil 71: 963, 1990

20. Blaustein DM, Zafonte RD, Thomas D et al: Predicting recovery of motor complete quadriplegic patients: 24-hour vs. 72-hour motor index scores. Am J Phys Med Rehabil 72:306, 1993

21. Kiwerski JE: Neurological outcome from conservative or surgical treatment of cervical spinal cord injured patients. J Paraplegia 31:192, 1993

22. Brunette DD, Rockswold GL: Neurologic recovery following rapid spinal realignment for complete cervical spinal cord injury. J Trauma 27:445, 1987

23. Jeanneret B, Magerl F, Ward JC: Overdistraction: a hazard of skull traction in the management of acute injuries of the cervical spine. Arch Orthop Trauma Surg 110:242, 1991

24. Cotler JM, Herbison GJ, Nasuti JF et al: Closed reduction of traumatic cervical spine dislocation using traction weights up to 140 pounds. Spine 18:386, 1993

25. Weinshel SS, Maiman DJ, Baek P, Scales L: Neurologic recovery in quadriplegia following operative treatment. J Spinal Disord 3:244, 1990

26. Bose B, Northrup BE, Osterholm JL et al: Reanalysis of central cervical cord injury management. Neurosurgery 15:367, 1984

27. Krengel WF, Anderson PA, Henley MB: Early stabilization and decompression for incomplete paraplegia due to a thoracic-level spinal cord injury. J Spine 18:2080, 1993

28. Lemons VR, Wagner FC Jr, Montesano PX: Management of thoracolumbar fractures with accompanying neurological injury. J Neurosurg 30:667, 1992

29. Hu SS, Capen DA, Rimoldi RL, Zigle JE: The effect of surgical decompression on neurologic outcome after lumber fractures. J Clin Orthop Related Res 288:166, 1993

30. Yashon D, Jane JA, White RJ: Prognosis and management of spinal cord and cauda equina bullet injuries in sixty-five civilians. J Neurosurg 32:163, 1970

31. Simpson RK Jr, Venger BH, Narayan RK: Treatment of acute penetrating injuries of the spine: a retrospective analysis. J Trauma 29:42, 1989

32. Waters RL, Adkins RH: The effects of removal of bullet fragments retained in the spinal canal. A collaborative study by the National Spinal Cord Injury Model Systems. J Spine 16:934, 1991

33. Wagner FC, Chehrazi B: Early decompression and neurologic outcome in acute cervical spinal cord injuries. J Neurosurg 56:669, 1982

34. Marshall LF, Knowlton S, Garfin SR et al: Deterioration following spinal cord injury. J Neurosurg 66:400, 1987

35. Levi L, Wolf A, Rigamonti D et al: Anterior decompression in cervical spine trauma: Does timing of surgery affect the outcome? Neurosurgery 29:216, 1991

36. Young JS, Dexter WR: Neurologic recovery distal to the zone of injury in 172 cases of closed, traumatic spinal cord injury. Paraplegia 16:39, 1978

37. Heiden JS, Wiess MH, Rosenberg AW et al: Management of cervical spinal cord trauma in Southern California. J Neurosurg 43:732, 1975

38. Anderson PA, Bohlman HH: Anterior decompression and arthrodesis of the cervical spine: long-term motor improvement. Part II. Improvement in complete traumatic quadriplegia. J Bone Joint Surg 74: 683, 1992

39. Katoh S, El Masri WS: Neurological recovery after conservative treatment of cervical cord injuries. J Bone Joint Surg (Br) 760B:225, 1994

40. Aebi M, Mohler J, Zach GA, Morscher E: Indication, surgical technique and results of 100 surgically-treated fractures and fracture-dislocations of the cervical spine. Clin Orthop 203:244, 1986

41. Donovan WH: Operative and nonoperative management of spinal cord injury: a review. Paraplegia 32: 375, 1994

42. Blight AR, DeCrescito V: Morphometric analysis of experimental spinal cord injury in the cat: the relation of injury intensity to survival of myelinated axons. Neuroscience 19:321, 1986

43. Demoupoulos HB, Flamm ES, Pietronigro DD, Tomasula J: The free radical pathology and the microcirculation in the major central nervous system disorders. Acta Physiol Scand, Suppl. 492:91, 1980

44. Hall ED, Braughler JM: Central nervous system trauma and stroke: II. Physiological and pharmacological evidence for the involvement of oxygen radical and lipid peroxidation. Free Radic Biol Med 6:303, 1989

45. Feurstein G, Rabinovici R: Recent advances in the pharmacology of spinal cord injury. Traum Q 9:53, 1993

46. Hall ED, Yonkers PA, Andrus PK et al: Biochemistry and pharmacology of lipid antioxidants in acute brain and spinal cord injury. J Neurotrauma, suppl. 2, 9:S425, 1992

47. Hall ED: The role of oxygen radicals in traumatic injury: clinical implications. J Emerg Med 11:31, 1993

48. Young W: Secondary injury mechanisms in acute spinal cord injury. J Emerg Med 11:13, 1993

49. Bracken MB, Shepard MJ, Collins WF et al: A randomized, controlled trial of methylprednisolone or

naloxone in the treatment of acute spinal-cord injury. N Engl J Med 322:1405, 1990

50. Bracken MB, Shepard MJ, Hellenbrand KG et al: Methylprednisolone and neurological function one year after spinal cord injury. J Neurosurg 63:704, 1985

51. Braughler JM, Hall ED: Lactate and pyruvate metabolism in injured cat spinal cord before and after a single large intravenous dose of methylprednisolone. J Neurosurg 29:256, 1983

52. Bracken MB, Holford TR: Effects of timing of methylprednisolone or naloxone administration on recovery of segmental and long-tract neurological function in NASCIS 2. J Neurosurg 79:500, 1993

53. Barletta E, Bremer EG, Culp LA: Neurite outgrowth in dorsal root neuronal hybrid clones modulated by ganglioside GM-1 and disintegrins. Exp Cell Res 193: 101, 1991

54. Gorio A, Diguilio AM, Young W et al: GM-1 effects on chemical, traumatic and peripheral nerve induced lesions to the spinal cord. In Goldberger ME, Gorio A, Murray M (eds): Development and Plasticity of Mammalian Spinal Cord. Padova, Liviana, 1986

55. Geisler FH, Dorsey FC, Coleman WP: Recovery of motor function after spinal cord injury—a randomized, placebo-controlled trial with GM-1 ganglioside. N Engl J Med 324:1829, 1991

56. Geisler FH, Dorsey FC, Coleman WP: GM-1 ganglioside in human spinal cord injury. J Neurotrauma, suppl. 2, 9:S517, 1992

57. Geisler FH, Dorsey FC, Coleman WP: Past and current clinical studies with GM-1 gangliosice in acute spinal cord injury. Ann Emerg Med 22:1041, 1993

58. Hall ED, Yonkers PA, Andrus PK et al: Biochemistry and pharmacology of lipid antioxidants in acute brain and spinal cord injury. J Neurotrauma, suppl. 2, 9:S425, 1992

59. Althaus JS, Williams CM, Andrus PK et al: In vitro and in vivo analysis of tirilazad mesylate (U-74006F) as a hydroxyl radical (-OH) scavenger. Soc Neurosci Abst 17:164, 1991

60. Anderson DK, Braughler JM, Hall ED et al: Effect of treatment with U-74006F on neurological recovery following experimental spinal cord injury. J Neurosurg 69:562, 1988

61. Stover SL, Lloyd LK, Waites KB, Jackson AB: Urinary tract infection in spinal cord injury. Arch Phys Med Rehabil 70:47, 1989

62. The National Institute on Disability and Rehabilitation Research: The prevention and management of urinary tract infections among people with spinal cord injuries. J Am Paraplegia Soc 15:194, 1992

63. Kass EJ, Koff SA, Diokno AC, Lapides J: The significance of bacilluria in children on long-term intermittent catheterization. J Urol 126:223, 1981

64. Diokno AC, Sonda LP, Hollander JB, Lapides J: Fate of patients started on clean intermittent self-catheterization therapy 10 years ago. J Urol 129:1120, 1983

65. McGuire EJ, Savastano JA: Long-term follow-up of spinal cord injury patients managed by intermittent catheterization. J Urol 129:775, 1983

66. de la Hunt MN, Deegan S, Scott JE: Intermittent catheterization for neuropathic urinary incontinence. Arch Dis Child 64:821, 1989

67. Sutton G, Shah S, Hill V: Clean intermittent self-catheterization for quadriplegic patients—a five year follow-up. Paraplegia 29:542, 1991

68. Yadav A, Vaidyanathan S, Panigrahi D: Clean intermittent catheterization for the neuropathic bladder. Paraplegia 31:380, 1993

69. Bakke A, Irgens LM, Malt UF, Hoisaeter PA: Clean intermittent catheterization—performing abilities, aversive experiences and distress. Paraplegia 31:288, 1993

70. Perkash I, Giroux J: Clean intermittent catheterization in spinal cord injury patients: a follow-up study. J Urol 149:1068, 1993

71. King RB, Carlson CE, Mervine J et al: Clean and sterile intermittent catheterization methods in hospitalized patients with spinal cord injury. Arch Phys Med Rehabil 73:798, 1992

72. Kuhn W, Rist M, Zaech GA: Intermittent urethral self-catheterization: long term results (bacteriological evolution, continence, acceptance, complications). Paraplegia 29:222, 1991

73. Maynard FM, Glass J: Management of the neuropathic bladder by clean intermittent catheterization. Paraplegia 25:106, 1987

74. Peterson JR, Roth EJ: Fever, bacteriuria, and pyuria in spinal cord injured patients with indwelling urethral catheters. Arch Phys Med Rehabil 70:839, 1989

75. Mudgal KC, Gupta R, Singh S et al: Bladder rehabilitation in spinal cord injury patients. J Indian Med Assoc 90:52, 1992

76. Menon EB, Tan ES: Bladder training in patients with spinal cord injury. Urology 40:425, 1992

77. Timoney AG, Shaw PJ: Urological outcome in female patients with spinal cord injury: the effectiveness of intermittent catheterization. Paraplegia 28:556, 1990

78. Hall MK, Hackler RH, Zampieri TA, Zampieri JB: Renal calculi in spinal cord-injured patient: association with reflux, bladder stones, and foley catheter drainage. Urology 34:126, 1989

79. McGuire EJ, Savastano J: Comparative urlogical outcome in women with spinal cord injury. J Urol 135: 730, 1986

80. Lloyd LK, Kuhlemeier KV, Fine PR, Stover SL: Initial bladder management in spinal cord injury: does it make a difference? J Urol 135:523, 1986

81. Barkin M, Dolfin D, Herschorn S et al: The urologic care of the spinal cord injury patient. J Urol 129:335, 1983

82. Dewire DM, Owens RS, Anderson GA et al: A comparison of the urological complications associated with long-term management of quadriplegics with and without chronic indwelling urinary catheters. J Urol 147:1069, 1992

83. Noll F, Russe O, Kling E et al: Intermittent catheterization versus percutaneous suprapubic cystostomy in the early management of traumatic spinal cord lesions. Paraplegia 26:4, 1988

84. Cardenas DD, Mayo ME: Bacteriuria with fever after spinal cord injury. Arch Phys Med Rehabil 68:291, 1987

85. Barnes DG, Shaw PJ, Timoney AG, Tsokos N: Management of the neuropathic bladder by suprapubic catheterization. Br J Urol 72:169, 1993

86. Chao R, Clowers D, Mayo ME: Fate of upper urinary tracts in patients with indwelling catheters after spinal cord injury. Urology 42:259, 1993

87. Jackson AB, DeVivo M: Urological long-term follow-up in women with spinal cord injuries. Arch Phys Med Rehabil 73:1029, 1992

88. Viera A, Merritt JL, Erickson RP: Renal function in spinal cord injury: a preliminary report. Arch Phys Med Rehabil 67:257, 1986

89. Yanagita T, Iwatsubo E, Haraoka M, Osada Y: The value of an aseptic intermittent catheterization program in the early management of spinal cord injury patients. Nippon Hinyokika Gakkai Zasshi 84:1954, 1993

90. Killorin W, Gray M, Bennett JK, Green BG: The value of urodynamics and bladder management in predicting upper urinary tract complications in male spinal cord injury patients. Paraplegia 30:437, 1992

91. Biering-Sorensen F, Hoiby N, Nordenbo A, Ravnborg M: Ciprofloxacin as prophylaxis for urinary tract infection: prospective, randomized, cross-over, placebo controlled study in patients with spinal cord lesion. J Urol 151:105, 1994

92. Gribble MJ, Puterman ML: Prophylaxis of urinary tract infection in persons with recent spinal cord injury: a prospective, randomized, double-blind, placebo-controlled study of trimethoprim-sulfamethoxazole. Am J Med 95:141, 1993

93. Banovac K, Wade N, Gonzalez F et al: Decreased incidence of urinary tract infections in patients with spinal cord injury: effect of methenamine. J Am Paraplegia 14:52, 1991

94. Mohler JL, Cowen DL, Flanigan RC: Suppression and treatment of urinary tract infection in patients with an intermittently catheterized neurogenic bladder. J Urol 138:336, 1987

95. Kuhlemeier KV, Stover SL, Lloyd LK: Prophylactic antibacterial therapy for preventing urinary tract infections in spinal cord injury patients. J Urol 134:514, 1985

96. Maynard FM, Diokno AC: Urinary infection and complications during clean intermittent catheterization following spinal cord injury. J Urol 132:943, 1984

97. Merritt JL, Erickson RP, Opitz JL: Bacteriuria during follow-up in patients with spinal cord injury: II. Efficacy of antimicrobial suppressants. Arch Phys Med Rehabil 63:413, 1982

98. Lindan R, Joiner E: A prospective study of the efficacy of low dose nitrofurantoin in preventing urinary tract infections in spinal cord injury patients, with comments on the role of *Pseudomonas*. Paraplegia 22:61, 1984

99. Donovan WH, Stolov WC, Clowers DE, Clowers MR: Bacteriuria during intermittent catheterization following spinal cord injury. Arch Phys Med Rehabil 59:351, 1978

100. Bakke A: Clean intermittent catheterization. A valuable treatment regimen? Abstract IMSOP Meeting, Oslo, 1986

101. Lewis RI, Carron HM, Lockhart JL, Politano VA: Significance of asymptomatic bacteriuria in neurogenic bladder disease. Urology 23:343, 1984

102. Sotolongo JR Jr, Koleilat N: Significance of asymptomatic bacteriuria in spinal cord injury patients on condom catheter. retraction J Urol 143:979, 1990

103. Sotolongo JR Jr, Koleilat N: Significance of asymptomatic bacteriuria in spinal cord injury patients on condom catheter retraction. J Urol 148:898, 1992

104. Yarkony GM, Roth EJ, Cybulski GR, Jaeger RJ: Nuromuscular stimulation in spinal cord injury. II: Prevention of secondary complications. Arch Phys Med Rehabil 73:195, 1992

105. Stein RB, Belanger M, Wheeler G et al: Electrical systems for improving locomotion after incomplete spinal cord injury: an assessment. Arch Phys Med Rehabil 74:954, 1993

106. Granat MH, Ferguson AC, Andrews BJ, Delargy M: The role of functional electrical stimulation in the rehabilitation of patients with incomplete spinal cord injury—observed benefits during gait studies. Paraplegia 31:207, 1993

107. Granat MH, Heller BW, Nicol DJ et al: Improving limb flexion in FES gait using the flexion withdrawal response for the spinal cord injured person. J Biomed Eng 15:51, 1993

108. Granat M, Keating JF, Smith AC et al: The use of functional electrical stimulation to assist gait in patients with incomplete spinal cord injury. Disabil Rehabil 14:93, 1992

109. Kralj A, Bajd T, Turk R, Benko H: Posture switching for prolonging FES standing in paraplegic patients. Paraplegia 24:221, 1986

110. Kralj A, Bajd T, Turk R: Enhancement of gait restoration in spinal injured patients by FES. Clin Orthop 233:34, 1988

111. Rattay F, Mayr W: Quantitative assessment of electrically activated fiber populations exemplified by rotating stimulation. Biomed Tech (Berlin) 32:184, 1987

112. Phillips CA: FES and lower extremity bracing for ambulation exercise of the SCI individual: a medically prescribed system. Phys Ther 69:842, 1989

113. Bajd T, Kralj A, Turk R et al: Use of FES in the rehabilitation of patients with incomplete SCI. J Biomed Eng 11:96, 1989

114. Yarkony GM, Jaeger RJ, Roth E et al: Functional neuromuscular stimulation for standing after SCI. Arch Phys Med Rehabil 71:201, 1990

115. Betz RR, Mulcahey MJ, Smith BT et al: Bipolar latissimus dorsi transposition and functional neuromuscular stimulation to restore elbow flexion in an individual with C4 quadriplegia and C5 denervation. J Am Paraplegia Soc 15:220, 1992

116. Nathan RH, Ohry A: Upper limb functions regained in quadriplegia: a hybrid computerized neuromuscular stimulation system. Arch Phys Med Rehabil 71:415, 1990

117. Gorman PH, Peckham PH: Upper extremity functional neuromuscular stimulation J Neuro Rehab 5:3, 1991

118. Peckham PH, Creasey GH: Neural prostheses: clinical applications of functional electrical stimulation in spinal cord injury. Paraplegia 30:96, 1992

119. Wijman CA, Stroh KC, Van Doren CL et al: Functional evaluation of quadriplegic patients using a hand neuroprosthesis. Arch Phys Med Rehabil 71:1053, 1990

120. Little JW, Micklesen P, Umlauf R, Britell C: Lower extremity manifestations of spasticity in chronic spinal cord injury. Am J Phys Med Rehabil 68:32, 1989

121. Maynard FW, Karunas RS, Waring WP: Epidemiology of spasticity following traumatic spinal cord injury. Arch Phys Med Rehabil 71:566, 1990

122. Whyte J, Robinson KM: Pharmacologic management. In: Glen MB, Whyte J (eds): The Practical Management of Spasticity in Children and Adults. Lea & Febiger, Philadelphia, 1990

123. Davidoff RA: Mode of action of antipasticity drugs. Neurosurgery: State of the Art Reviews 4:315, 1989

124. Wilson LA, McKechnie AA: Oral diazepam in the treatment of spasticity in paraplegia. A double blind trial and subsequent impressions. Scott Med J 11:46, 1966

125. Cocchiarella A, Downey JA, Darling RC: Evaluation of the effect of diazepam on spasticity. Arch Phys Med Rehabil 49:393, 1967

126. Corbett M, Frankel HL, Michaelis L: A double blind, cross-over trial of valium in the treatment of spasticity. Paraplegia 10:19, 1972

127. Verrier M, Ashby P, MacLeod S: Diazepam effect on reflex activity in patients with complete spinal lesions and in those with other causes of spasticity. Arch Phys Med Rehabil 58:148, 1977

128. Cook JB, Nathan PW: On the site of action of diazepam in spasticity in man. J Neurol Sci 5:33, 1967

129. Jones RF, Burke D, Marosszeky JE, Gillies JD: A new agent for the control of spasticity. J Neurol Neurosurg Psychiatry 33:464, 1970

130. Basmajian JV, Yucel V: Effects of a GABA-derivative (BA-34647) on spasticity. Am J Phys Med 53:223, 1974

131. Duncan GW, Shahani BT, Young RR: An evaluation of baclofen treatment for certain symptoms in patients with spinal cord lesions. Neurology 26:441, 1976

132. Hinderer SR, Lehmann JF, Price R: Spasticity in spinal cord injured persons: quantitative effects of baclofen and placebo treatments. Am J Phys Med Rehabil 69:311, 1990

133. Merritt JL: Management of spasticity in spinal cord injury. Mayo Clin Proc 56:614, 1981

134. Basmajian JV, Super G: Dantrolene sodium in the treatment of spasticity. Arch Phys Med Rehabil 54:60, 1973

135. Monster AW: Spasticity and the effect of dantrolene sodium. Arch Phys Med Rehabil 55:373, 1974

136. Weiser R, Terenty T, Hudgson P, Weightman D: Dantrolene sodium in the treatment of spasticity in chronic spinal cord disease. The Practitioner 221:123, 1978

137. Luisto M, Moller K, Nuutila A, Palo J: Dantrolene sodium in spasticity of varying etiology. Acta Neurol Scand 65:355, 1982

138. Chan CH: Dantrolene sodium and hepatic injury. Neurology 40:1427, 1990

139. Maynard FM: Early clinical experience with clonidine in spinal spasticity. Paraplegia 24:175, 1986

140. Donovan WH, Carter E, Rossi D, Wilkerson MA: Clonidine effect on spasticity: a clinical trial. Arch Phys Med Rehabil 69:193, 1988

141. Nance PW, Shears AH, Nance DM: Reflex changes induced by clonidine in spinal cord injured patients. Paraplegia 27:296, 1989

142. Davies J: Selective depression of synaptic transmission of spinal neurons in the cat by a new centrally acting muscle relaxant, 5-chloro-4-(2-imidazolin-2-yl-

amino)-2,1,3-benzothiodazole (DS103-282). Br J Pharmacol 76:473, 1982

143. Mathias CJ, Luckitt J, Desai P et al: Pharmacodynamics and pharmacokinetics of the oral antispastic agent tizanidine in patients with spinal cord injury. J Rehabil Res Dev 26:9, 1989

144. Cartlidge NEF, Hudgson P, Weightman D: A comparison of baclofen and diazepam in the treatment of spasticity. J Neurol Sci 23:17, 1974

145. Roussan M, Terrence C, Fromm G: Baclofen versus diazepam for the treatment of spasticity and long-term follow-up of baclofen therapy. Pharmatherapeutica 4:278, 1985

146. Glass A, Hannah A: A comparison of dantrolene sodium and diazepam in the treatment of spasticity. Paraplegia 12:170, 1974

147. Newman PM, Nogues M, Newman PK et al: Tizanidine in the treatment of spasticity. Eur J Clin Pharmacol 23:31, 1982

148. Corston RN, Johnson F, Godwin-Austen RB: The drug treatment of spastic gait. J Neurol Neurosurg Psychiatry 44:1035, 1981

149. Penn RD, Savoy SM, Corcos D et al: Intrathecal baclofen for severe spinal spasticity. N Engl J Med 320:1217, 1989

150. Loubser PG, Narayan RK, Sandin KJ et al: Continuous infusion of intrathecal baclofen: long-term effects on spasticity in spinal cord injury. Paraplegia 29:48, 1991

151. Penn RD: Intrathecal baclofen for spasticity of spinal origin: seven years of experience. J Neurosurg 77:236, 1992

152. Erickson DL, Lo J, Michaelson M: Control of intractable spasticity with intrathecal morphine sulfate. Neurosurgery 24:236, 1989

153. Freeman LW, Heimburger RF: The surgical relief of spasticity in paraplegic patients. I. Anterior rhizotomy. J Neurosurg 4:435, 1947

154. Dujovny M, Laha RK, Yonas H: Surgical management of spasticity. Curr Probl Surg 17:249, 1980

155. Barolat G: Surgical management of spasticity and spasms in spinal cord injury: an overview. J Am Paraplegia Soc 11:9, 1988

156. Fogel JP, Waters RL, Mahomar F: Dorsal myelotomy for relief of spasticity in spinal injury patients. Clin Orthop Related Res 192:137, 1985

157. Freeman LW, Heimburger RF: The surgical relief of spasticity in paraplegic patients. II. Peripheral nerve section, posterior rhizotomy, and other procedures. J Neurosurg 5:555, 1948

158. Kasdon DL, Lathi ES: A prospective study of radiofrequency rhizotomy in the treatment of posttraumatic spasticity. Neurosurgery 15:526, 1984

159. Herz DA, Looman JE, Tiberio A et al: The management of paralytic spasticity. Neurosurgery 26:300, 1990

160. Dimitrijevic MM, Dimitrijevic MR, Illis LS et al: Spinal cord stimulation for the control of spasticity in patients with chronic spinal cord injury: I. Clinical observations. Cent Nerv Syst Trauma 3:129, 1986

161. Dimitrijevic MR, Illis LS, Nakajima K et al: Spinal cord stimulation for the control of spasticity in patients with chronic spinal cord injury. II. Neurophysiologic observations. Cent Nerv Syst Trauma 3:145, 1986

162. Barolat G, Myklebust JB, Wenninger W: Effects of spinal cord stimulation on spasticity and spasms secondary to myelopathy. Appl Neurophysiol 51:29, 1988

163. Siegfried J, Lazorthes Y, Broggi G: Electrical spinal cord stimulation for spastic movement disorders. Appl Neurophysiol 44:77, 1981

164. Campos RJ, Dimitrijevic MM, Faganel J, Sharkey PC: Clinical evaluation of spinal cord stimulation on motor performance in patients with upper motor neuron lesions. Appl Neurophysiol 44:141, 1981

4

Traumatic Brain Injury

Scott H. Garner
M. Alan J. Finlayson

Rehabilitation is an ongoing process that enables individuals to find solutions for their problems in living. Ultimately, success will be determined by improvement of functioning in the community (reduction of handicap). Rehabilitation management of individuals with impairments from traumatic brain injury (TBI) is especially complex, spanning multiple clinical environments and domains. Clinical issues are usually multidimensional and challenge the problem-solving capabilities of the clinicians who cannot easily refer to scientific support or well-established precedents for any of their solutions. Adjustment is more difficult both because the individual's learning skills can be impaired and because the community is often poorly informed and not always sympathetic to difficulties encountered by individuals after brain trauma, especially when it involves behavioral control.

CONFOUNDING PROBLEMS

The levels of evidence used to evaluate the efficacy of brain injury treatments is marred not only by the lack of actual studies in the Level I or Level II class, but also by fundamental difficulties in this field of study which make the possibility of completing Level I or II studies unachievable. These difficulties include the following categories:

A Lack of Agreement About Outcome Criteria

A recent review based on work by the Head Injury Interdisciplinary Special Interest Group (HI SIG) of the American Congress of Rehabilitation Medicine attempts to address these difficulties.[1] According to their report, current outcome monitoring systems are widely perceived as technically inadequate, leaving rehabilitation professionals with nagging scientific questions about the effectiveness of TBI rehabilitation.

Outcome is perceived differently by different clients, therapists, and third-party payers. Clients of rehabilitation programs may wish to achieve particular goals (e.g., ability to work, drive, relate to others). These goals may or may not correspond to those of the rehabilitation providers who may establish different priorities for short-term goals, even though they may value and respect the client's point of view. For example, independent wheelchair capability may be viewed as a practical mobility solution by the health professional, but the client may highly value walking. Rather than seeing the wheelchair as representing independence, clients may see this outcome as a failure of the treatment system.

Third-party payers play an important part in rehabilitation. They usually value fiscal "efficiency" and are more concerned with cost containment than in meeting social and legal obligations. The payer may also urge the rehabilitation provider to focus on rehabilitation goals that are conspicuous and obtainable in a short time span. They may promote concentration on skills that will result in community survival, but not necessarily on quality of life (as viewed by the client or even the rehabilitation provider). Thus, public agreement on the value of certain outcomes is lacking. This puts into question the goals and treatment set by the rehabilitation providers if these goals are not of demonstrable value.

Heterogeneity of Client Problems

Individuals usually enter the rehabilitation system after an acute injury, and severe injuries may result in multiorgan impairments. Basic survival is often the first goal set by the treatment team. Therefore, medical stability could be viewed as a successful outcome and is often achieved by traditional surgical and medical interventions.

Mild head injury, on the other hand, may result in subjective difficulties that often are not perceived or acknowledged by the traditional medical system or by the public. Difficulty with pain and cognition can create significant functional limitations.

In the postconcussive situation, symptom relief and social outcomes (e.g., return to work, quality of life) may be more important as outcome measures.

The wide range of physical, cognitive, and behavioral difficulties encountered by rehabilitation clinicians makes it difficult to assemble homogeneous groups for clinical study based on premorbid functional differences. Additionally, specific variables such as lesion size, location, and chronicity can influence behavioral outcome.[2]

Involvement of Multiple Disciplines in a Variety of Environments

Patients may receive treatment in multiple environments during the course of recovery. For example, they may be treated in the emergency room, intensive care unit, neurosurgical ward, rehabilitation ward, skilled nursing home, day clinics, home, or community setting. Interventions, or lack thereof, at any of these locations may have a positive or negative influence on outcome without identifying the source.

Treatment is delivered by a plethora of health and rehabilitation disciplines, by family, and inadvertently by others in the environment. Defining and describing the richness and subtleties of treatment intervention are thus incomplete, particularly when it involves the teaching of functional skills.

Natural Recovery Occurs for a Prolonged Time After Injury

Improvement in functioning (irrespective of the outcome measure used) is usually seen after traumatic injury as a result of central nervous system (CNS) repair mechanisms, recovery of old skills, and development of new adaptive behaviors. The process cannot be put on hold; it can only be influenced positively or negatively. Initially, it was argued that most recovery following TBI occurred within the first 2 years, generally in the early part of that time frame.[3] However, recent evidence suggests that recovery can occur over a much longer interval, at least 10 years.[4,5]

Biologic Constraints

Biologic constraints may limit recovery, and environmental and biologic treatments may influence these constraints to an unknown degree. Predictive outcome variables are important biologic and social factors that may influence recovery. Variables include age, premorbid psychosocial characteristics, and indices of injury severity. Much of the literature on treatment effectiveness fails to consider these potential constraints. Conversely the literature on prognostic outcome variables ignores the effect of treatment methods and their possible impact on outcome.

Appropriate Experimental Design

In Chapter 1, Sackett proposed the random clinical trial as the main clinical decision-making tool in rehabilitation. However, the question was posed in an either/or fashion. One either conducted randomized trials or were left with the vagaries of clinical observation. In fact, there is ample evidence to support single-case experimental designs as a valid scientific enterprise.[6] Properly conducted single-case methodologies permit conclusions to be drawn about the unit of utmost importance to the practicing clinician—the individual patient. Such an undertaking does not devalue the role of randomized group trials in determining the magnitude of treatment effect or the comparison of two treatment approaches. Because the unit of study is, indeed, the individual, however, alternative procedures must be found. For example, in a sample (N = 8) in which the individual values are 1, 2, 3, 4, 6, 7, 8, 9, respectively, the arithmetic mean is 5, although such a data point was not in the original sample. Thus, individual cases are represented by a value that was not obtained by any of them.

Hersen and Barlow[6] raise five classes of objections that can be raised against group comparisons:

1. Ethical objectives
2. Practical problems in collecting large numbers of patients
3. Averaging of results over the group
4. Generality of findings
5. Intersubject variability

Of these, the question of variability has been rarely addressed. In a recent investigation, Hetherington et al.[4] showed that variability in performance differentiated groups of individuals with traumatic brain injury at 5 and 10 years postinjury. This variability has implications not only for experimental design, but also in the choice of statistical methods of inference. Reitan[7] demonstrated that "clinical inference" could order the data when statistical inference was inadequate.

Thus if the unit of concern is the individual, the complexity of variables involved in the assessment and treatment of brain injury is such that it is premature to consider the assignment of this richness to randomness. Many of these variables have an impact on data. Rather than conducting randomized clinical trials, perhaps the appropriate application of other experimental designs will narrow the scope of the question so that clinically relevant, intergroup comparisons can be made.

CLINICAL DECISIONS

This chapter focuses on reported studies and divides them into three well-known areas according to the World Health Organization (WHO) classification: impairments, disability, and handicap. Impairments are the focus of most early treatment (medical management), and some rehabilitation disciplines are oriented to treatment of impairments. Disabilities are traditionally treated in rehabilitation settings (often with multiple disciplines). An example of a disability measure is Functional Independence Measure (FIM), which targets independence in areas of basic activities of daily living (ADL) functioning (e.g., mobility, hygiene, communication).

Handicap is seen as interfering with fulfillment of a social role typical for that individual. An example

of a handicap outcome measure is the Community Integration Questionnaire.[8] Interventions in this area are usually community based and specific to certain aspects of community living (e.g., family counseling, vocational rehabilitation).

Research in Clinical Decision Making in Rehabilitation

To review some of the points in Chapter 1 regarding research in the area of clinical effectiveness in brain injury rehabilitation:

1. There is a regression of abnormal clinical situations toward the mean, therefore, any therapy that is initiated can appear efficacious.
2. Clinical practice is never "blind," patients, families, and clinicians know when active treatment is underway. There is a desire for patients and clinicians to succeed and thus overestimate efficacy.

The consensus approach to treatment using uncontrolled clinical experience often results in widespread application of treatments that are useless, or even harmful. When these same treatments are evaluated using a double-blind, randomized methodology, the results are often less encouraging.

Literature Review

Several recurrent problems become apparent when reviewing the literature on TBI:

1. There is almost a complete absence of randomization trials.
2. A wide variety of clinical outcome measures is reported, some of which may not be clinically relevant.
3. There is an absence of studies that have prospective bias and a high incidence of nonrandomized historical cohort comparisons between current patients and former patients who receive rehabilitation.

Thus, the evidence for efficacy tends to fall into either Level IV or Level V in terms of a grading scale.

Coma and Vegetative State

The entry point into the health care system is usually the emergency department and intensive care unit where severe injuries are classified by the Glasgow Coma Scale. This scale measures responsiveness to the environment in terms of eye, verbal, and motor responses. The score is 8 or less in severe head injuries, 9 to 12 in moderate head injury, and 13 to 15 in mild head injury. In general, a coma that exists in the early period after the injury usually lasts no longer than 3 to 4 weeks and is characterized by unconsciousness in which there is neither arousal nor awareness.

Early Treatment

Preservation of life involves the stabilization of medical problems, neurosurgical evaluation and intervention if required, and concurrent life support.

Sensory Stimulation

From a rehabilitation point of view, sensory stimulation has been proposed as an early treatment intervention. The goal of sensory stimulation is to shorten the duration of the unconscious state and to counteract unstructured environmental stimulation or sensory deprivation. The issue of treatment at this stage also requires adequate distinction between early coma and prolonged nonresponsiveness (formerly termed a "vegetative state").

In "prolonged nonresponsiveness," the patient usually demonstrates no signs of cognition, but returns to wakefulness with eyes open in response to verbal stimuli. Sleep/wake cycles, normal blood pressure, and normal respiration are present. However, patients are usually not able to show organization of responsiveness and are not able to engage in verbal interactions. The term "persistent" is usually used after 1 year has elapsed.

Sensory stimulation is often applied to patients at a variety of times from onset of injury, and research to some extent has been hampered by inadequate descriptions of responsiveness. For this reason, Rader and Ellis[9] developed a more structured methodology of assessment called The Sensory Stimulation Assessment Measure (SSAM) to more clearly define responsiveness to sensory stimulation.

Little definitive research is available in the area of sensory stimulation, and the effectiveness of sensory stimulation remains in question. Studies by LeWinn and Dimancescu,[10] Mitchell et al.,[11] Hall et al.,[12] Wood et al.,[13] and Pierce et al.,[14] differ in their opinions about diagnosis, time since onset, and outcome measures. In most cases, little information is given about the control group. Thus, the study designs in all cases would be graded as Level IV or Level V. Results were favorable in the four studies,[10–13] but there was no evident difference in the outcomes of patients undergoing sensory stimulation in the protocols of Rader and Ellis[9] and Pierce et al.[14] The grading of recommendations for treatment would thus be a Grade C. Definitive treatment approaches must be evaluated further.

A review article by Sandle and Horn[15] outlines the pros and cons of treatment and reasons either to continue to provide sensory stimulation or to abandon it. They point out the ongoing need to treat this group appropriately and to prevent the occurrence of treatable conditions such as decubiti ulcers, contractures, and pain. Although treatment of medical conditions is appropriate and needed during this stage of recovery, it presents a huge challenge to clinicians. They must provide treatment effectively and efficiently to meet the needs of both the patients and families, but they must not be irresponsible in terms of costly treatments that are of questionable benefit. The actual efficacy of the early stimulation approach beyond that provided by hospital staff in the early care units is unclear.

Arguments for providing sensory stimulation include the benefit of consistent contact and understanding of the responsiveness of the patient. It offers techniques to families of patients emerging from coma, can engage the family in the rehabilitation process, and provide them with a sense of purpose. It also provides opportunity for education and support at this time of emotional crisis for the family. The underlying biology of coma and possible biologic interventions such as brain stimulation or pharmacologic intervention may be a more productive area of inquiry in the long run, in that there is likely to be a biologic ceiling through which environmental methodologies are unable to break.

Acute Rehabilitation

Recovery from brain injury typically follows the pattern of moving from a coma to the community (i.e., moving from an inability to participate to more participatory stages with more traditional forms of rehabilitation and then being discharged into the community). In-patient TBI rehabilitation services are time honored and widely applied, but surprisingly little research has been performed into their effectiveness. In addition, the components that make up a typical rehabilitation program have not been well substantiated. A comprehensive treatment team in rehabilitation is an accepted norm, but Keith[16] has called for reevaluation. Keith challenges the traditional time-honored interdisciplinary model and the lack of literature to support its effectiveness. The three options for multiple team members range from a multidisciplinary approach, in which there is little communication between care providers, to an interdisciplinary team model, and then to a mediator model, which Leland et al.[17] have described as a transdisciplinary model. The literature that describes the impact of rehabilitation care recognizes that there are multiple disciplines, but usually provides little description about the way in which health professionals work with the patient and with each other.

TRADITIONAL MULTIDISCIPLINARY PROGRAMS

Actual models of traditional multidisciplinary programs vary from center to center, and no clear definition of what constitutes a comprehensive team has ever been widely accepted.

Basic Questions

Three questions address the process of rehabilitation:

1. Does involvement with rehabilitation professionals have an advantage over a similar, unstructured involvement with other personnel who are not as qualified?
2. Does providing more structured time, either with qualified professional personnel or unqualified personnel, have a greater impact on rate of recovery or ultimate functional outcome?
3. Is the timing of access to therapeutic interaction with a trained professional important? Is it better to begin rehabilitation treatment earlier, and is it ever too late to begin rehabilitation treatment?

The most basic question about whether rehabilitation care is beneficial is difficult to answer when one compares participation with professionals and nonparticipation or unstructured access to help. This question was most definitively asked by Aronow,[18] who studied people with severe brain injury who had participated in a comprehensive inpatient rehabilitation program in an acute rehabilitation hospital. This group was compared to a nonrehabilitation group in a general neurosurgical unit who did not have access to comprehensive rehabilitation services. The two groups were thought to be comparable in injury criteria, and in fact the rehabilitation treatment group on the whole had longer durations of post-traumatic amnesia (PTA). There was an attempt to control for systematic differences in groups using analysis of covariant and grouping patients based on duration of PTA. Although the average level of cost outcome was better for rehabilitation patients of comparable severity, there was no actual difference in functional outcome between groups.

Early Rehabilitation

Cope and Hall[19] described the benefits of early rehabilitation. They studied 36 severely head-injured patients, 16 of whom were admitted early (less than 35 days postinjury), and 20 patients who were admitted late (greater than 35 days postinjury). Although the actual functional outcome was similar in the two groups, the average stay for the late admission group was much longer than the early admission group.

The ultimate early intervention is of course at the coma state. In a careful study by MacKey et al.,[20] a group of 38 severely head injured patients had been admitted from two different programs, one with an early trauma rehabilitation program (17 patients). This group was compared to 21 patients who had received acute care services at 10 different hospitals without formalized early trauma rehabilitation programs. All patients in the rehabilitation program received similar care, and service was initiated within 24 hours of admission. The outcome measures showed reduced length of coma, reduced acute length of stay, and reduced rehabilitation length of stay. A greater percentage of the early formal program patients were discharged to their homes, when compared to the nonformal treatment group.

Intensity

Work by Blackerby et al.[21] attempted to look at the difference in outcome between an intense program and a less intense program based on hours of treatment per day. Although there was no statistical analysis, there was a reduction in length of stay for patients in the more intense programs.

Complex Factors in Acute Rehabilitation

In evaluating the literature on acute rehabilitation effectiveness, one again encounters the lack of studies that can be classified as Level I or Level II. No patients were randomized either into a study group or into a placebo group. However, there was evidence of Level III to suggest the benefit from early access to rehabilitation, intensive rehabilitation, and presumably from access to some type of formal structured program. Overall, the level of support is Grade III in quality.

Many questions continue about acute hospital-based rehabilitation. The nature of the interventions and the composition of professionals are often not described. Interventions vary from center to center. The type and style of interaction between professionals in hospital-based programs also vary widely.

Outcome Measures

Whether health professionals who have a high knowledge base actually make a difference in outcome when compared to less knowledgeable care providers is a more basic question that has not been formally addressed.

Johnston and Hall[22] have argued that TBI rehabilitation is threatened unless its scientific validity can be established. The first step is developing better outcome and better patient description measures. These measures need to be relevant to the individual and appropriate to their stage of recovery. By improving these descriptors, individual components of treatment programs can be broken down and possibly reassembled, as it is clear that the current literature is describing something that may vary widely from team to team. The development of appropriate measurement tools will be hastened by the increasing need to be accountable for resources used in rehabilitation.

SPECIFIC IMPAIRMENTS AND INTERVENTIONS

A variety of pathologic changes occur from TBI which result in physical, cognitive, and behavioral sequelae. Spasticity, heterotopic ossification, seizures, and behavioral problems are commonly encountered during accute rehabilitation.

Seizures

The one area that has benefited from a controlled clinical trial is that of post-traumatic seizure treatment. Prophylaxis with phenytoin has commonly been a standard treatment, and it was never certain as to when this treatment should end.

A rigorous study by Tempkin et al.[23] provided Level I evidence with a randomized trial that demonstrated statistical significant benefit from an experimental treatment in the first week, but subsequent lack of effect thereafter. Clinical seizures that occur after the first week should be managed with anticonvulsants, as has been the practice.

Commonly used medications thereafter include phenytoin, carbamazepine, and valproic acid. The usual preference in rehabilitation has been to use medication that lessens the impact on neurobehavioral performance. The use of carbamazepine and valproic acid has reduced the number of cognitive side effects. This issue led Massagli[24] to review the literature in populations other than TBI. She noted the lack of convincing studies within the population of brain injury to support the choice of medication, and all three anticonvulsants may be of clinical benefit in different situations.

Medication for Behavioral Problems

Many reported case studies imply benefit from a variety of medications for agitation. These medications include amitriptyline, β-blockers, benzodiazepines (such as lorazepam and clonazepam), amantadine, anticonvulsants carbamazepine, and sodium valproate. No study groups of sufficient size beyond that of case studies have justified the use for any one agent in a given clinical situation. It would appear that an "N of 1" study design is appropriate to isolate medications of most use in a particular situation and the context of treatment is just as important, given the ongoing evidence of benefit from behavioral methodology, as suggested by Gaultieri.[25]

Spasticity

In the area of spasticity, management is similar to treatment used for other patient groups (e.g. spinal cord injury). Appropriate physical care is likely of significant importance and can include appropriate skin care, normalization of bladder and bowel function, adequate and nonforceful passive range of motion, administration of temperature modalities, use of other physical modalities such as vibration and functional electrical stimulation, appropriate use of static and dynamic splints, and carefully planned orthopedic or neurosurgical interventions in a few cases.[26]

Management of spasticity with medication is problematic, but usually includes the medications diazepam, baclofen, and dantrolene. At this time no agent has been definitively proven to be useful in any subgroup of patients with brain injury or in the larger patient group.

Heterotopic Ossification

Another physical problem commonly encountered in patients with severe brain injury is that of heterotopic ossification, which overlaps with problems also encountered in individuals with spinal cord injury. It can occur at a frequency of 11 to 20 percent, and treatment options include anti-inflammatory medications (e.g., indomethacin or ibuprofen), etidronate disodium, or surgical removal.[27] There may be a role for other interventions such as low-dose radiotherapy, but this option has not been for-mally addressed in the acquired brain injury populations. The level of evidence for these impairments is Grade C.

COGNITIVE REMEDIATION

The process of cognitive remediation is aimed at therapies directed at cognitive deficits observed after TBI. A number of individual tasks and systematic programs have been developed or proposed for the remediation of such deficits. Pioneering efforts in ameliorating neuropsychological deficits were begun by Diller and Gordon.[28] Other examples of systematic remediation programs include REHABT by Reitan and Wolfson[29] and Alfano and Finlayson[30] and the process approach of Sohlberg and Mateer.[31] The procedures also have been adapted for computer use.[32-34] Programmatic studies have been undertaken using these techniques, by Goldstein and Rutvan,[35] Prigatano et al.,[36] and Ben-Yishay.[37] Although these procedures are generally thought effective, there have been many challenges to them, as for example, Ponsford and Kinsella.[38] However, the bulk of research, both pro and con, has been conducted at Levels III, IV, and V.

Several principles underlying cognitive remediation have been developed. These were recently detailed by Gordon and Hibbard.[39] Additionally, efforts to tie remedial processes to underlying brain functions have reached a high level of sophistication.

Investigations

Despite the effort expended on the development of cognitive remedial procedures, little in the way of systematic investigation has occurred. Proponents of these procedures generally recognize this weakness (e.g., Gordon and Hibbard[39]). The studies that have been conducted typically include few patients with limited descriptors. Several sources of selection bias have been present, often dictated by rigid selection criteria or referral pattern. Studies have varied in technique, length of training time, outcome criteria, and choice of control subjects. In his reviews of the effectiveness of cognitive remediation, Benedict[40] cited a number of methodologic problems. Many of the investigations involved case study designs, and there has been a dirth of between-group comparisons. With some exceptions (e.g., Stuss et al.[41]), single-case investigations have failed to use adequate baselines. Samples have been poorly selected, making study comparisons and broader generalizations impossible. The measures used for training and the tasks selected for evaluation are often incompatible.

Ben-Yishay and Prigatano[42] recently summarized the literature on these interventions. They concluded that there was insufficient evidence to claim that cognitive remediation can restore functioning to preinjury levels. They cited a lack of evidence to support the use of direct remediation exercises with memory disorders. However, they did note that remediation may be helpful for circumscribed deficits and that it may lead to improvement through a reduction of general deficits. Finally, they expressed some optimism about the use of strategies to improve attention and problem-solving abilities. Citing their own work,[42] they underlined the greater value of psychological factors (acceptance, mood control, and social involvement) relative to neurologic and cognitive variables in the prediction of successful employment after TBI.

This study highlights one of the greatest concerns about cognitive remediation—the lack of generalization (e.g., Wood and Fussey[43]). Maintenance of treatment gains and transfer of training are also problematic. Generalization is often confined to gains on the actual procedures. Occasionally, improvement on related neuropsychological measures is seen. Often, however, procedures appear to have been developed based on "the basis of train and hope" generalization strategies (Stocks and Baer[43a]).

Functional Models

Fordyce[44] has questioned the value of traditional cognitive remedial strategies and argued for a more functional approach to remediation of problems arising after TBI. Greater effort is being expended on the application of behavioral technologies to the remediation of cognitive deficits.[45,46]

Recently, models for the systematic application of behavioral technologies to problems arising after TBI have been developed (e.g., see Giles[47] and Wesolowski and Zencius[48]). As these approaches are applied more systematically, the challenge to traditional cognitive remedial procedures will resemble the earlier debate on the efficacy of perceptual training processes in reading disability.

Questions To Be Answered

As the field of cognitive remediation develops, several critical questions must be addressed. For example, is it more beneficial to restore or remediate underlying impairments, or should training of substitute or alternative mechanisms be the treatment goal? Regardless of whether a remedial or compensatory strategy has been selected, should treatment target specific neuropsychological and other impairments, or address only functional skills? Should treatment focus on improving or changing the individual with brain injury, or should the modification of society and the reduction of barriers in the environment be targeted?

Secondary questions involve the timing of these efforts (i.e., impairment training early in rehabilitation, disability or functional training at a moderate stage, and handicap or barrier reduction at a later phase). In addition, there will be increasing challenges to demonstrate the effectiveness of training of underlying impairments (mechanisms) rather than addressing functional problems in "the real world." Does training on a hierarchy of mental processes equate with shaping procedures or chaining paradigms based on functional behavioral analysis? These questions and others await empirical study. At present, there is no Level I or Level II evidence to guide the clinician in making decisions about cognitive remedial procedures.

As trials on remedial efficacy are conducted, it will be important to recognize the complexity of issues involved in brain injury. The interaction of factors relating to the actual injury (e.g., location, severity, age at onset), variation in individual functional neuroanatomy, individual psychological differences, and variations in the context or environment in which these injuries occur all contribute to the complexity of the problem and limit the researcher's ability to establish homogeneous groups. It is unlikely that assigning these variables to chance in randomized clinical trials will advance our knowledge. Systematic evaluation of these factors in isolation or in combination is needed. Better use of single case design and other methodologies arising from behavioral analysis will also advance our knowledge and assist in decision making about the use of these procedures.

COMMUNITY REHABILITATION AS AN ALTERNATIVE TO HOSPITALIZATION

Earlier in this chapter, we reviewed the research on hospital-based rehabilitation. Unfortunately, the question of alternatives to hospitalization is rarely considered, other than in the context of reduced expenses. However, several clinical arguments can be raised for an early return home once medical stability has been achieved. A much earlier return home with nursing/medical support can also be defended.

Going home is certainly perceived as relevant and meaningful by patients in rehabilitation centers. Their single-minded insistence on this goal frequently detracts from therapeutic objectives, as clients often fail to see how institutional treatments are relevant in their lives. Giving in to the client on this issue may be the best thing that rehabilitation practitioners can do.

The brain is the organ of adaptive behavior or learning. Consequently, skill acquisition in rehabilitation, the subsequent maintenance of these gains, and the transfer of these skills to other situations are invariably compromised after acquired brain injury. Cognitive functions, singularly or in combination, can slow the learning process and impede, or even prevent, generalization.[49] In traditional rehabilitation programs, artificial or analog situations are created for training purposes.[47] The behavioral literature emphasizes the importance of natural contingencies in maintaining behavior.[50] It follows, therefore, that treatment in the individual's own "community" will not only enhance the acquisition of skill but also improve skill retention and, most important, generalization. Thus, both treatment effectiveness and treatment efficiency are improved. The use of natural antecedents and consequences has additional economic benefit. By using "local" contingencies, existing resources are accessed, thereby reducing the cost associated with the creation of new methods.

An institution, by definition, has its own set of rules, code of conduct, and culture. They can be as simple as learning to locate toilets or as complicated as understanding the subtleties of "who's who" on the rehabilitation team. A critical component of rehabilitation success and incident-free behavior is the patient's mastery of these rules and regulations. A community also has its own code and culture. Rarely, are brain-injured individuals familiar with the culture of a hospital or rehabilitation center, but they are familiar with the culture of their own community. Yet we insist that survivors of brain injury grasp a new culture when their learning and memory problems are most pronounced. Despite this period of intense, overlearning of new rules, the knowledge acquired is rarely needed in the person's life after discharge. The task of building or rebuilding a life would be more easily accomplished if this new and short-lived culture did not have to be acquired simultaneously.

"My long-term memory is OK" is an often heard self-description after TBI. On further inquiry, patients relate that their memory for people, places, things, and events before onset is often retained. This fact is rarely used to advantage in rehabilitation. Often items from the patient's home are brought to the bedside, but these are limited samples of the richness of the individual's past. Relearning can be accomplished most easily in the familiar environment of an individual's own community. Natural cues and prompts are available there to enhance the relearning of old skills or the acquisition of new ones.

Although cognitive retraining has face validity as "cerebral weight lifting," patients often balk at cognitive retraining exercises in hospital with comments such as "what's this got to do with my job ... driving ... raising kids, etc?" They frequently fail to see the relevance of hospital-based programs, no matter how cleverly contrived. Cognitive limitations associated with frontotemporal dysfunction make comprehension and appreciation of the therapist's rationale difficult. The most relevant learning experiences occur in the real world. An overflowing sink or a burning pot is a far more salient reminder than a therapist's admonition. By being in the client's "home," therapists are forced to focus on the individual characteristics of the client and the activities and skills needed for success in the environment. Therapists can no longer rely on "canned" or "textbook" approaches to rehabilitation. Creativity and customization are encouraged. On the other hand, exposing the person early in the recovery process to real world consequences for real world failure may reduce denial and increase self-awareness.

When individuals with brain injury are transferred to centers distant from their community, it disturbs their pattern of social and family relationships. No doubt this disturbance contributes to the increase in social isolation after brain injury. All too often, friends stop visiting as shared interests, abilities, and experiences diverge, thus increasing the density of the remaining social network, which places a greater burden on families and contributes to burnout. If the person can remain at home or return early, however, friends are less likely to lose the habit of visiting. By seeing the early phases of spontaneous recovery, friends develop a sense that "this can change" and are more likely to remain optimistic about recovery and also to develop a tolerance for the cognitive and behavioral changes in their friend.

Perhaps the greatest advantage of being on the person's own "turf" is that the person's own rules, routines, and schedules are followed. By preserving this sense of mastery and control, confidence and self-image are enhanced, and dependence and feelings of helplessness can be avoided. Familiar surroundings can reduce anxiety, facilitate success, and help maintain a positive self-image after TBI.

Several factors can limit home-based or community rehabilitation. For example, skill and performance deficits may be such that behaviors occur either too infrequently or too frequently in the natural environment. Under these conditions, analog situations or controlled environments may be more useful. Second, distances involved and limited access to professional services or appropriate supports may preclude community involvement. Third, individuals may not have a home to which they can return. Finally, their age and stage of life may be a factor, or the symptoms may be of sufficient severity (physical or psychological) to preclude a return to their premorbid environment. Although accommodations may need to be made for these individuals, the majority of persons with brain injury would likely benefit from an early return to home and family. Unfortunately, this discussion consists primarily of logical argument with total absence of Level I and Level II evidence. Thus, recommendations regarding early return home can only receive Grade C support.

RETURN TO WORK AFTER BRAIN INJURY

We have said earlier that the reduction of handicap should be the main goal of rehabilitation. One of the more critical social rules in our society is that of wage earner. Thus, a return to competitive employment after brain injury is generally considered a major goal and the ultimate challenge for rehabilitation professionals. Several investigators have studied the rate of return to work in samples of individuals with severe brain injury. The success rates range from 19 to 50 percent.[51-54] For example, McMordie et al.[55] surveyed a group of 177 individuals with acquired brain injury. Time since onset varied from 9 months to 27 years. In response to the questionnaire, 45 percent of the sample were judged to be engaged in some type of work-related activity. However, only 19 percent of the sample were thought to be engaged in competitive employment and they were usually in occupations that required less functioning than their premorbid occupations.

Several barriers to successful employability after TBI have been identified and are summarized here:

1. Cognitive/communication difficulties including cognitive slowing, memory difficulties, and limited expressive skill
2. Social/emotional difficulties including behavioral discontrol, reduced tact, and swearing
3. Poor social skills including insubordination, inability to accept criticism, and reduced personal interaction
4. Psychological issues including depression, hopelessness, and isolation
5. Comorbidity such as drug and alcohol abuse.

Earlier investigators attempted to use psychological test procedures to identify and predict those who are most likely to return to work. For example, Heaton et al.[56] conducted a retrospective evaluation of 381 subjects. They looked at the role of neuropsychological and personality measures in predicting employment status. A global measure of neuropsychological dysfunction and personality variables were strong predictors of employment status. In fact, the variables arising from the Minnesota Multiphasic Personality Inventory correctly classified 78.6 percent of the subjects. In more recent investigation Ezrachi et al.[57] investigated employability following a program of neuropsychological rehabilitation in 59 clients. They noted that length of coma was a significant predictor. Neuropsychological functioning also contributed to the predictive equation. However, the concept of acceptance was a significant predictor of employment status. In their study, awareness was not identified as a vague psychological construct, but was operationally defined on the basis of functioning within the treatment group. A single person's qualities could be classified as "the right attitude" but, nevertheless, were highly related to vocational success.

The literature indicates that both biologic and psychological variables contribute to the success of return to work programs. Variables relating to injury severity and neuropsychological dysfunction may well place physical constraints on outcome, but personality and social variables certainly influence the direction and end point of return to work strategies.

As in the case of remediation of neuropsychological deficits, return to employment strategies have focused on remedial efforts to improve the functioning of the individual with brain injury. For example, Pareneté et al.[58] outlined several approaches to supporting the cognitive limitations encountered in an individual's brain injury. These strategies included compensatory techniques, habit training, and the use of technologies. Collectively, these strategies served as cognitive prosthetic devices. Although there are anecdotal reports of success, little systematic investigation of their utility has been undertaken.

Somewhat higher rates of return to work after brain injury have been reported after systematic rehabilitation efforts. Ben-Yishay et al.[59] reported that 84 percent of the sample of 94 patients successfully returned to productive and diverse employment after rehabilitation, with 63 percent of these individuals being employed at a competitive level. These findings are quite encouraging, but the generalizability of the findings is limited. Entry into the program was selective, and the candidates do not truly reflect the population of individuals with a brain injury.

Further optimism can be derived from efforts with a supported work model for individuals following brain injury.[60] Supported employment provides support services at the client's place of employment. Acting as a coach or trainer, the support person provides on-the-job training, facilitates interpersonal interactions, and essentially serves as a surrogate frontal lobe for the client. The process involves gradual weaning of support, but ongoing evaluation and follow-up are routinely conducted to ensure job retention. Success in the program is also highly dependent on initial evaluation of both client and employer in order to ensure suitable job placement. Again, although support employment is a promising line of endeavor, its efficacy has not been validated except by case study reporting (e.g., Wehman et al.[61]).

The studies of vocational rehabilitation in TBI consists of Level III, Level IV, and Level V evidence. Thus, care must be taken in applying these recommendations to clinical practice, as only Grade C support is available.

REFERENCES

1. Johnston MV: Outcomes evaluation in traumatic brain injury rehabilitation. Arch Phys Med Rehabil 75:SC2, 1994
2. Reitan RM: Problems and prospects in studying the psychological correlates of brain lesions. Cortex 2:127, 1966
3. Bond MR, Brooks DN: Understanding the process of recovery as a basis for the investigation of rehabilitation for the brain injured. Scand J Rehabil Med 8:127, 1976
4. Hetherington CR, Stuss DT, Finlayson MAJ: Reaction time and variability 5 and 10 years after traumatic brain injury. Brain Inj (in press)
5. Sbordone RJ, Liter JC, Pettler-Jennings P: Recovery of function following severe traumatic brain injury. A retrospective 10 year follow-up. Brain Inj 9:285, 1995
6. Hersen M, Barlow DH: Single-case Experimental Designs: Strategies for Studying Behavior Change. Pergamon Press, Toronto, 1976
7. Reitan RM: Psychological deficits resulting from cerebral lesions in man. In Warrend JM, Akert KA (eds): The Frontal Granular Cortex and Behavior, McGraw-Hill, New York, 1964

8. Willer B, Linn R, Allen K: Community integration and barriers to integration for individuals with brain injury. In Finlayson MAJ, Garner SH (eds): Brain Injury Rehabilitation: Clinical Considerations, Williams & Wilkins, Baltimore, 1994

9. Rader MA, Ellis DW: The sensory stimulation assessment measure (SSAM): a tool for early evaluation of severely brain injured patients. Brain Inj 8:309, 1994

10. LeWinn EB, Dimancescu MD: Environment deprivation and enrichment in coma. Lancet 156, 1978

11. Mitchell S et al: Coma arousal procedure: a therapeutic intervention in the treatment of head injury. Brain Inj 4:273, 1990

12. Hall ME, McDonald S, Young GC: The effectiveness of directed multisensory stimulation versus non-directed stimulation in comatose CHI patients: pilot study of a single subject design. Brain Inj 6:435, 1992

13. Wood RL, Winkowski TB, Miller JL et al: Evaluating sensory regulation as a method to improve awareness in patients with altered states of consciousness: a pilot study. Brain Inj 6:411, 1992

14. Pierce JP et al: The effectiveness of coma arousal intervention. Brain Inj 4:191, 1990

15. Sandle ME, Horn LA: Sensory stimulation: accepted practice or expected practice? J Head Trauma Rehabil 7:115, 1992

16. Keith RA: Comprehensive treatment team in rehabilitation. Archiv Phys Med Rehabil 72:269, 1991

17. Leland M, Leurs FD, Henman S et al: Rehab counseling bulletin 31:89, 1988

18. Aronow HU: Rehabilitation effectiveness with severe brain injury: translating research into policy. Head Trauma Rehabil 2:24, 1987

19. Cope N, Hall K: Head injury rehabilitation: benefit of early intervention. Arch Phys Med Rehabil 63:433, 1982

20. MacKey L, Bernstein B, Chapman P et al: Early intervention in severe head injury: long-term benefits of a formalized program. Arch Phys Med Rehabil 73:635, 1992

21. Blackerby WF et al: Intensity of rehabilitation and length of stay. Brain Inj 4:1967, 1990

22. Johnston MV, Hall KM: Part 1. Overview in systems principles. Arch Phys Med Rehabil 75:SC2, 1994

23. Tempkin NR, Dikmen SS, Wilensky HA et al: A randomized double-blind study of phenytoin for the prevention of post-traumatic seizures. N Engl J Med 323: 497, 1990

24. Massagli TL: Neurobehavioral effects of phenytoin, carbamazepine, and valproic acid: implications for use in traumatic brain injury. Arch Phys Med Rehabil 72: 219, 1991

25. Gualtieri T: Pharmacological interventions for cognitive and behavioral impairments. In Finlayson MAJ, Garner SH (eds): Brain Injury Rehabilitation: Clinical Considerations. Williams & Wilkins, Baltimore, 1994

26. Glen MB, Whyte J: The Practical Management of Spasticity in Children and Adults. Lea and Febiger, Philadelphia, 1990

27. Spielman G, Generallia TA, Rogers CR: Disodium etidronate: Its role in preventing heterotopic ossifications in severe head injury. Arch Phys Med Rehabil 64:539, 1983

28. Diller L, Gordon WA: Intervention for cognitive deficits in brain-damaged adults. J Consul Clin Psychol 49:822, 1981

29. Reitan RM, Wolfson D: The Halstead-Reitan Neuropsychological Test Battery: Theory and Clinical Interpretation. 2nd Ed. Neuropsychology Press, Tucson, 1993

30. Alfano DP, Finlayson MAJ: Clinical neuropsychology in rehabilitation. The Clinical Psychologist 1:105, 1987

31. Sohlberg M, Mateer CA: Introduction to Cognitive Rehabilitation: Theory and Practice. Guilford Press, New York, 1989

32. Bracey OL: Cognitive Rehabilitation: a Process Approach. Cognit Rehabil 4:210, 1986

33. Gianutsos R: Cognitive rehabilitation: a neuropsychological specialty comes of age. Brain Inj 5:353, 1991

34. Finlayson MAJ, Alfano DP, Sullivan JF: A neuropsychological approach to cognitive remediation: microcomputer applications. Can Psychol 28:180, 1987

35. Goldstein G, Rutvan GL: Rehabilitation of the Brain-Damaged Adult. Oxford University Press, New York, 1983

36. Prigatano GP, Fordyce DJ, Zeiner HK et al: Neuropsychological rehabilitation after closed head injury in young adults. J Neurol Neurosurg Psychiatry 47:505, 1984

37. Ben-Yishay Y (ed): Working Approaches to Remediation of Cognitive Deficits in Brain-Damaged Persons, (Rehabilitation Monograph No. 62). NYU Institute of Rehabilitation Medicine, New York, 1981

38. Ponsford JL, Kinsella G: Evaluation of a remedial programme for attentional deficits following closed-head injury. J Clin Exp Neuropsychol 10:693, 1988

39. Gordon WA, Hibbard MR: Critical issues in cognitive remediation. Neuropsychology 6:361, 1992

40. Benedict RHB: The effectiveness of cognitive remediation strategies for victims of traumatic brain-injury: a review of the literature. Clin Psychol Rev 9:605, 1989

41. Stuss DT, Mateer CA, Sohlberg MM: Innovative approaches to frontal lobe deficits. In Finlayson MAJ, Garner SH, (eds): Brain Injury Rehabilitation: Clinical Considerations, Williams & Wilkins, Baltimore, 1994

42. Ben-Yishay Y, Prigatano GP: Cognitive remediation. In Rosenthal M, Griffith ER, Bond MR et al (eds). Rehabilitation of the Adult and Child with Traumatic Brain Injury. (2nd Ed). FA Davis, Philadelphia, 1990

43. Wood RL, Fussey I: Cognitive Rehabilitation in Perspective. Taylor & Francis, London, 1990

43a. Stokes TF, Baer DM: An implicit technology of generalization. J Appl Behav Anal 10:349, 1977

44. Fordyce DJ: Neuropsychologic assessment and cognitive rehabilitation: issues of psychologic validity. p. 187. In Finlayson MAJ, Garner SH (eds): Brain Injury Rehabilitation: Clinical Considerations. Williams & Wilkins, Baltimore, 1994

45. Foxx RM, Martella RC, Marchand-Martella NE: The acquisition, maintenance, and generalization of problem-solving skills by closed head-injured adults. Behav Ther 20:61, 1989

46. Lloyd LF, Cuvo AJ: Maintenance and generalization of behaviors after treatment of persons with traumatic brain injury. Brain Inj 8:529, 1994

47. Giles GM: Functional assessment and intervention. p. 124. In Finlayson MAJ, Garner SH (eds): Brain Injury Rehabilitation: Clinical Considerations. Williams & Wilkins, Baltimore, 1994

48. Wesolowski MD, Zencius AH: A Practical Guide to Head Injury Rehabilitation: A Focus on Postacute Residential Treatment. Plenum Press, New York, 1994

49. Alfano DP: Recovery of function following brain injury. p. 34. In Finlayson MAJ, Garner SH (eds): Brain Injury Rehabilitation: Clinical Considerations, Williams & Wilkins, Baltimore, 1994

50. Martin G, Pear J: Behavioral Modification: What It Is and How To Do It. Prentice Hall, Englewood Cliffs, New Jersey, 1992

51. Weddell R, Oddy M, Jankins D: Social adjustment after rehabilitation: a two year follow-up of patients with severe head injury. Psychol Med 10:257, 1980

52. Stapleton MB: Maryland Rehabilitation Center closed head injury study: a retrospective survey. Cognit Rehabil 4:34, 1986

53. Brooks N, McKinlay W, Symington C et al: Return to work within the first seven years of severe head injury. Brain Inj 1:5, 1987

54. Haffey WJ, Abrams DL: Employment outcomes for participants in a brain injury work re-entry program: preliminary findings. J Head Trauma Rehabil 63:24, 1991

55. McMordie WR, Barker SL, Paolo TM: Return to work (RTW) after head injury. Brain Inj 4:57, 1990

56. Heaton R, Chelune G, Lehman R: Using neuropsychological and personality tests to assess the likelihood of patient employment. J Nerv Ment Dis 166:408, 1978

57. Ezrachi O, Ben-Yishay Y, Kay T et al: Predicting employment in traumatic brain injury following neuropsychological rehabilitation. J Head Trauma Rehabil 6:71, 1991

58. Parenté R, Stapleton ML, Wheatley CJ: Practical strategies for vocational re-entry after traumatic brain injury. J Head Trauma Rehabil 6:35, 1991

59. Ben-Yishay Y, Silver SM, Piasetsky E et al: Relationship between employability and vocational outcome after intensive holistic cognitive rehabilitation. J Head Trauma Rehabil 2:35, 1987

60. Wehman P, Kreutzer J, Wood W et al: Supported work model for persons with traumatic brain injury: toward job placement. Rehabil Counseling Bull 31, 298, 1988

61. Wehman P, Kreutzer J, Wood W et al: Arch Phys Med Rehabil 70:109, 1989

5

Low Back Pain

Diagnostic Approach

Ralph Bloch

Low back pain figures among the common complaints in general practice in industrialized countries.[1-3] It is a major source of occupational morbidity and disability.[4,5] Economic losses due to low back pain are staggering.[6,7] Yet, its clinicopathologic classification is fuzzy and its pathophysiology poorly understood.[4] Diagnoses tend to be nonspecific, and therapeutic results are disappointing.[8,9] Prognostic indicators, although statistically significant in large groups, are of little use when faced with individual patients.[10,11]

Although the incidence of low back pain in most industrialized countries is similar,[12-15] loss of productivity, compensation rates, clinical taxonomy, use of diagnostic methods and choice of therapeutic modalities show large geographic variations.[16] Low back pain exemplifies the complexity of medicine with its intricate interactions of biologic disturbance, psychological traits, and social determinants in patients' environment.[17] Overly simplistic and reductionist approaches are at least partially to blame for our limited therapeutic successes.

When faced with a low back patient, a clinician is confronted by conflicting expectations: the patient wants relief from pain and affirmation of disability; the employer demands speedy restoration to full work capacity; and the insurer requires diagnostic, therapeutic, and compensation cost containment. It may, for example, not be efficient to perform an expensive and possibly risky diagnostic test of high accuracy just to demonstrate a disorder for which no effective treatment exists.

Despite these qualifications, I first discuss the various diagnostic entities thought to be associated with low back pain. I then consider different diagnostic tests and their sensitivity and specificity. Major spinal trauma with associated fracture dislocation is not considered here. Circumstances are usually sufficiently obvious to avoid confusion. Local malignancy and abscess, primary inflammatory diseases, and metabolic disorders were touched on, but their detailed discussion would exceed the scope of this chapter.

The aim of this chapter is not to present a cookbook "how to" approach. Rather, it attempts to provide the rational clinician with an aid to the critical appraisal of currently practiced diagnostic approaches to low back pain. I try to discriminate between that which has been clearly established at present, that which is plausible, and that which is merely conjecture. However, we must not forget that simple lack of proof does not equate disproof.

LITERATURE SEARCH

This chapter is based on an extensive review of the clinical literature. Using MEDLINE, I searched for articles that simultaneously met criteria for clinical conditions, types of intervention, and research methodology. The medical subject headings (MeSH), indicating specific conditions associated with low back pain, are given in Table 5-1.

55

Table 5-1. Clinical Conditions Used in MEDLINE Search (MeSH)

Backache
Back pain
Disc displacement
Intervertebral disc
Spinal stenosis
Spondylitis
Spondylolisthesis
Spondylolysis

I included all clinical interventions that carried a tag of "*DI" (diagnostic), "*RA" (radiologic), "*TH" (therapeutic), "*TU" (therapeutic use), or "*SU" (surgery). The tag "human" was mandatory to exclude nonclinical research.

The methodologic search terms applied are given in Table 5-2.

The EBSCO CD-ROM database was searched for the period 1966 to 1992. Subsequent publications were collected prospectively directly from appropriate journals. A total of 1,051 references was found. Relevant articles were selected from these references depending on title, abstract (where available), and language of publication (English, French, or German).

Available time and space does not permit a comprehensive analytic review of the literature or meta-analysis. Rather, I have selected references from those noted above that appear pertinent.

CLINICOPATHOLOGIC TAXONOMY

The classical clinical sequence proceeds from presenting complaint through history taking, physical examination, and investigation to establishing a pathophysiologic diagnosis as basis for treatment and prognosis. Medical students are taught that a diagnostic label represents a clinicopathologic entity, whereby a given clinical presentation is associated with a well-defined pathology and pathophysiology, requiring a specific therapy and carrying a presumptive prognosis.

Unfortunately, we have not reached this state of perfect knowledge in disorders associated with low back pain. A variety of different evolutions and distributions of pain can be attributed to the same pathologic process, whereas identical clinical presentations may result from a multitude of dissimilar causes.

Although some clinical and paraclinical findings appear more frequently in association with a certain demonstrable pathologic process or in symptomatic patients, they can also occur in otherwise healthy individuals. Often, diagnostic labels are based on theoretic constructs, lacking solid confirmatory evidence. Few of the available therapeutic interventions are specifically directed at unique causes of low back pain. Attempting to predict the clinical course of a given back pain patient resembles a black art more than a logical science.

Clinical taxonomies of low back pain disorders tend to be exercises in tautology. Clinical or paraclinical findings may be declared "pathognomonic" for a certain disorder, thus endowing them with instant sensitivity and specificity. Surgical confirmation of a diagnosis also leads to a quandary. Thus, only patients suspected of requiring an operation are subjected to the knife. Others may well suffer from the same condition, a fact that can neither be confirmed nor refuted. Surgical confirmation of a diagnostic test may determine its specificity although not its sensitivity. Nevertheless, the quest for establishing a firm diagnosis still occupies a central place in the management of patients with low back pain.

Clinical Syndromes

Low back pain generally manifests itself initially as a clinical syndrome. Clinical syndromes are recognized by sufficiently distinct clusters of reliable clinical findings (Table 5-3).

Occasionally, it is possible to clearly attribute a syndrome to a specific disease category or structural

Table 5-2. Research Methodology Terms Used for MEDLINE Search (MeSH)

Case-control studies
Comparative studies
Evaluation studies
Follow-up studies
Longitudinal studies
Meta-analysis
Prospective studies
Retrospective studies
Review

Table 5-3. Clinical Syndromes

Acute lumbago without referred pain
Acute lumbago with referred pain
Sciatica without neurologic deficits
Sciatica with neurologic deficits
Recurrent (mechanical) back pain
Chronic back pain
Failed back
Spinal claudication

Table 5-4. Clinical Syndromes: Structural Diagnosis

Arachnoid and epidural scar
Arteriovenous malformation
Disc herniation and/or extrusion
Metabolic bone disease
Neoplasm
Primary neurologic diseases
Rheumatologic disorders
Spinal stenosis
Spinal arthrosis (spondylosis)
Spinal fracture
Spinal abscess, osteomyelitis, discitis
Spondylolysis and spondylolisthesis

diagnosis (Fig. 5-1). Structural diagnoses are confirmed ultimately by abnormal findings on microscopic or macroscopic examination of tissue. Because of the invasiveness of this diagnostic standard, sensitivity of specific clinical diagnostic tests may be difficult or ethically objectionable to establish (Table 5-4).

Heuristic Diagnosis

As a rationale for a diagnostic trial, one seeks to demonstrate the presence of a heuristic diagnosis (Table 5-5). Heuristic diagnoses are established by the reliable reproduction of specific symptom sets through anatomically precise nociceptive maneuvers or by the abolition of symptoms through specific application of local anesthetic or segmental immobilization. I extend this group to diagnoses with a plausible etiology, for which a specific causal therapeutic modality exists. A therapeutic trial then establishes or refutes that diagnosis. Such a definition has its dangers when the therapy used carries significant risks, as is the case with surgery.

At present, no diagnostic standard exists for tests purporting to diagnose these heuristic conditions

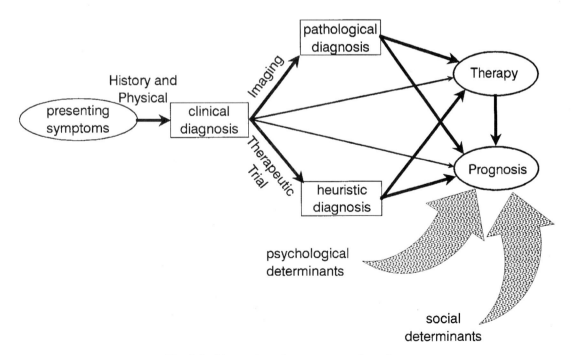

Fig. 5-1. Diagnosis and management flow chart.

Table 5-5. Heuristic Diagnoses

Disc degeneration
Facet syndrome
Muscle spasm
Piriformis syndrome
Sacroiliac joint syndrome
Sclerotomal pain[18]
Segmental instability

that relates them to objective pathologic changes. In the future, possibly, definite symptomatic relief can be used as a diagnostic standard. It may then be possible to determine specificity and, less likely, sensitivity of the various reproductive and abolitional tests.

Hypothetical Conditions

Frequently, patients are said to suffer from a hypothetical condition. Hypothetical conditions are diagnostic labels lacking a clearly defined and widely accepted operational definition and/or plausible pathophysiologic explanation. Their diagnosis depends on esoteric diagnostic features or tests, characterized by a systematic lack of inter-rater reliability. I do not provide a list of conditions that I deem to be hypothetical, and Tables 5-4 and 5-5 are not complete. I leave it to the reader to categorize diagnostic labels not mentioned here.

Most of these diagnostic categories can be superimposed by a variety of psychosocial behavior patterns. Patients' subjective responses to pain and discomfort depend on mood, culture, experience, personality, and primary and secondary gains. There are no good studies on the prevalence of true malingering, but most clinicians would agree that it is rare.

CLINICAL SYNDROMES

Acute Lumbago

The expression, although common in Europe and among laymen, is used rarely in the North American medical literature. It corresponds to the "back strain" in the orthopedic literature. Yet it is an apt term, describing a condition, usually of acute onset, with a deep aching pain in the back, which may or may not radiate into buttocks, thighs, and occasionally, legs (referred pain). Patients describe difficulty moving their back or trunk. Commonly, there are palpable contractions of paraspinal muscles. New neurologic deficits should not be demonstrable.

Sciatica

Sciatica may show many of the features of lumbago. The characteristic difference is the character of leg or thigh pain. Whereas in lumbago the thigh or leg pain is described as diffuse, dull, and aching, in true sciatica the pain tends to be sharp and localized.[19] Another hallmark of sciatica is a truly positive *straight leg raising test*. Limitation of straight leg raising in itself is not a sign of nerve involvement, rather it parallels the severity of backache. Straight leg raising must be limited due to aggravation of leg pain, rather than back pain.[20] Associated with sciatica may be other sensory, motor, or reflex signs of nerve or root impairment.

Recurrent Mechanical Back Pain

The pain distribution in recurrent mechanical back pain is similar to that in lumbago, although usually less incapacitating. It is characterized by asymptomatic periods alternating with episodes of back pain, usually triggered by certain movements or efforts. As a clinical diagnosis, without specific attributable pathologic causes, it presumably constitutes the bulk of low back pain patients both in primary and referred care. Because the pathophysiology is poorly understood, there are no specific treatments. Standard texts on low back pain cite recovery rates of 90 percent.[21] Careful studies in primary care draw a more somber picture,[22] with only one-third of initially dysfunctional patients showing good results at 1 year; 69 percent of patients with recent-onset low back pain still report painful episodes after 1 year.

Chronic Back Pain

The pain is more or less continuous, although there may be aggravations and improvements. Pain distribution and character tend to be more diffuse than in lumbago or sciatica. Psychologic and social epiphenomena are common.[23]

Failed Back

"Failed back" or "failed, failed back" indicates severe chronic back pain despite or resulting from one or more attempts at surgical cure. The diagnosis implies physicians' resignation and patients' desperation.[24,25]

Spinal Claudication

Spinal claudication is a distinct clinical syndrome, apart from the groups mentioned above. Patients complain of increasing pain in buttocks, thighs, or legs on walking any distance and on prolonged standing. Discomfort is relieved by rest or lumbar flexion. In contrast to true claudication, circulation in the lower limbs is usually normal and pain also occurs on prolonged standing.[26]

PATHOLOGICAL ENTITIES

I do not discuss arteriovenous malformation, metabolic bone disease, neoplasm, primary neurologic diseases, spinal fracture, abscess, osteomyelitis, and discitis although there is no doubt as to their existence. They are rare but should be thought of when history and examination are suggestive. Even though these are important diagnoses to make and, more important, not to miss, epidemiologic and health-economic reality advises against routine imaging of every patient with back pain on the off chance that one of these conditions may be present. There are excellent texts available on these topics.[27]

Arachnoid and Epidural Scar

Direct involvement of lumbosacral nerve roots with intradural or extradural scar tissue is a cause for distressing chronic back pain for which no effective therapy is available at present. Clinically, the term *arachnoiditis* is also applied to this condition, even when inflammation no longer exists. The process can progress all the way to osseous metaplasia (arachnoiditis ossificans).[28,29] From a purely neurophysiologic point of view, a radicular pain distribution with nerve root traction signs is expected. Variable distributions and characterizations of pain result

from chronification. Epidural scar formation, one of the causes for "failed back" is the result of surgery.[30,31] It has also been reported after radiculography.[32] The long-term prognosis of arachnoid and epidural scar formation is unclear.

Disc Herniation and/or Extrusion

Disc herniation was first described 60 years ago as a cause of low back pain.[33] Although approximately 90 percent of back pain episodes have causes other than disc herniation, the public associates pain in the back invariably with the lay diagnosis of "slipped disc." Disc herniation is a frequent cause of acute sciatica (see above). However, asymptomatic disc extrusion is possible in the presence of a large spinal canal. The disc levels at L4-L5 and L5-S1 account for approximately 98 percent of all herniations.[34] Rarely, other discs herniate as well. The neurologic symptoms and signs usually relate to neurotomes and myotomes of the lower level. The first step in the pathogenesis of disc herniation is degeneration of the annular ring with formation of defects in the posterolateral part of the annulus. The nucleus pulposus deteriorates more slowly. Thus, herniation is more common between the ages of 20 and 40, while the nuclear material is still gelatinous. In a series of postmortem examinations, 11.5 percent of men and 18.7 percent of women had some evidence of posterior displacement of disc material.[35] The presence of true acute sciatica, particularly when associated with signs of root irritation and impairment, should raise the suspicion of disc herniation.[36] Confirmation is based on appropriate imaging.

In the absence of neurologic deficits, disc herniation is not an absolute indication for surgery because the prognosis is benign.[37]

Rheumatologic Causes of Back Pain

Most rheumatologic causes of low back pain are associated with radiologic and/or clinical evidence of sacroiliitis. They include ankylosing spondylitis, Reiter syndrome, Behçet syndrome, psoriatic arthritis, enteropathic arthritis, and Whipple's disease and are best differentiated on the basis of concurrent symptomatology.

Rheumatoid arthritis can involve almost any joint including sacroiliac joints.[38] Vertebral osteochondritis (Scheuermann's disease) is a condition of unknown pathogenesis. Its onset is gradual during childhood and adolesence. Diagnosis is based on pathognomonic radiologic changes. Fibromyalgia (fibrositis) is another idiopathic disorder, characterized by pain amplification, discrete tender points, and sleep disorder.[39] Polymyalgia rheumatica, a diffuse inflammatory disease of advanced age with elevated sedimentation rate and giant cell arteritis, can manifest itself with generalized back pain and stiffness.

Diffuse idiopathic skeletal hyperostosis is another idiopathic disorder with characteristic radiologic changes and occasional thoracolumbar aching.

Comprehensive discussions of rheumatologic causes of low back pain are available in textbooks on rheumatology.

Degenerative Disease of the Spine

A useful classification of spinal degeneration in the lumbar spine is given by Resnick and Niwayama.[40] They distinguish between arthritis of synovial joints (apophyseal and costovertebral), osteochondrosis (involving the nucleus pulposus) and spondylosis deformans (involving the annulus fibrosus) of the discovertebral joint, and degenerative changes of fibrous joints and entheses (ligamento-osseous junctions). Radiologically, each of these processes can manifest itself through sclerosis of adjacent bone, loss of joint space, deformation, and vacuum phenomenon—that is, the collection of free gas in the joint (excluding fibrous joints and entheses). These degenerative processes are normal concomitants of aging but are modulated by heredity, mechanical loading, and a variety of specific metabolic disorders such as ochronosis and crystal deposition. Congenital structural abnormalities such as transitional vertebrae may accelerate degeneration, possibly due to abnormal loading.

Postmortem and radiologic studies demonstrate degenerative changes in 60 to 80 percent of normal individuals by the age of 50 to 60 and in practically everyone older than the age of 70.[41] Generally, comparative radiologic studies of normal individuals and back pain patients show little difference.[42] The likelihood ratio of finding specific radiologic changes in

back pain patients is 2.5 for disc space narrowing and 1.2 for osteophytosis,[43] suggesting that degeneration of the nucleus pulposus may be a direct cause of back pain, but degeneration of the annulus is not. Other studies show inconsistent correlations of back pain with radiologic changes.[44–46] In view of this marginal correspondence between the presence of symptoms and degenerative radiologic changes, one can doubt the usefulness of looking for tell-tale signs of spondylosis in mature patients with back pain.

Spinal Stenosis

A common cause of spinal claudication is stenosis of the spinal canal. It can be caused by degenerative changes of the intervertebral disc and of the facet joints and, after surgery, superimposed on previously limited dimensions of the spinal canal. The typical positional and exertional exacerbations are thought to be related to geometry and engorgement of the venous plexus resulting from an increased venous return from the lower extremities. Even though one should properly consider the relationship between the cross-section of the spinal cord and the cross-sectional area of the spinal canal, in practice values of 15 mm for the midsagittal and 20 mm for the transverse diameter are accepted as lower limits of normal for both men and women.[47] A meta-analysis of the literature suggests that magnetic resonance imaging (MRI) studies have the highest accuracy for the diagnosis of spinal stenosis when compared with conventional myelography and computed tomography (CT).[48] Because of the large cost differential, decision analytical studies are needed to determine the most efficient way of investigating suspected spinal stenosis. Spinal stenosis does not seem to progress,[49] and surgical results are variable.

Spondylolysis and Spondylolisthesis

Spondylolysis represents a defect in the pars interarticularis of a vertebra, usually lower lumbar. Spondylolysis is uncommon in infancy and rarely develops after skeletal maturity has been reached.[50] In 3 to 7 percent of asymptomatic individuals, radiologic evidence of spondylolysis can be found.[51] The incidence varies according to gender and race. Familial clustering has been described.[52] Congenital abnormalities of the spine are more frequent in proximity to spondylolytic defects. Young athletes appear at increased risk.[53] It has been proposed that spondylolysis is caused by stress fractures in predisposed individuals.[54] Spondylolisthesis is the displacement of one vertebra on another. Spondylolisthesis usually only occurs in the presence of spondylolysis, although it can exist in isolation.[55] The degree of slippage is graded, according to Meyerding,[56] from I to IV, as the number of quarters of the vertebral diameter of displacement. In addition, spondylolisthesis is recognized in association with osteoarthritis and as retrolisthesis with degeneration of the nucleus pulposus.

Only about 10 percent of spondylolistheses progress significantly without surgery.[57] Patients with spondylolisthesis suffer more frequent episodes of recurrent mechanical low back pain[58] and sciatica.[59]

HEURISTIC CONDITIONS

Facet Syndromes

The spinal facet syndrome has been brought into prominence by Mooney and Robertson.[60] It is argued that pseudoradicular pain may be caused by arthritis of one or more specific facet joints. Initial tests are by intra-articular injection of local anesthetic under radiographic control. Both reproduction and abolition of pain are thought to be diagnostic. Subjective diagnostic accuracy of this method seems to depend greatly on the operator. In fact, significant doubt exists as to the usefulness of this diagnostic test.[61]

Segmental Instability

Abnormal segmental mobility may be both the cause and the result of degenerative changes.[62] Instability is defined as "loss of stiffness."[63] Whether and how it is a direct cause of pain remain to be determined. Various static and dynamic radiologic tests have been proposed to detect segmental instability.[64–66] The accuracy of radiologic methods, including stereoroentgenography to detect instability is being questioned.[67] Implanted metallic markers seem to improve the accuracy of radiologic diagnosis but appear too invasive for routine clinical use. A single-

blind trial of external skeletal fixation of the involved segment has been somewhat successful in predicting the outcome of surgical fusion in 35 patients.[68]

Disc Degeneration

It is unclear whether the simple presence of "disc degeneration" is a direct cause of back pain. Few clinicians today would subscribe to the existence of the "isolated disc resorption syndrome."[69] Radiologic methods have low specificity for clinically relevant disc degeneration, showing abnormalities both in symptomatic and nonsymptomatic individuals[70–72] even when the pain response to intradiscal injection is considered.[73] Because "disc degeneration" and implied "segmental instability" are, in the opinion of some surgeons, indications for discectomy and/or fusion, it seems important to develop a better understanding of these conditions.

Sacroiliac Joint Syndrome

Although a pathologically plausible cause of low back pain, degeneration and instability of the sacroiliac joints are similarly difficult to define clinically.[74,75]

Piriformis Syndrome and Bursitis (e.g., Trochanteric)

Piriformis syndrome and bursitis are diagnosed clinically, apparently mimicking back pain. No systematic prospective studies are available.

DIAGNOSTIC METHODS

As in other clinical encounters, the workup of the patient with low back pain starts with a comprehensive history. Based on some key features, clinical suspicions arise. The physical examination serves, on the one hand, to reject or confirm such suspicions, and on the other hand, to screen for as-yet-undeclared possibilities. Auxilliary investigations should be used primarily to confirm or reject a strong clinical suspicion. Routine screening procedures, be they biochemical, imaging, provocatory, electrophysiologic, or psychologic, should be discouraged. Not only do they contribute to the high cost of low back pain care,[76,77] but because of their generally low specificity they lead to unnecessary, possibly risky therapeutic interventions.

The role of a thorough and systematic approach to the patient with low back pain as a therapeutic measure should not be underestimated, because it signals to patients that they and their complaints are being taken seriously by the physician.[78,79] Excessive investigation, however, may confirm the patients in their sick role.

It is possible to compile the accumulated clinical experience in the form of algorithms[80] or even computer programs.[81] Such methods seem to have attained an accuracy comparable with that of a good clinician. Such methods may turn out to be quite problematic, because they might encourage a transfer of responsibility for the care of the back pain patient to lesser-skilled clinicians.

Comprehensive History

Although the use of evaluation forms encourages collecting a systematic and complete history,[80] it tends to focus the physician's attention away from the patient to the form. Subtle hints may be missed. The patient's agenda becomes subjugated to the sequence of items on the form. There are currently no studies available comparing overall outcome depending on the use of history forms. It is clear that the reliability of the elicited history is enhanced by the use of closed question formats.[82] Validated questionnaires,[83,84] to be completed by literate patients themselves or with the aid of a trained assistant, facilitate evaluating the course of illness. None of these formal methods of collecting history have been shown to enhance sensitivity and specificity of the history in regard to the organic diagnosis.

The exact circumstance of minor back injuries adds little to the diagnosis; changes in general bodily function before and after onset of pain, however, are crucial in alerting the clinician to nonmechanical or progressive causes of pain.

The character and distribution of pain are moderately reliable. A clear history of shooting sciatic pain is suggestive of nerve root involvement. A very flowery epic description of suffering, however, would point more toward a strong psychogenic component. Three psychosocial factors have been found to carry a poor functional prognosis: previous episodes of low back pain, less than 9 years of education, and "feeling sick all the time."[85]

Besides the usual items elicited in a clinical history, information about the situation at home and, above all, at work is crucial in arriving at a prognosis.[86] Social stress in the workplace seems to affect outcome more than many purely organic factors.

Physical Examination

A systematic physician-controlled sequence is advantageous. Various protocols have been published[80] and validated.[82] Reliable signs include operative scars, loss of lordosis (< 2 cm on modified Schober test), list (> 1 cm), limited flexion (< 5 cm),[87] catch, limited lateral flexion (< 3 cm),[86] lumbar and buttock tenderness, straight leg raising (< 75°) root irritation,[19] and compression signs.[82] Tests for sacroiliac pain, which have been shown in some hands to be reliable, include distraction, compression thigh thrust, and pelvic torsion left and right.[88] Unreliable tests are sacral thrust and cranial shear. Even though the test results can be reproduced reliably, their relationship to actual sacroiliac joint pathology has not been adequately demonstrated.

A variety of eponymic tests are recommended for the workup of low back pain patients including the Brudzinski/Kernig, Cram, Hoover, Milgram, and Naffziger tests and Stooptest. Sensitivity and specificity of these tests have not been established. By using a sufficiently large number of low specificity tests, any clinical suspicion can be confirmed.

There are clinical tests for somatic amplification that have been validated.[89] Subsequently, some of these tests were found not to be reliable in other hands.[90] Tests that discriminate between organic and nonorganic causes of low back pain include superficial tenderness (skin folds), distraction tests (e.g., distracted straight leg raising), nonanatomic sensory or motor deficits, and over reaction. However, simulation tests such as axial loading and hip rotation did not reproduce well. These findings also discriminate between patients in whom anticipated financial compensation is or is not involved.[91]

Plain Radiographs

When deciding whether a low back pain patient should be x-rayed, one not only should consider what diagnoses the radiographs may reveal that would have been missed otherwise but also whether this finding will alter therapy and outcome. When screening patients with low back pain at the initial visit in primary care, the population would have to be subjected to a 0.03 Gy of radiation at an additional cost of $2,000 (1982) to prevent one patient day of suffering.[92]

Observer variability is surprisingly high when reading lumbosacral radiographs,[93] particularly regarding the common findings of degeneration and congenital lesions. But even compression fractures and lytic lesions show only slight-to-moderate agreement. Even though the addition of oblique films improves the sensitivity of lumbar radiographs, it does not appear to alter the incidence of clinically consequential findings significantly.[94]

Patients with low back pain do not exhibit findings of spondylosis or disc degeneration more frequently than asymptomatic subjects, but wedge-shaped vertebral bodies are somewhat more common in symptomatic patients younger than 40 years old.[95] Transitional vertebrae, Schmorl's nodes, disc narrowing at L3-L4 and L5-S1, vacuum sign, lumbar sacralization,[96] and claw spurs do not discriminate between symptomatic and asymptomatic subjects. Traction spurs and narrowing at L4-L5, however, are more common in symptomatic patients, as well as being associated with clinical findings of nerve compression.[97]

In older subjects, findings of disc degeneration seems to be more strongly associated with symptoms.[98]

The presence of clinically unsuspected findings that will alter outcome are extremely rare.[99]

How Much Radiology?

Routine use of radiographs in traditional primary care seems to increase patient satisfaction.[100,101] This effect, however, can be abolished by specific patient education.[102] Criteria that suggest the need for radiographs on initial contact include age older than 50, temperature greater than 37.8°C, significant trauma, neuromotor deficits, unexpected weight loss, abuse of alcohol or parenteral drugs, and history of cancer or corticosteroid use.[103] When a specific policy is implemented, requiring explicit justification of every lumbar radiograph on the requisition form, a 47 percent reduction of routine lumbar films seems possible.[104] The impact of such a policy appears to be dependent on local customs. In a study from Duke University, in which the rate of initial radiographs for low back pain was 21.1 percent, applying the criteria mentioned above would actually have increased the ordering of radiographs.[105] Even in this study, low radiograph use did not appear deleterious.

In summary, only a fraction of patients presenting with low back pain require radiographs at the initial contact. Good patient education is necessary if trust is to be maintained. Institutions with a radiograph rate greater than 30 percent should consider instituting a restrictive policy.

CT Scan and MRI

When there is a high suspicion of intraspinal nerve compression, computer-enhanced imaging can be useful. MRI seems to exhibit a slightly superior sensitivity and specificity than CT.[106,107] Availability and cost may neutralize this advantage. Careful decision-analytical studies are needed before optimal choices are possible. Both methods, however, are vastly superior to conventional radiology.

The mere presence of root irritation signs is no absolute indication for imaging studies, because natural history of disc herniation is generally benign.[37]

Myelography and Epidural Venography

Before the availability of CT and MRI, these positive contrast studies were used for the delineation of intraspinal mass lesions or nerve root impingement. Because venography is technically more demanding than myelography, it can be argued that in facilities where computer-assisted imaging is not available, myelography is usually the method of choice if signs of nerve compression or cauda equina impairment exist.

Discography

Discography is recommended by some orthopedic surgeons to identify patients likely to profit from lumbar fusion, but this method remains unproven[108] for the evaluation of the low back pain patient.

Electromyography

Electromyography is commonly used in the evaluation of the back pain patient seeking compensation when there are no objective findings on physical examination. The physician attempts to demonstrate subliminal signs of active or chronic denervation or slowed proximal conduction velocity. No adequate studies were found demonstrating sensitivity and specificity in these circumstances. Somatosensory-evoked potentials have been shown to be neither sensitive nor specific.[109] H-reflex latency has a sensitivity for "the presence of back pain" of about 68 percent, but specificity is not quoted.[110] Electromyographic methods should be further investigated for sensitivity and specificity before routine use in back pain can be recommended.

Thermography

It is plausible that pain and nerve root irritation should cause alterations of autonomic activity. Thermographic changes can therefore be expected. Yet, sensitivity and specificity of thermography have not been demonstrated.[111]

REFERENCES

1. Cunningham LS, Kelsey JL: Epidemiology of musculoskeletal impairments and associated disabilty. Am J Public Health 74:574, 1984
2. Cypress BK: Characteristics of physician visits for back symptoms: a national perspective. Am J Public Health 73:389, 1983
3. Deyo RA, Tsui-Wu YJ: Descriptive epidemiology of low-back pain and its related medical care in the United States. Spine 12:264, 1987
4. Spitzer WO, LeBlanc FE, Dupuis M et al: Scientific approach to the assessment and management of activity-related spinal disorders. (The Quebec Task Force Report.) Spine 12:S1, 1987
5. Deyo RA, Tsui-Wu YJ: Functional disability due to back pain. A population based study indicating the importance of socioeconomic factors. Arthritis Rheum 30:1247, 1987
6. Bonica JJ: The nature of the problem. p. 1. Management of Low Back Pain. In Carron H, McLaughlin RE (eds): John Wright PSG, Boston, 1982
7. Cats-Baril WL, Frymoyer JW: The economics of spinal disorders. In Frymoyer JW (ed): The Adult Spine: Principles and Practice. Raven Press, New York, 1991
8. Deyo RA: Conservative therapy for low-back pain. Distinguishing useful from useless therapy. JAMA 250:1057, 1983
9. Von Korff M, Deyo RA, Cherkin D, Barlow W: Back pain in primary care—outcomes at 1 year. Spine 18:855, 1993
10. Burton AK, Tillotson KM: Prediction of the clinical course of low-back trouble using multivariable models. Spine 16:7, 1991
11. Deyo RA, Diehl AK: Psychosocial predictors of disability in patients with low back pain. J Rheumatol 15:1557, 1988
12. Svenson HO: Low back pain in 40–47 year old men: II. Socioeconomic factors and previous sickness absence. Scand J Rehabil Med 14:55, 1982
13. Horal J: The clinical appearance of low back disorders in the city of Gothenberg Sweden: comparison of incapacitated probands with matched controls. Acta Orthop Scand, suppl. 118:1, 1969
14. Gibson ES, Martin RH, Terry CW: Incidence of low back pain and pre-placement x-ray screening. J Occup Med 22:515, 1980
15. Klein BP, Jensen RC, Sanderson LM: Assessment of workers compensation claims for back strain/sprains. J Occup Med 26:443, 1984
16. Cherkin DC, Deyo RA, Loeser JD et al: An international comparison of back pain surgery rates. Spine 19:1201, 1994
17. Waddell G, Main CJ, Morris EW et al: Chronic low back pain. Psychological distress and illness behaviour. Spine 9:209, 1984
18. Kellgren JN: On the distribution of pain arising from deep somatic structures with charts of somatic pain areas. Clin Sci 4:35, 1939
19. Waddell G: Clinical diagnosis of leg pain and nerve root involvement in low back disorders. Acta Orthop Belg 53:152, 1987
20. Edgar MA, Park WM: Induced pain patterns on passive straight leg raising in lower lumbar disk protrusion. J Bone Joint Surg [Br] 56:658, 1974
21. American Academy of Orthopaedic Surgeons: Orthopaedic Knowledge Update 3: Home Study Syllabus.

American Academy of Orthopaedic Surgeons, Park Ridge, IL, 1990

22. Von Korff M, Deyo RA, Cherkin D, Barlow W: Back pain in primary care—outcomes at 1 year. Spine 18:855, 1993

23. Wadell G, Main CJ, Morris EW et al: Chronic low back pain, psychological distress and illness behaviour. Spine 9:209, 1984

24. Young A, Wynn Parry CB: The assessment and management of the failed back. Parts I and II. Int Disabil Stud 10:21, 1988

25. Waddell G, Kummel EG, Lotto WN et al: Failed lumbar disc surgery and repeat surgery following industrial injuries. J Bone Joint Surg [Am] 61:201, 1979

26. Hall S, Bartlesow JD, Onofrio BM et al: Lumbar spinal stenosis. Ann Intern Med 103:271, 1985

27. Borenstein DG, Wiesel SW: Low Back Pain—Medical Diagnosis and Comprehensive Management. WB Saunders, Philadelphia, 1989

28. Slager VT: Arachnoiditis ossificans. Report of a case and a review of the subject. Arch Pathol 70:322, 1960

29. Barthelemy CR: Arachnoiditis ossificans. J Comput Assist Tomogr 6:809, 1982

30. Mirowitz SA, Shady KL: Gadopentate dimeglumine-enhanced MR imaging of the postoperative lumbar spine: comparison of fat-suppressed and conventional T1-weighted imaging. AJR 159:385, 1992

31. Tullberg T, Rydberg J, Isaacson J: Radiographic changes after lumbar discectomy. Spine 18:843, 1992

32. Dullerud R, Morland TJ: Adhesive arachnoiditis after radiculography with Dimer-X and Depo-Medrol. Radiology 119:153, 1976

33. Mixter WJ, Barr JS: Rupture of the intervertebral disc with involvement of the spinal canal. N Engl J Med 211:210, 1934

34. Spangfort EV: The lumbar disk herniation: a computer-aided analysis of 2,504 operations. Acta Orthop Scand, suppl. 142:1, 1972

35. Andrae R: Ueber Knorpelknötchen am hintern Ende der Wirbelbandscheibe im Bereich des Spinalkanals. Beitr Path Anat 82:464, 1929

36. Morris EW, DiPaola M, Valance R, Waddell G: Diagnosis and decision making in lumbar disk prolapse and nerve entrapment. Spine 11:436, 1986

37. Weber H: Lumbar disk herniation: a controlled prospective study with ten years of observation. Spine 8:131, 1984

38. Graudal H, de Carvalho A, Lassen L: The course of sacro-iliac involvement in rheumatoid arthritis. Scand J Rheumatol, suppl. 32:34, 1979

39. Moldofsky H, Scarisbrick P, England R, Smythe H: Musculoskeletal symptoms and non-REM sleep disturbance in patients with "fibrositis syndrome" and healthy subjects. Psychosom Med 37:341, 1975

40. Resnick D, Niwayama G: Degenerative disease of the spine. p. 1480. In Resnick D (ed): Diagnosis of Bone and Joint Disorders. Vol. 3. WB Saunders, Philadelphia, 1988

41. Schmorl G, Junghanns H: The Human Spine in Health and Disease. 2nd Ed. Grune & Stratton, Orlando, FL, 1971

42. Splithoff CA: Lumbosacral junction. Roentgenographic comparison of patients with and without backaches. JAMA 152:1610, 1953

43. Torgerson WR, Dotter WE: Comparative roentgenographic study of the symptomatic and asymptomatic spine. J Bone Joint Surg [Am] 58:850, 1976

44. Lawrence JS, Bremner JM, Bier F: Osteoarthrosis: prevalence in the population and relationship between symptoms and ray changes. Ann Rheum Dis 25:1, 1966

45. Witt I, Vestergaard A, Rosenklitt A: A comparative analysis of x-ray findings of the lumbar spine in patients with and without lumbar pain. Spine 9:298, 1984

46. Frymoyer JW, Newberg A, Pope MH et al: Spine radiographs in patients with low back pain. An epidemiological study in men. J Bone Joint Surg [Am] 66:1048, 1984

47. Eisenstein S: The morphometry and pathological anatomy of the lumbar spine in South African negroes and caucasoids with specific reference to spinal stenosis. J Bone Joint Surg [Br] 59:173, 1977

48. Kent DL, Haynor DR, Larson EB, Deyo RA: Diagnosis of lumbar spinal stenosis in adults: a metaanalysis of the accuracy of CT, MR, and myelography. AJR 158:1135, 1992

49. Johnsson KE, Rosen I, Uden A: The natural course of lumbar spinal stenosis. Clin Orthop 279:82, 1992

50. Roche MB, Rowe GG: The incidence of separate neural arch and coincidental bone variations. Anat Rec 109:233, 1951

51. Fredrickson BE, Baker D, McHolick WJ et al: The natural history of spondylolysis and spondylolisthesis. J Bone Joint Surg [Am] 66:699, 1984

52. Shahriaree H, Sajadi K, Rooholamini SA: A family with spondylolisthesis. J Bone Joint Surg [Am] 61:1256, 1979

53. Jackson DW, Wiltse LL, Dingeman RD, Hayes M: Stress reactions involving the pars interarticularis in young athletes. Am J Sports Med 9:304, 1981

54. Wiltse LL, Widell EH Jr, Jackson DW: Fatigue fracture: the basic lesion in isthmic spondylolisthesis. J Bone Joint Surg [Am] 57:17, 1975

55. Junghanns H: Spondylolisthesen ohne Spalt im Zwischengelenkstueck. Arch Orthop Unfallchir 29:118, 1930

56. Meyerding HW: Low backache and sciatic pain associated with spondylolisthesis and protruded intervertebral disc. J Bone Joint Surg 23:461, 1941

57. Fredrickson BE, Baker D, Mcholick WJ et al: The natural history of spondylolysis and spondylolisthesis. J Bone Joint Surg [Am] 66:699, 1984

58. Saraste H: Longterm clinical and radiological followup of spondylosis and spondylolisthesis. J Pediatr Orthop 7:631, 1987

59. Frennered K: Isthmic spondylolisthesis among patients receiving disability pension under the diagnosis of chronic low back pain syndrome. Spine 19:2766, 1994

60. Mooney V, Robertson J: The facet syndrome. Clin Orthop 115:149, 1976

61. Jackson RP: The facet syndrome—myth or reality? Clin Orthop 279:110, 1992

62. Kirkaldy-Willis WH, Farfan HF: Instability of the lumbar spine. Clin Orthop 165:110, 1982

63. Pope MH, Frymoyer JW, Krag MH: Diagnosing instability. Clin Orthop 279:60, 1992

64. Morgan FP, King T: Primary instability of lumbar vertebrae as a common cause of low back pain. J Bone Joint Surg [Br] 39:6, 1957

65. Weiler PJ, King GJ, Gertzbein SD: Analysis of sagittal plane instability of the lumbar spine in vivo. Spine 15:1300, 1990

66. Friberg O: Lumbar instability: a dynamic approach by traction-compression radiography. Spine 12:119, 1987

67. Dvorak KJ, Panjabi MM, Novotny JE et al: Clinical validation of functional flexion-extension roentgenograms of the lumbar spine. Spine 16:943, 1991

68. Esses SI, Botsford DJ, Kostuik JP: The role of external spinal skeletal fixation in the assessment of low-back disorders. Spine 14:594, 1989

69. Crock HV: Internal disc disruption: a challenge to disc prolapse fifty years on. Spine 11:650, 1986

70. Dabbs VM, Dabbs LG: Correlation between disk height narrowing and low-back pain. Spine 15:1366, 1990

71. Frymoyer JW: Predicting disability from low back pain. Clin Orthop 279:101, 1992

72. Magora A, Schwartz A: Relation between low back pain and x-ray changes. Scand J Rehabil Med 12:47, 1980

73. Nachemson A: Editorial comment: lumbar discography—where are we today? Spine 14:555, 1989

74. Potter NA, Rothstein JM: Intertester reliability for selected clinical tests of the sacroiliac joint. Phys Ther 65:1671, 1985

75. Walheim GG, Selvik G: Mobility of the pubic symphysis. In vivo measurements with an electromechanic method and a roentgen stereo-photogrammetric method. Clin Orthop 191:129, 1984

76. Frymoyer JW, Cats-Baril WL: An overview of the incidence and costs of low back pain. Orthop Clin North Am 22:263, 1991

77. Spengler DM, Bigos SJ, Martin NA et al: Back injuries in industry: a retrospective study. 1. Overview and cost analysis. Spine 11:241, 1986

78. Roter DL, Hall JA: Studies of doctor–patient interactions. Annu Rev Public Health 10:163, 1989

79. Bass MJ: The physician's actions and the outcome of illness in family practice. J Fam Pract 23:43, 1986

80. Wiesel SW: A standardized approach to the diagnosis and treatment of low back pain. In Borenstein DG, Wiesel SW (eds): Low Back Pain—Medical Diagnosis and Comprehensive Management. WB Saunders, Philadelphia, 1989

81. Mathew B, Norris D, Hendry D, Waddell G: Artificial intelligence in the diagnosis of low-back pain and sciatica. Spine 13:168, 1988

82. Waddell G, Main CJ, Morris EW et al: Normality and reliability in the clinical assessment of backache. BMJ 284:1519, 1982

83. Melzack R: The McGill pain questionnaire: major properties and scoring methods. Pain 1:277, 1975

84. Main CJ, Waddell G: The detection of psychological abnormality in chronic low back pain using four simple scales. Curr Concepts Pain 2:10, 1984

85. Deyo RA, Diehl AK: Psychosocial predictors of disability in patients with low back pain. J Rheumatol 15:1557, 1988

86. Frymoyer JW: Predicting disability from low back pain. Clin Orthop 279:101, 1992

87. Moll J, Wright V: p. 218. In Jayson MI (ed): The Lumbar Spine and Back Pain. Churchill Livingstone, Edinburgh, 1987

88. Laslett M, Williams M: The reliability of selected pain provocation tests for sacro-iliac joint pathology. Spine 19:1243, 1994

89. Waddell G, McCullogh JA, Kummel E, Venner RM: Non-organic physical sign in low back pain. Spine 5:117, 1980

90. Korbon GA, DeGood DE, Schroeder ME et al: The development of a somatic amplification scale for low-back pain. Spine 12:787, 1987

91. Hayes B, Solyom CA, Wing PC, Berkowitz J: Use of psychometric measures and nonorganic signs testing in detecting nomogenic disorders in low back pain patients. Spine 18:1254, 1993

92. Liang M, Komaroff AL: Roentgenograms in primary care patients with acute low back pain: a cost-effectiveness study. Arch Intern Med 142:1108, 1982

93. Deyo RA, McNiesh LM, Cone RO: Observer variability in the interpretation of lumbar spine radiographs. Arthritis Rheum 28:1066, 1985

94. Gehweiler JA, Jr, Daffner RH: Low back pain: the controversy of radiologic evaluation. AJR 140:109, 1983

95. Witt I, Vestergaard A, Rosenklint A: A comparative analysis of x-ray findings of the lumbar spine patients with and without lumbar pain. Spine 9:298, 1984

96. Magora A, Schwartz A: Relation between the low back pain syndrome and x-ray findings. 2: Transitional vertebra (mainly sacralization). Scand J Rehabil Med 10:135, 1978

97. Frymoyer JW, Newberg A, Pope MH et al: Spine radiographs in patients with low-back pain: an epidemiological study in men. J Bone Joint Surg [Am] 66:1048, 1984

98. Biering-Sorensen F, Hansen FR, Schroll M, Runeborg O: The relation of spinal x-ray to low back pain and physical activity among 60-year-old men and women. Spine 10:445, 1985

99. Knudsen L, Philipson T: Radiography of the lumbar spine: analysis of 1494 conventional examinations. [Danish] Ugeskr Laeger 147:3898, 1985

100. Rockey PH, Tompkins RK, Wood RW, Wolcott BW: The usefulness of x-ray examinations in the evaluation of patients with back pain. J Fam Pract 7:455, 1978

101. Kaplan DM, Knapp M, Romm FJ, Velez R: Low back pain and x-ray films of the lumbar spine: a prospective study in primary care. South Med J 79:811, 1986

102. Deyo RA, Diehl AK, Rosenthal M: Reducing roentgenography use: can patient expectations be altered? Arch Intern Med 147:141, 1987

103. Deyo RA, Diehl AK: Lumbar spine films in primary care: current use and the effects of selective ordering criteria. J Gen Intern Med 1:20, 1986

104. Baker SR, Rabin A, Lantos G, Gallagher EJ: The effects of restricting the indications for lumbosacral spine radiography in patients with acute back symptoms. Am J Roentgenol 149:535, 1987

105. Frazier LM, Carey TS, Lyles MF et al: Selective criteria may increase lumbosacral spine roentgenogram use in acute low-back pain. Arch Intern Med 149:47, 1989

106. Kent DL, Haynor DR, Longstreth WT, Larson EB: The clinical efficacy of magnetic resonance imaging in neuroimaging. Ann Intern Med 120:856, 1994

107. Kent DL, Haynor DR, Larson EB, Deyo RA: Diagnosis of lumbar spinal stenosis in adults: a metaanalysis of the accuracy of CT, MR and myelography. Am J Roentgenol 158:1135, 1992

108. Nachemson A: Editorial comment: lumbar discography—where are we today? Spine 14:555, 1989

109. Rodriquez AA, Kanis L, Rodriquez AA, Lane D: Somatosensory evoked potentials from dermatomal stimulation as an indicator of L5 and S1 radiculopathy. Arch Phys Med Rehabil 68:366, 1987

110. Humphreys CR, Triano JJ, Brandl MJ: Sensitivity study of H-reflex alterations in idiopathic low back pain patients vs. a healthy population. J Manipulative Physiol Ther 12:71, 1989. [published erratum appears in J Manipulative Physiol Ther 12, no. 5, 1989]

111. Hoffman RM, Kent DL, Deyo RA: Diagnostic accuracy and clinical utility of thermography for lumbar radiculopathy: a meta-analysis. Spine 16:623, 1991

Nonsurgical Treatment of Acute Low Back Pain

Sikhar N. Banerjee

Low back pain is experienced by most people at some time in their lives, and it is estimated that general yearly prevalence in the United States is between 15 and 20 percent.[1]

Many treatment methods have been introduced through the years that claimed effectiveness. Many treatment methods continue to be popular despite proven lack of efficacy. In recent years, two task forces have reviewed the efficacy of various treatment methods and suggested practice guidelines based on critical review of available literature. In 1987, the Quebec Task Force report[2] recommended a critical pathway emphasizing early diagnosis of potentially life-threatening or seriously disabling diseases and limited bed rest and early mobilization of patients requiring nonsurgical treatment. The Agency for Health Care Policy and Research at the US Department of Health and Human Services recently published a similar clinical practice guideline for acute low back problems in adults.[3]

This chapter discusses the most commonly used nonsurgical treatments of acute low back pain and reviews the levels of evidence regarding their efficacy. To assist the clinician in making diagnostic and treatment decisions, algorithms based on efficacious treatment methods are presented in Appendices 5-1 to 5-4.

BED REST

Bed rest has remained the most common treatment modality for acute low back pain until recently, when several clinical trials have shown deleterious effects of prolonged bed rest.

Wiesel et al.[4] studied 80 army combat trainees with acute nonradiating low back pain and normal neurologic straight leg raising testing and radiologic examination. They were admitted to the hospital and randomly assigned to a bed rest and an ambulatory group with restricted duties. Both groups received acetaminophen, one tablet twice daily, and the trial was discontinued after 14 days even if the patients continued to have pain and disability. The bed rest group returned to full activity significantly earlier than the ambulatory group ($P < .001$). The bed rest group also had significantly less pain ($P < .005$). The major drawback of this study is that the outcome assessments were not blinded and the pain reporting was on an arbitrary scale. The patients were forced to undergo a specific treatment, and as such, the findings may not be generalizable to the civilian population.

Gilbert et al.[5] conducted a randomized trial involving 252 eligible patients with acute low back pain with or without radiation to the legs and no neurologic deficit or any other significant spinal or pelvic pathology.

The patients were randomized to one of four treatment groups: (1) bed rest for at least 4 days; (2) bed rest, physiotherapy, and education; (3) physiotherapy and education; or (4) control group with analgesics only. The patients were followed for 3 to 44 days. At the end of the trial period, there was no significant difference between groups on the main outcomes measure of activity discomfort scale and the mean recovery period. However, the bed rest group experienced a significant but small increase of restrictions of daily activities ($P < .034$), took longer to achieve a normal level of activities; and consumed more analgesics. Deyo et al.[6] studied the effects of 2 and 7 days of bed rest involving 203 patients with mechanical low back pain without neurologic deficits, and 78 percent had acute pain (30 days or less). Patients were randomly assigned to 2 days or 7 days of bed rest, and all patients received a recommendation regarding local heat application, exercise, and weight loss.

At the 3-week follow-up, there was no significant difference between groups on all outcome measures (functional status, perceptions, symptoms, signs, and use of services) except the group with 2 days at bed rest missed significantly less time from work ($P = .01$).

Even though it is methodologically sound, the study did not address the issue of bed rest versus no bed rest. Also, the generalizability of the study is open to question because only 203 of the 450 eligible patients were randomized to treatment groups, and 189 and 179 patients were available at 3-week and 3-month follow-up.

Malmivaara et al.[7] studied the efficacy of three treatment methods: bed rest for 2 days, back mobilization exercise, and continuation of ordinary activities as tolerated (control group). One hundred eighty-six subjects with acute or acute on chronic low back pain without neurologic deficit or sciatic syndrome were randomly assigned to three treatment groups. The outcomes were assessed at 3 and 12 weeks after randomization and included return to work, straight leg raising, lumbar flexion, and Oswestry back disability index. At 3 weeks, the control group was significantly better than the bed rest group regarding absence from work and ability to work. When compared with the exercise group, the control group recovered better in terms of number of sick days, duration of pain, and scores on Oswestry index. At 12 weeks, the bed rest group had recovered more slowly than the control groups.

The recovery was also slower in the exercise group when compared with the control group. The authors concluded that avoidance of bed rest and continuing with ordinary activity as tolerated provided the most rapid recovery in patients with acute low back pain without neurologic deficits or sciatic syndrome.

Recommendations

Most patients with acute low back pain without significant spinal pathology or neurologic deficit will achieve progressive satisfactory recovery without bed rest or a very limited period (2 days) of bed rest.

NON-NARCOTIC ANALGESICS AND NSAIDS

Non-narcotic analgesics (i.e., acetaminophen) and nonsteroidal anti-inflammatory drugs (NSAIDs) are used frequently for symptom control in patients with acute low back pain. Several controlled studies have compared NSAIDs with placebos, but no controlled trial exists comparing acetaminophen with a placebo.

Amlie et al.[8] evaluated the efficacy of piroxicam in a double-blind placebo-controlled randomized trial involving 287 patients with acute low back pain without radicular symptoms or inflammatory spondylitis.

The experimental group received 40 mg piroxicam once daily for 2 days and 20 mg once daily for the remaining 5 days. Treatment started 48 hours after the onset of pain and continued for 7 days. They were allowed to take additional analgesics (paracetamol up to 1,000 mg two to three times a day) if necessary. At the end of 3 days, the piroxicam group experienced significantly greater pain relief as measured by a visual analog scale in lying ($P < .001$), sitting ($P < .01$), and standing ($P < .01$). At the end of 1 week, there was no significant difference in pain relief between the groups even though the control group used more additional analgesics. More patients in the piroxicam group returned to work after 1 week ($P < .05$) than the control group.

Postacchini et al.[9] studied 168 patients with acute low back pain with or without neurologic deficits. Patients were randomized to one of five treatment groups: manipulation (for 4 weeks), drug therapy (Declofenac, full dosage for 10 to 14 days), physiotherapy (for 2 to 3 weeks), placebo, or bed rest (for 8 days). All patients were assessed at 3 weeks, 2 months, and 6 months after initiation of treatment.

The outcome measures consisted of two subjective (pain perception, ability to perform daily activities) and four objective measurements (spinal flexion, abdominal muscle strength, positive straight leg raising degrees, pain on palpation on lumbar spinous process). At the 3-week follow-up, patients treated with manipulation had maximal improvement, and the drug therapy groups had more improvement than the placebo group. At 2 months, the drug therapy group had the best outcome ($P < .01$), and at 6 months, there was no significant difference between the treatment groups.

Basmajian[10] studied the efficacy of two drugs, diflunisal and cyclobenzaprine, in a randomized double-blind parallel-controlled trial involving 18 centers. The 175 patients were randomized to (1) cyclobenzaprine 5 mg and diflunisal 500 mg twice a day, (2) cyclobenzaprine 5 mg twice a day, (3) diflunisal 500 mg twice a day, or (4) placebo. The total treatment time was 7 to 10 days. Outcome measures were local pain, tenderness, range of motion, and activities of daily living, and measurements were taken at baseline, day 2, 4, 7, and 10. On day 4 the combined drug group made significant gains (P = .006) over the other three groups. By day 10, almost all patients had recovered, and there were no significant differences between the groups.

Recommendations

Three controlled trials have demonstrated the efficacy of NSAIDs compared with placebos in relieving acute low back pain discomfort from 1 week to 2 months of symptom duration. Even though manufacturers claimed better efficacy of their product, there is no evidence that one NSAID is better than another.[11] However, individual patients may prefer one NSAID over another, and Brooks et al.[12] suggested a change to a different NSAID if no relief is experienced within 2 weeks. When using NSAIDs for acute back pain, one should consider potential side effects of dyspepsia, gastric erosion and bleeding (which can be controlled with misoprostol), and interference in controlling hypertension and cardiac failure especially in older patients.

MUSCLE RELAXANTS

Muscle relaxants are frequently used in the treatment of acute back pain and soft tissue injuries. The rationale of using muscle relaxants is to reduce involuntary muscle spasm, thereby reducing pain. Several randomized clinical trials have been reported comparing muscle relaxants with placebos, with conflicting outcomes.

Diazepam

Hingorani[13] reported a randomized double-blind controlled trial involving 50 patients with acute low back pain requiring hospital admission. The patients were divided at random into two groups, each consisting of 25 patients. The experimental group received diazepam 10 mg intramuscularly (IM) every 6 hours for 24 hours and then 2 mg orally (PO) every 6 hours for 5 days. The control group received sterile water injections. All patients were put on bed rest and given Ca aspirin 10 g three times a day. Some patients were given supportive therapy in the form of pelvic traction, sedation, and supplementary analgesics.

The outcome measures consisted of a subjective report of pain and tenderness and objective measures of range of motion, straight leg raising, and neurologic signs. All patients were assessed for outcome after 24 hours and 5 days. At the end of the treatment program, there was no difference in the outcome between groups.

This study has many methodologic deficiencies. The author does not indicate how randomization was carried out, and various supportive therapies may mask the treatment effect of the experimental treatment. No statistical analysis was given.

Carisoprodol (Soma)

Boyles et al.[14] compared the effectiveness of carisoprodol (Soma) and diazepam in a double-blind randomized study involving 71 patients with acute thoracolumbar strain of less than 7 days' duration. One group received carisoprodol 350 mg and the second group received diazepam 5 mg four times a day for 7 days. All patients were reviewed by participating physicians after 3 and 7 days of treatment. Carisoprodol demonstrated a consistent pattern of superiority over diazepam.

Hindle[15] compared the effectiveness of carisoprodol, butabarbital, and a placebo in a double-blind study involving 43 patients with acute low back pain of 12 to 48 hours' duration. The patients in each group were given carisoprodol 350 mg or butabarbital 15 mg or a placebo four times a day for 4 days. Carisoprodal was found to be significantly more effective than butabarbital or the placebo in reducing discomfort and improving range of motion of the lumbar spine.

Orphenadrine (Norflex)

Gold[16] reported the results of a randomized trial involving 60 patients with moderate-to-severe low back pain. The patients were randomized into three treatment groups: (1) orphenadrine (Norflex) 100 mg PO bid, (2) phenobarbital 32 mg bid, or (3) placebo 1 bid. After 48 hours, the orphenadrine group experienced significantly more pain relief ($P \leq .001$). However, only 9 of 20 patients in the experimental group experienced significant pain relief. Neither investigators nor patients were blinded.

Klinger et al.[17] studied the effects of intravenous orphenadrine (60 mg) compared with a placebo in a group of 80 patients with acute low back pain with paravertebral muscle spasm and limited range of motion of the lumbar spine. The trial design was randomized double-blind placebo controlled. Forty-five minutes after drug/placebo administration the orphenadrine group experienced significantly higher pain relief, increased range of motion, and reduced muscle spasm ($P \leq .001$). Thirty-four of forty patients in the orphenadrine group experienced symptom relief as opposed to 4 in the placebo group.

Cyclobenzaprine (Flexeril)

Baratta[18] reported the results of a randomized double-blind placebo-controlled trial involving 117 patients with acute low back pain of 3 to 5 days' duration.

The experimental group received cyclobenzaprine (Flexeril) 10 mg PO tid, and the control group received a placebo one tablet PO tid. The patients were evaluated by a physician 2 to 3 hours after the first dose and then 2 to 4, 5 to 7, and 8 to 12 days after initiation of treatment. All patients improved in the course of time, but the Flexeril group experienced significantly more pain relief ($P < .05$), less muscle spasm ($P < .01$), improved range of motion ($P < .05$), and improved global measure by the physician ($P < .05$). Seventy-one percent of the Flexeril group and 25 percent of the placebo group experienced moderate-to-marked improvement, and 43 percent of patients in the Flexeril group and 17 percent in the placebo group experienced one or more adverse reactions (i.e., drowsiness, dizziness, nausea, etc.) ($P < .01$).

Basmajian[10] studied a combination therapy with cyclobenzaprine (5 mg bid) and diflunisal (500 mg bid) compared with each drug alone or with a placebo. One hundred seventy-five patients from 18 centers were allocated to each treatment group in a randomized double-blind controlled fashion. Combined therapy was found to be superior ($P = .006$) on day 4 of treatment, and after 7 to 10 days, most patients improved and there was no significant difference between groups.

Baclofen (Lioresal)

Baclofen is commonly used for the relief of spinal spasticity. Dapas et al.,[19] in a study of 200 patients with moderate-to-severe low back pain, reported that baclofen (20 mg PO bid) significantly reduced discomfort and muscle spasm ($P < .01$) compared with placebo.

Patients with tumors, infection, fractures, or herniated discs were excluded from the study. The design was randomized double-blind placebo controlled. All patients were advised on bed rest and local heat. The dosage of baclofen was adjusted depending on side effects and symptom relief. The total duration of treatment was 10 days, and they were gradually weaned off the drug in the next 3 days. Patients in both groups improved in all parameters, but the baclofen group experienced significantly more improvement. As expected, the baclofen group experienced increased adverse reaction (i.e., fatigue, dizziness, and nausea), which subsided with dose adjustment.

Dantrolene Na (Dantrium)

Dantrolene Na is an antispastic drug that reduces muscle spasm primarily by inhibiting release of Ca^{2+} from sarcoplasmic reticulum and has been commonly used for relief of cortical spasticity.

Casale[20] studied 20 patients with acute exacerbation of chronic back pain and without radiculopathy, and patients were randomly assigned in a double-blind fashion to receive either dantrolene Na 25 mg PO daily or placebo for 4 days.

At the end of the treatment, patients receiving dantrolene Na experienced significantly reduced pain and spasm ($P < .001$) and improvement in electromyographic parameters of muscle spasm ($P < .01$). There were no side effects in the drug-treated group.

Tetrazepam (Myolastan)

Tetrazepam is a benzodiazepine with a muscle-relaxant property at lower dosage than used for sedation. Arbus et al.[21] studied the analgesic and muscle-relaxing effects of tetrazepam in a group of 50 patients with chronic and subacute low back pain associated with electromyographically (EMG) proven muscle spasm. After excluding placebo responders, 50 patients were randomly assigned to receive either progressively increasing dosage of tetrazepam up to 150 mg daily (50 mg tid) or one tablet of placebo tid. The patients were kept on the full dosage of the drug for 10 days. At the end of 4 days, the tetrapezam group was significantly better in all parameters (pain, spasm, Schober index, EMG activity). By day 14, the level of significance was lower, most likely due to spontaneous recovery. Side effects of drowsiness and nausea were minimal in both groups.

Recommendations

Of the ten randomized trials regarding the efficacy of muscle relaxants, seven compared a muscle relaxant with placebo and all eight trials demonstrated significant improvement in pain and spasm. One trial[13] compared diazepam injection with placebo and did not detect any difference between groups. Another trial[14] compared two muscle relaxants, and one was found to be superior. Only one trial compared combined therapy of NSAIDs and muscle relaxant[10] with NSAID muscle relaxants and placebo alone, and the combined therapy provided better symptom relief. It appears from these trials that muscle relaxants are better than placebos in relieving symptoms of pain and spasm of acute low back pain primarily during the first 4 to 5 days after the onset of symptoms. There is no good evidence that muscle relaxants are better than NSAIDs or one muscle relaxant being superior to others. All muscle relaxants have side effects, especially drowsiness, fatigue, and weakness.

NARCOTIC ANALGESICS

Oral narcotic analgesics such as morphine derivatives (codeine) or synthetic opioids (hydrocodone) are frequently prescribed for alleviation of back and other musculoskeletal pain. No control trial has been reported comparing narcotic analgesics with placebo for acute low back pain.

Wiesel et al.[4] reported the results of treatment of acute back pain in 75 combat trainees who were randomly assigned to three treatment groups: acetaminophen one tablet bid, codeine 60 mg qid, or oxycodone with acetylsalicylic acid one tablet qid. All patients were treated with bed rest. The patients experienced maximal pain relief in the first 3 days of treatment, and patients taking the narcotic analgesics took the same amount of time to return to work as those taking acetaminophen. The author claims that patients taking narcotic analgesics experienced less pain, but no statistical analysis was provided.

Brown et al.[22] compared the analgesic effects of diflunisal (Dolobid) and acetaminophen with codeine in a group of 47 patients with mild-to-moderate low back pain. This was an open-label 15-day randomized double-blind controlled trial.

One group received 1,000 mg of diflunisal followed by 500 mg bid, and the second group received 300 mg of acetaminophen with 30 mg codeine—two tablets initially followed by one tablet every 4 hours until the pain was relieved. All patients were on bed rest for 24 hours, followed by gradual mobilization exercise.

The outcome consisted of patient and investigator's assessment of pain intensity on an arbitrary scale of 1 to 4. All patients taking diflunisal had complete pain relief by day 12, and patients taking acetaminophen with codeine had almost complete pain relief by day 12 and mild rebound pain between day 12 and 15. No statistical analysis was given.

Muncie et al.[23] randomly assigned 42 patients with soft tissue injuries including mild-to-moderate low back pain to two groups: 100 mg diflunisal initially followed by 500 mg bid, or acetaminophen (650 mg) with codeine (60 mg) two tablets initially followed by one or two tablets every 4 to 6 hours. The outcomes were based on the patient's report of pain and limitation of motion on a scale of 0 to 4. At the end of the treatment period, both groups reported similar pain relief and reduction of limitation of motion. The diflunisal group experienced less side effects from the drugs.

Recommendations

The use of narcotic analgesics in the treatment of low back pain of moderate severity cannot be justified on the basis of available data. The three controlled trials reviewed here demonstrated equal efficacy of narcotic analgesics and NSAIDs in relieving pain, except the narcotic analgesics produced significantly more side effects.

ORAL STEROIDS

Oral steroids are sometimes used in the treatment of acute low back pain especially for patients with radicular symptoms. Only very limited information is available in the literature regarding the use of oral steroids in acute low back pain.

Haimovic et al.[24] reported a prospective double-blind trial comparing oral dexamethasone (7-day course starting with 64 mg in a sliding scale to 8 mg) with placebo. Thirty-three patients with acute low back pain and monoradiculopathy were eligible for the study, but only 27 were available for a 1- to 4-year follow-up. All patients were kept on bed rest for 7 days and given narcotic and non-narcotic analgesics. Patients were evaluated after 7 days and at 1 and 4 years regarding intensity of pain on a scale of 0 to 6.

Dexamethasone was not found to be better than placebo, both for short- and long-term relief of lumbosacral radicular pain.

Recommendations

Based on these limited data, an oral steroid cannot be recommended for the treatment of patients with acute low back pain, especially considering the potential serious side effects.

TRACTION

Pelvic traction has been used for many years in the treatment of acute low back pain with or without sciatica, and its mechanism of action remains unclear. The rationale of traction treatment is that it causes spinal elongation and reduction of muscle spasm, thereby reducing discomfort.

Mathews et al.[25] compared the effects of pelvic traction (range between 80 and 135 lb) in a group of 27 patients with sciatica randomly assigned to the treatment group or control group who received pelvic traction not exceeding 20 lb. All patients received traction treatment for 30 minutes, 5 days a week for 3 weeks. At the end of the treatment period, there was no significant difference between the groups in pain relief or increase in straight leg raising angle.

Larsson et al.[26] studied the effects of pelvic autotraction and corset and rest in 82 patients with sciatica and positive straight leg raising of 2 weeks' to 3.5 months' duration. The patients were randomly assigned to either three sessions of 1 hour autotraction or corset and rest. At 1 and 3 weeks, all patients were assessed by an independent investigator regarding pain relief, straight leg raising, spinal mobility, and neurologic status. At the end of 1 and 3 weeks, the autotraction group achieved significantly more complete and partial recovery than the corset group. All patients were surveyed through questionnaires after 3 months, and there was no difference between groups.

Weber et al.[27] reported a summary of four randomized trials carried out during a period of 11 years using four different types of traction equipment. A total of 215 patients with herniated lumbar discs were randomized to one of the traction methods and a control group before surgery. At the end of treatment, there was no significant difference between the two groups as measured by pain relief, improved range of motion, straight leg raising, or motor or sensory function. No statistical analysis was available.

Pal et al.[28] reported the results of a randomized trial in 39 hospitalized patients with back pain and sciatica who were treated with continuous pelvic traction of 5.5 to 8.2 kg or 1.4 to 1.8 kg. All patients were assessed for pain score on visual analog scale, analgesic intake, straight leg raising angle, and neurologic deficits. At the end of 1 to 2 weeks, there was a significant reduction in pain score and analgesic intake and an increase in straight leg raise angle in all patients. There was no significant difference between groups.

Coxhead et al.[29] compared four treatment methods (traction, manipulation, exercise, and corset) in a randomized factorial-designed trial involving 334 patients with sciatic symptoms. Traction was given with a motor-driven *True Trac* apparatus intermittently and daily during the first week, and treatment frequency gradually reduced in the subsequent 3 weeks. At the end of the 4-week trial period, patients who received traction were no better than those who did not get traction based on four outcome measures—patient's own assessment, pain, return to work, and 16-month follow-up questionnaires.

Van den Heijden et al.,[30] in a recent publication, reviewed 17 randomized control trials (RCTs) for neck and back pain, and 11 of these trials evaluated lumbar traction for acute low back pain. Only one trial reported a beneficial effect of lumbar traction.

Recommendations

Even though pelvic traction has been used for treatment of acute low back pain for many years, available evidence does not support its use in the treatment of acute low back pain. Only one trial found traction to be beneficial in relieving pain and improving spinal mobility, but after 3 weeks, the traction was no longer superior to other treatments. Pelvic traction for prolonged periods may force the patient to be confined to bed and suffer the debilitating effects of bed rest.

MANIPULATION

Spinal manipulation has been used for the treatment of neck and back pain for centuries. However, in the past 40 to 50 years, spinal manipulation has been primarily identified with osteopathic and chiropractic physicians and created controversy regarding its efficacy. In recent years, several well-designed RCTs have been carried out comparing spinal manipulation with other conservative treatments.

Shekelle et al.,[31] in a review of spinal manipulation treatment for low back pain, identified 25 controlled trials comparing spinal manipulation with sham manipulation or other conservative measures. The authors identified nine control trials for acute low back pain, of which two of the highest-quality trials showed statistically significant benefit of manipulation for patients whose back pain has lasted 2 to 4 weeks. A meta-analysis of the remaining seven trials showed that spinal manipulation increased the probability of recovery at 2 to 3 weeks after the start of treatment by 0.17 (95 percent prob-

ability limits, 0.07 to 0.28). This difference in probability means that if the underlying recovery rate at 2 to 3 weeks is 50 percent (the rate of recovery in the control groups), then 67 percent of the patients treated with manipulation will recover during the same period. Anderson et al.[32] carried out a meta-analysis of 23 RCTs comparing manipulation or mobilization with other conservative treatments and concluded that patients with acute low back pain without radiculopathy derive consistent short-term (1 month) benefit from manipulation therapy. There are considerable differences between different types of manipulation used in these trials, and therefore, it is difficult to generalize their results.

The chiropractic/osteopathic manipulation is usually a high-velocity short-lever manipulation directed toward a specific spinal segment. Long-lever manipulation, however, is more nonspecific, using the pelvis, shoulder, or head to manipulate the spine.

Hadler et al.[33] carried out a stratified RCT comparing mobilization with long-lever high-velocity manipulation of lumbar spine involving 54 patients with acute low back pain of less than 1 month's duration. The patients were stratified into two groups: those who had pain less than 2 weeks, and those who had pain for 2 to 4 weeks. After randomization, a patient was treated by single mobilization or manipulation treatment. Immediately after the treatment, each patient was asked to indicate treatment effect on a horizontal analog scale. Subsequently, all subjects were contacted by telephone every 3 days for 12 days to answer the 24-item Ronald-Morris questionnaire. Most subjects made rapid recovery during the 2-week follow-up period. Subjects whose duration of symptoms was less than 2 weeks recovered at the same rate irrespective of treatment group. However, those subjects whose pain duration was between 2 to 4 weeks and had manipulation treatment improved to a greater degree in the first week ($P = .009$). At the end of the 2-week follow-up period, both groups had almost identical recovery.

MacDonald et al.[34] compared the effects of osteopathic manipulation and "control" treatment on 95 subjects with thoracolumbar pain of varied durations. Osteopathic manipulation consisted of direct pressure and stretching of affected muscles, low-velocity high-amplitude movement to hypomobile joints, and high-velocity low-amplitude thrusts to hypomobile vertebral segments. The control group, like the experimental group, was advised on posture and exercise and to avoid occupational stress. The manipulation treatment was given twice weekly until the subject recovered or the manipulator thought that further treatment would not derive any benefit. The outcome of this trial was very similar to the trial conducted by Hadler et al.[33] Subjects with a pain duration of 14 to 28 days derived significant benefit from manipulation lasting 1 to 2 weeks. At the end of 4 weeks, there was no significant difference between groups.

Recommendations

Several RCTs have demonstrated the effectiveness of spinal manipulation in relieving discomfort in patients with acute low back pain without radiculopathy. The manipulation treatment is most effective in those patients with a pain duration of 14 to 28 days. The effectiveness of manipulation in patients with a pain duration of more than 1 month or with radiculopathy remains unproven.

EXERCISE

Various types of exercise programs have been recommended as part of an overall conservative treatment for acute low back pain. Specific exercise programs are expected to achieve specific treatment goals (i.e., improved spinal mobility, strengthening of paraspinal and abdominal muscles, and overall strength and endurance). Unfortunately, there have been very few controlled clinical trials to assess the effectiveness of an exercise program.

Lindstorm et al.[35] reported the results of a randomized trial with 62 patients with acute low back pain of more than 1 month's duration. The patients were randomized to three treatment groups: (1) conventional treatment—hot pack, massage, and mobilization and strengthening exercise versus (2) alternative treatment—intermittent pelvic traction and isometric exercise of abdominal muscles and hip extensors versus (3) control group—hot pack and rest. Patients received ten treatments during a month. At the end of the trial, all patients were evaluated by a physician who was unaware of the treatment group to which the patient belonged.

The patient group treated with pelvic traction and isometric exercise of abdominal and gluteal muscles achieved significantly better improvement.

Coxhead et al.[29] conducted a multicenter randomized trial involving 292 patients with back pain and sciatica with an average duration of 14.3 weeks. The patients were assigned to one of four treatment groups in a factorial design: (1) traction, (2) exercise at physiotherapists' discretion, (3) manipulation, or (4) corset. At the end of 4 weeks, 78 percent of all patients improved irrespective of the specific treatment.

Davies et al.[36] studied the effects of extension and isometric flexion exercise and short-wave diathermy in 43 patients with low back pain of 3 weeks' to 6 months' duration. All patients were treated for 4 weeks, and the outcome assessment was blind. Even though a larger number of patients in the extension exercise group experienced improved symptoms, the difference was not statistically significant, most likely due to the small sample size. There was a significant reduction of pain and an increase in spinal mobility in each treatment group, and the period to resume work and sport was similar in each group.

Evans et al.[37] evaluated the effects of Kendall's flexion exercise routine involving 242 patients with acute low back pain with or without radiation to the legs. The duration of pain was less than 30 days, and patients were randomized to one of four treatment groups: (1) flexion exercise, education, and bed rest for 4 days, (2) flexion exercise and education, (3) bed rest only, or (4) control group—analgesics only. Subjects were instructed on a 20-minute exercise program to be performed daily for 2 months, or longer if necessary. At 6- and 12-week and 1-year follow-up, there was no significant difference between the groups as regards self-reported level of pain or restriction of activities.

Stankovic et al.[38] compared the effects of the McKenzie method of extension exercise with attendance for 45 minutes in a mini-back school in a group of 100 patients with acute low back pain with or without radiation to the legs. The duration of pain in most patients was less than 1 week, even though some patients had pain for 4 weeks. The patients received the McKenzie treatment for 20 minutes daily for 2 weeks and were then allowed to assume flexion posture in sitting and standing. Outcome assessment was performed by an independent observer after 3 weeks and by one of the authors after 1 year.

The patients in the McKenzie treatment group returned to work earlier ($P < .001$), had less recurrences ($P < 001$), had lower pain scores ($P < .001$), and had better spinal movement ($P < .001$).

Lindstorm et al.[39] reported a randomized trial involving 103 Swedish auto workers who had been out of work for 6 weeks because of subacute non-specific mechanical low back pain. The subjects were randomized to either a graded activity program or traditional therapy of rest, analgesics, and physiotherapy. The graded activity program consisted of a functional capacity assessment, workplace visit, attendance in back school, and individualized submaximal gradual-increase exercise program using operant conditioning principles as outlined by Fordyce. The subjects were followed for 3 years. At the 1-year follow-up, the rate of return to work in the graded activity program was significantly faster ($P = .03$) than the control group. At the 2-year follow-up, the average duration of sick leave was significantly less in the activity group ($P = .05$).

Faas et al.[40] studied the efficacy of exercise therapy involving 473 patients with acute low back pain with or without radiation to the upper leg and duration of less than 3 weeks.

The patients received standardized information about back pain and then randomized to one of three groups: (1) exercise therapy—20 minutes twice a week for 5 weeks, (2) usual care—analgesics and information about back pain—importance of heat and physical activity, or (3) placebo therapy—ultrasound therapy by a physiotherapist twice a week for 5 weeks.

All patients were followed up to 1 year. There was no difference between groups as regards recurrences, functional health status, or medical care usage.

Gundewall et al.[41] evaluated the effects of a supervised exercise program in the prevention of low back pain among a group of 60 nursing personnel. The subjects were randomized to either supervised exercise program during work six times per month for 13 months or no intervention. The exercise program consisted of isometric and dynamic exercises to strengthen back extensor muscles. The exercise group experienced less new episodes of back pain (4 percent compared with 38 percent for the control group), fewer days of lost work time, and a lower average duration of back pain.

Kellett et al.[42] studied the effects of an exercise program on 60 cabinet manufacturing company workers with current or past back pain. The workers were randomly assigned to an exercise or control group.

The exercise group participated in an exercise program at work, once a week, consisting of 30 minutes of aerobic exercise and 10 minutes of relaxation. They were advised to participate in 30 minutes of walking, jogging, or cycling once a week on their own. Before the introduction of the exercise program, there was no difference in the incidence of back pain between the exercise and control group. The incidence and days lost from work were reduced in the exercise group during the 1.5-year intervention period.

Recommendations

There is conflicting evidence regarding the effectiveness of exercise programs in reducing discomfort and lost time from work. During the first 4 weeks after the onset of acute low back pain, low-stress aerobic exercise can be helpful in preventing debilitation from inactivity. Subsequently, a conditioning program to improve strength of trunk muscles can be helpful. A behaviorally oriented exercise program guided by prescribed quotas rather than pain may result in an improved outcome. Also, an exercise program has been found to be effective in preventing the incidence and duration of episodes of back pain among nursing personnel and factory workers.

MODALITIES

Many physical modalities such as heat, ice, and electricity have been used for centuries for symptomatic relief of pain. The evidence for their efficacy in treatment of acute low back pain is controversial.

Waterworth et al.[43] reported an RCT comparing the effects of diflunisal (1,000 mg PO and then 500 mg PO bid for 10 days), physiotherapy (short-wave diathermy 15 to 20 minutes, ultrasound 5 to 10 minutes, flexion extension exercise for 5 days a week for 45-minute sessions), and manipulation by physiotherapist. A total of 104 patients with acute low back pain with or without radiation to the leg of less than 1 month's duration were randomized into three treatment groups. Patients' physicians assessed the outcome (pain, return to work, spinal movement) after 10 to 12 days of treatment, and the physicians were not blinded. At the end of the trial, most patients improved and returned to work, but there was no statistically significant difference between the groups.

Postacchini et al.[9] evaluated the effects of manipulation, physiotherapy (massage, infrared daily for 2 to 3 weeks), drug therapy (diclofenac), placebo (antiedema gel for application to back), bed rest (20 to 24 hours for 4 to 6 days and 15 to 20 hours for 2 days), attendance in back school (four 1-hour sessions and exercise daily), on a group of 159 patients with acute low back pain (with or without radiation to the legs) of less than 4 weeks' duration. Outcomes were measured at 3 weeks, 2 months, and 6 months after the start of the treatments. At the 3-week follow-up, the maximal improvements were observed in the group treated by manipulation ($P < .001$), as indicated by patients' report of pain, restriction of daily activities, spinal mobility, muscle strength, degree of positivity of straight leg raising, and local tenderness. At 2 and 6 months' follow-up, there were no significant differences between groups.

Gibson et al.[44] reported a randomized trial involving 109 patients with low back pain (without neurologic symptoms) of 2 to 12 months' duration; they were assigned to osteopathic manipulation, short-wave diathermy, and detuned short-wave diathermy. Short-wave diathermy treatments were given three times a week, and osteopathic treatment was once a week for 4 weeks.

Blind outcome assessments were performed at 2, 4, and 12 weeks after the start of the treatments regarding pain, spinal mobility, local tenderness, and work status. There were immediate improvements in more than half of the patients in each treatment group, and improvements were maintained at the 12-week follow-up. However, there was no significant difference between treatment groups regarding pain, tenderness, or spinal mobility.

Recommendations

There have been only two reports of controlled trials assessing the efficacy of physical modalities in the treatment of acute low back pain. In one trial, modalities with exercise were equally as effective as NSAIDs or manipulation. The second trial found manipulation to be more effective than modalities and NSAIDs, but modalities were more efficacious than placebo. Similarly, modalities were equally effective in the treatment of chronic back pain but not superior to other treatment. Modalities can provide temporary symptom relief in patients with acute or chronic low back pain and can be an adjunct to other treatment methods.

TRANSCUTANEOUS ELECTRICAL NERVE STIMULATION

Transcutaneous electrical nerve stimulation (TENS) has been widely used for the treatment of acute and chronic pain. Both high-frequency and low-frequency acupuncture, like electrical stimulation, have claimed efficacy based on uncontrolled nonrandomized trials.

Fox et al.[45] treated 12 patients with chronic low back pain with acupuncture and low-frequency electrical stimulation in a balanced crossover trial. Each patient received two acupuncture treatments followed by two electrical stimulation treatments. Treatments were given 1 week apart, and pain relief was measured by the McGill Pain Questionnaire. Both treatments provided more than 33 percent pain relief in 75 percent of acupuncture and 66 percent of electrical stimulation patients. The difference was not statistically significant.

Lehman et al.[46] studied the efficacy of high-frequency electrical stimulation in a randomized trial involving 53 patients with low back pain of more than 3 months' duration who were admitted to an inpatient rehabilitation program. On admission, the patients were randomly assigned to one of three treatment groups: (1) low-intensity high-frequency electrical stimulation, (2) dead battery electrical stimulation (placebo), or (3) electro-acupuncture.

The treatment program was of 3 weeks' duration. At the end of the treatment period, the patients in all treatment groups made significant gains on most outcome measures, but there was no significant difference between the groups based on a global measure of low back rating scale. However, at the 6-month follow-up, the acupuncture group had significantly less pain ($P = .04$).

Deyo et al.[47] reported a randomized trial involving 145 subjects with chronic low back pain of mean duration of 4.1 years. The subjects were assigned to one of four treatments groups: (1) TENS plus exercise, (2) TENS alone, (3) exercise and sham TENS, or (4) sham TENS alone. The treatment duration was 4 weeks. The TENS treatment was of both high- and low-frequency types. All four study groups demonstrated significant improvement in all outcome measures, but at the 3-month follow-up, the outcome measures had returned toward baseline. At 4 weeks, no significant treatment effect of TENS was demonstrated on all outcomes together, but exercise had a significant treatment effect overall and four individual outcome measures. There was no clinically or statistically significant difference between true and sham TENS groups.

Hackett et al.[48] compared the treatment effects of pulsed electrical stimulation with surface electrodes ("electro-acupuncture") in a group of 37 patients with acute low back pain of less than 3 days' duration. Patients were randomly assigned to one of two treatment groups: (1) electro-acupuncture and placebo tablets, or (2) Paracetamol and placebo electro-acupuncture. At the end of 1 and 2 weeks, there was no significant difference between groups, but at 6 weeks, the electro-acupuncture group had significantly less pain.

Hermann et al.[49] studied the effects of TENS (Codetron) on 58 injured workers with acute low back pain of 3 to 10 weeks' duration. The subjects were randomly assigned to one of two treatment groups: active TENS/Codetron and exercise, or placebo TENS/Codetron and exercise. The active TENS/Codetron group received 15 minutes of high-frequency, followed by 15 minutes of low-frequency, TENS/Codetron treatments approximately 30 minutes before an exercise program. The program duration was 4 weeks. There was a significant reduction of disability and pain in each treatment group when compared with baseline values, but there was no significant difference between groups on these outcome measures. Similarly, there was no difference in return to work between the groups.

Recommendations

Although TENS is commonly used for the management of patients with acute and chronic back pain, the five clinical trials reviewed here indicate that addition of TENS does not provide any added treatment effects. TENS may be tried for symptom relief when other measures fail to relieve pain in patients with acute or chronic low back pain.

ACUPUNCTURE

Traditional Chinese acupuncture requires that needles be inserted into specific areas of the body (meridians) and rotated to produce noxious stimulus to the body. Electro-acupuncture adds electrical stimulation to these needles. All RCTs evaluating the efficacy of acupuncture involved patients with chronic back pain.

Hackett et al.[48] reported the results of a randomized trial in 37 patients with acute low back pain of less than 3 days' duration. The patients were randomized to one of two treatment groups: (1) two treatments of "electro-acupuncture" and two placebo Paracetamol tablets every 4 hours, or (2) placebo acupuncture and two tablets every 4 hours. Electro-acupuncture was carried out with surface electrodes applied to points and delivered low-amptitude pulsed-square waves.

At the end of the first and second week, there was no significant difference between the groups regarding pain or mobility. However, at 6 weeks the electro-acupuncture group had significantly less pain and more mobility.

Coan et al.[50] compared the effects of classical Chinese acupuncture in a group of 50 patients with chronic low back pain of more than 6 months' duration. The patients were randomized to receive immediate treatment (experimental group) or delayed treatment (control) after 8 weeks. All patients received ten or more treatments. At 10.3 weeks after enrollment, 89 percent of the immediate treatment group reported improvement in pain scores, use of analgesics, and limitation of activities. In the delayed treatment group (control), 32 percent reported improvement before the start of their treatment. At the 40-week follow-up, both groups reported reduction of symptoms.

Mendelson et al.[51] reported the results of a randomized crossover trial comparing traditional Chinese acupuncture with placebo acupuncture in a group of 77 patients with chronic low back pain with a mean duration of more than 12 years. The patients were crossed over to active treatment after a rest period of 4 weeks, and each group was treated for 4 weeks. Both groups reported significant reduction of discomfort, but the difference of pain reduction was not significant between the groups. The group receiving active treatment first is the group that experienced better pain relief.

Lehman et al.[46] reported a randomized trial involving 54 patients with chronic back pain who were treated in an inpatient rehabilitation program consisting of education, exercise, and one of electro-acupuncture, TENS, or sham TENS. All patients improved significantly in all outcome measures, but the electro-acupuncture group consistently reported less pain. However, there was no significant overall difference between the three treatment groups.

TerRiet et al.[52] reviewed 51 controlled clinical trials studying the effectiveness of acupuncture in chronic pain including back pain. The review was based on 18 predefined well-accepted methodologic criteria. Most studies were of poor quality, and only 11 studies scored more than 50 points of a maximum of 100. The highest score of 62 was achieved by one study. The authors concluded that the efficacy of acupuncture for the treatment of acute pain remains doubtful.

Recommendations

The efficacy of acupuncture in the treatment of acute back pain remains to be established as no controlled trial has been carried out. The effectiveness of acupuncture in chronic back pain remains controversial because of contradictory outcomes and poor quality of many studies.

CORSETS AND ORTHOSES

Lumbar corsets and various orthoses have been used for low back pain, especially for chronic low back pain. The mechanical effectiveness of an orthosis may result from restriction of intersegmental motion, reduction of intradiscal pressure, and unloading of the spinal column. Nachemson et al.[53] measured the intradiscal and intra-abdominal pressures and myoelectric activities of abdominal and paraspinal muscles in four able-bodied volunteers wearing three dif-

ferent types of orthoses (corset, Rainey flexion jacket, and Boston extension brace). The subjects were asked to carry out six different tasks wearing each brace. All braces unloaded the spine and reduced intradiscal pressure and myoelectric activities in two-thirds of the tasks. None of the orthoses raised intra-abdominal pressure significantly, and the mechanical effectiveness was not superior to the others.

Coxhead et al.[28] compared the treatment effects of lumbar corsets on a group of 292 patients with acute and chronic back pain with an average duration of 14.3 weeks. Lumbar corsets were not more efficacious than traction, manipulation, or exercise above or in combination.

Million et al.[54] assessed the effectiveness of lumbar corsets with or without rigid support in a randomized trial involving 19 patients with chronic back pain of at least 6 months' duration. Rigid corsets were found to be superior in relieving discomfort and also on several objective measures.

Walsh et al.[55] studied the effectiveness of lumbar corsets in preventing back injury and time loss from work in a group of 90 male warehouse workers not receiving treatment for back injury or pain. The subjects were randomly assigned to no intervention (control), 1-hour session on back pain prevention and body mechanics, or education and wearing of lumbosacral corsets during working hours. At the 6-month follow-up, the group with training and orthosis showed substantially less time lost even though there was no change in abdominal strength, productivity, or accident rate.

Reddell et al.[56] evaluated a weight-lifting belt in the prevention of back injury in 642 airline baggage handlers who were randomly assigned to one of four treatment groups: belt only during work activities, belt and 1-hour training class, training class only, or no intervention.

The study period lasted 8 months, and 58 percent of the workers who were issued belts stopped using them. There was no significant difference between treatment groups regarding back injury rate, lost or restricted work days, and worker's compensation rates.

Recommendations

Corset and lumbar braces have been found to be effective in restricting motion and reducing intradiscal pressure and myoelectric activity in healthy individuals. However, there is no evidence that corsets or braces are effective in the treatment of acute low back pain. There is conflicting evidence regarding the efficacy of corsets or belts in the prevention or reducing impact of back pain in workers who perform frequent lifting tasks.

BACK SCHOOL

Back school is a structured educational program in a group setting aimed at helping the sufferer to deal with pain effectively through proper posture, body mechanics, etc. Back school originated in Sweden in the early 1980s and has become popular especially in the treatment of chronic back pain.

Bergquist-Ullman et al.[57] reported a randomized trial involving 217 workers in an automotive plant who were suffering from acute or subacute low back pain of less than 3 months' duration. The subjects were randomized into three treatment groups: back school (four 45 minutes sessions in 2 weeks), combined physiotherapy (manual therapy), or placebo short-wave diathermy. The patients attending back school had a shorter duration of lost time from work from the initial episode compared with the other two treatment groups. At the end of 1 year, the numbers and length of lost time from work due to recurrences were not different between the treatment groups.

Lindequist et al.[68] studied the efficacy of a back school in a group of 56 patients suffering from acute low back pain with or without radiation to the legs. The subjects were randomized to either attend back school or given advice not to strain their backs and use analgesics when needed. In a 3- and 6-week follow-up and a 1-year follow-up questionnaire survey, there was no significant difference between the two groups regarding initial duration of symptoms, sick leaves, or number and duration of recurrences during the 1-year period. The back school group was more satisfied with the treatment.

Linton et al.[59] reviewed seven controlled and nine uncontrolled trials regarding the efficacy of back school in the treatment of acute and chronic back pain. One controlled trial[57] showed the effectiveness of back school in acute back pain, but the other three controlled trials did not find any difference between

groups. Three controlled trials involving patients with chronic back pain reached conflicting conclusions.

Keijsers et al.[60] critically reviewed eight controlled trials for the efficacy of the back school and concluded that the available studies do not suggest that back schools are particularly effective for the treatment of back pain.

Recommendations

There have been several trials claiming the effectiveness of the back school for the treatment of back pain, but only one controlled trial demonstrated short-term positive effects in a group of auto workers with acute or subacute back pain. Two critical reviews concluded that the efficacy of the back school is yet to be established. However, considering negligible potential harm and low cost, education programs similar to the back school may be helpful as an integral part of a comprehensive treatment program.

BIOFEEDBACK

The objective of biofeedback therapy is to reduce pain by the reduction of muscle tension through auditory and/or visual feedback. All reported controlled trials involved patients with chronic back pain of several years' duration.

Bush et al.[61] evaluated the effects of auditory feedback from paraspinal muscles in a group of 66 chronic low back pain patients and compared with placebo and no treatment. All groups demonstrated a small but statistically significant improvement in pain, depression, and anxiety, but there was no significant difference between the groups.

Asfour et al.[62] reported a randomized trial involving 30 patients with chronic back pain and compared the efficacy of EMG feedback with no feedback. All patients underwent comprehensive rehabilitation treatment, and experimental groups received EMG feedback to increase strength of back extensors. At the end of 2 weeks of study, the experimental group demonstrated a significant increase in back muscle strength, but there was no difference in pain level between the groups.

Flor et al.[63] studied the effects of EMG biofeedback in 18 patients with chronic back pain due to rheumatic diseases and concluded that biofeedback treatment is effective in reducing discomfort and utilization of health care systems. The control groups consisted of pseudotherapy and standard medical treatment.

Nouwen[64] reported the results of a controlled trial involving 20 patients with chronic back pain with high standing paraspinal EMG level. The experimental group received 15 biofeedback treatments during a 3-week period, and the control group was kept on the waiting list for 9 weeks. The experimental group showed significant reduction of standing paraspinal EMG level but no significant reduction of pain.

Recommendations

The effectiveness of EMG biofeedback treatment has not been studied in patients with acute low back pain. There is conflicting evidence of the efficacy of EMG biofeedback in chronic back pain patients.

EPIDURAL INJECTIONS

Epidural injections of local anesthetics with corticosteroids or narcotics have been used primarily for treatment of lumbar radiculopathy. The rationale for epidural injection is to reduce inflammation and swelling of affected lumbar roots, which in turn will relieve pain.

Dilke et al.[65] reported the results of a double-blind RCT involving 100 consecutive patients with a clinical diagnosis of nerve root compression of 1 week's to 2 years' duration. The experimental group received epidural injection of 80 mg of methylprednisolone in 10 ml of normal saline, and the control group received superficial injection of 1 ml of normal saline. All patients underwent graded rehabilitation with hydrotherapy and exercise. The experimental group experienced significantly better pain relief ($P < .01$) and a higher rate of return to work at 3 months ($P < .01$).

Sonek et al.[66] compared the effects of epidural injection of 80 mg of methylprednisolone (2 ml) and 2 ml normal saline in a group of 51 patients suffering from lumbar radiculopathy (12 days' to 36 weeks' duration) confirmed by myelography. Patients were randomly assigned to the two treatment groups, and outcome assessment was blinded.

There was no significant difference between the groups as regards pain relief or surgical intervention.

Cuckler et al.[67] treated 73 patients with lumbar radiculopathy (radiologically proven) due to herniated disc or spinal stenosis, in random order with epidural injection of either 7 ml of methylprednisolone (80 mg) and procaine or 5 ml of 1 percent procaine with 2 ml of sterile saline. At 24 hours, 41.6 ± 6.2 percent in the steroid-treated group and 43.6 ± 6.6 percent in the control group experienced 75 percent or more relief of symptoms. The difference was not statistically significant. Long-term follow-up at 20 months failed to demonstrate difference between the groups.

Ridley et al.[68] carried out a double-blind crossover trial involving 39 patients with clinical history and signs consistent with lumbosacral nerve root compression. Patients were treated with either epidural injection of 80 mg methylprednisolone in 10 ml of saline or injection of 2 ml of normal saline to interspinous ligaments. At the end of 1 and 2 weeks, the active treatment group experienced significantly more pain relief compared with the placebo group. However, after 24 weeks, 35 percent of the patients who experienced pain relief with active treatment suffered relapse.

Bush et al.[69] compared the effects of caudal epidural injection of 25 ml mixture of normal saline and 80 mg of triamcinolone, and 0.5 percent procaine HCl with 25 ml of normal saline. The study population consisted of 23 patients with symptoms and signs of lumbar root compression with a duration of pain ranging from 1 to 13 months. At the 4-week follow-up, the active treatment group had significantly less pain ($P = .02$), improved lifestyle ($P = .02$), and improved straight leg raising ($P = .01$). At 1 year, these differences in pain and lifestyle improvement were no longer significant.

Recommendations

There is no evidence in the literature that epidural steroid injection is efficacious in the treatment of acute low back pain without radiculopathy. Three of five trials reviewed here found epidural steroids effective in reducing pain in the short term, with a high rate of recurrence in one trial after 6 months. The results of these trials are difficult to generalize because of different injection methods and patient population with varying durations of pain and diagnosis. Epidural steroid injection may be helpful in relieving discomfort in patients with lumbar radiculopathy when other treatment methods have failed or surgery is not a desired option. Epidural injections are invasive, and the potential for serious side effects should be considered.

FACET INJECTIONS

Facet joint injections with local anesthetics and/or corticosteroid have been used for the treatment of primarily chronic low back pain of more than 3 months' duration. These patients are thought to be suffering from "facet syndrome" with primarily low back pain without neurologic signs or sciatica and pain aggravated by extension of the spine.

Jackson[70] treated 390 patients with low back pain (without neurologic signs or symptoms with a mean duration of 15 weeks) with facet joint (L4-L5-S1) injection with Marcaine (0.5 percent) and cortisone. All patients had facet arthrogram before injection treatment. Initial mean pain relief was only 29 percent, and 85 percent experienced some pain relief. In a second study, the author treated 25 patients with lidocaine or saline injection of the facet joints in random order. There was no significant difference in mean pain scores between the groups. In a third study, the author carried out facet joint injections in 36 patients undergoing spinal fusion. Twenty-six patients who responded favorably with facet joint injections did not have a better outcome after fusion than the 10 patients who did not experience pain relief from injections. The author concluded from these three studies that lumbar facet joint is not a common source of back pain, and injection of intra-articular saline is as effective as local anesthetics.

Lilius et al.[71] treated 109 patients with low back pain of more than 3 months' duration with injections of 8 ml mixture of Marcaine and 80 mg of methylprednisolone into the facet joint or pericapsular area or 8 ml of normal saline into the facet joints. Patients in all three treatment groups experienced significant reduction of pain, 1 hour, 2 weeks, 6 weeks ($P \le .001$), and 3 months after injections ($P \le .04$). There was no significant difference between the groups in work attendance or pain and disability scores. The authors concluded that facet joint injection is a nonspecific method of treatment.

Carette et al.[72] selected 110 patients out of 190 chronic low back pain patients without neurologic deficit who had 50 percent or more pain relief after a local anesthetic injection into L4-L5 and L5-S1 facet joints. These patients were then randomized to receive facet joint injections of a mixture of 20 mg methyl prednisolone (1 ml) and 1 ml normal saline or 2 ml of normal saline.

At the 1-month follow-up, 42 percent in the methylprednisolone group and 33 percent in the normal saline group reported marked improvement in pain ($P = .53$). In both groups, there was improvement in other outcome measures, but the difference was not statistically significant between the groups. The results were similar at the 3-month follow-up, but at the 6-month follow-up the methyl prednisolone group had significantly more improvement ($P = .02$). However, when concurrent interventions were taken into account, the difference was not significant. The author concluded that injections of methylprednisolone into the facet joints are of little value in the treatment of chronic back pain.

Nash[73] treated 66 patients with presumptive diagnosis of facet joint pain with either intra-articular injection of methylprednisolone (20 mg) and local anesthetic or blockade of the medial branch of the posterior rami with local anesthetics. The patients were treated in pairs, and the type of treatment was decided on by the toss of a coin. At the 1-month follow-up, both treatments were equally effective, but neither treatment was successful in reducing discomfort significantly.

Recommendations

There has been no adequate studies done assessing the efficacy of facet joint injections in acute low back pain. The four trials reviewed here studied the efficacy of facet injections in chronic back pain and found that neither type of the agent (steroid, saline, or local anesthetics) or the location of injection (intra-articular, pericapsular, or nerve block) made any significant difference in outcome. Based on this limited data, facet joint injection cannot be recommended for the treatment of acute or chronic low back pain.

TRIGGER POINT AND LOCAL INJECTIONS

Trigger point and local injections involve injections of local anesthetics with or without steroid into the painful soft tissues of the back (muscles or ligaments) to relieve discomfort.

Frost et al.[74] compared the effects of trigger point injection of 0.5 percent Carbocaine or normal saline in 53 patients with acute muscle pain in the neck, shoulder, and lower back. Twenty-eight patients received local anesthetic, and 25 received normal saline injections.

All patients received three injections at an interval of 2 to 3 days. No separate data analysis for back pain was given. After the first injection, the normal saline group had significantly more pain relief ($P \leq .05$), but after the second and third injections there was no significant difference between groups.

Garvey et al.[75] reported the results of a randomized double-blind controlled trial involving 63 patients with acute back pain who received one of four treatments: (1) trigger point injection with 1 percent lidocaine, (2) trigger point injection with lidocaine and steroid, (3) dry needling of trigger point, or (4) ethylchloride spray. All patients had 4 weeks of conservative treatment with NSAIDs and activity restriction before entry into the trial. At the end of 2 weeks after completion of treatment, there was no significant difference in pain perception between the groups receiving medication and those receiving needling or ethylchloride spray ($P \leq .093$). The authors concluded that trigger point therapy may be a useful adjunct in the treatment of acute back pain, and the sample size of this trial was too small (needed a sample size of 200 in each combined group to show a difference of 20 percent) to detect a 20 percent difference between medication and no medication group.

Collee et al.[76] compared the analgesic effects of injection of painful area with 5 ml of 0.5 percent lignocaine and 5 ml of normal saline in 41 patients with iliac crest pain syndrome. The patient population consisted of two groups—rheumatology clinic and general practice patients. Rheumatology patients were more chronic. At 10 minutes and day 7 there was no significant difference between the groups in pain score on a visual analog scale. However, at day 14, the pain score was significantly lower in the lignocaine group. In a subgroup analysis, the rheumatology clinic group of patients in the lignocaine group experienced more pain relief. In the general practice group of patients, with a shorter duration of pain, there was no significant difference in pain relief between the two treatments.

Ongley et al.[77] reported the results of a randomized double-blind trial comparing the treatment effects of a solution containing 25 percent dextrose and glycerine in 2.5 percent phenol and normal saline. Eighty-one patients with chronic low back pain of more than 1 year's duration (average, 10 years) were randomized to these two treatments and given 6 weeks of injections into the ligaments of the lower back at six sites.

One, three, and six months after completion of treatments, both treatment groups showed reduction of pain and disability (35 of 40 in experimental and 16 of 41 in normal saline group), but the experimental group treated with sclerosing solution experienced significantly more reduction of pain and disability ($P < .01$ to .04).

Recommendations

The efficacy of injection of local anesthetics with or without steroid in acute low back pain remains uncertain. Only one study has shown the effectiveness of injections of sclerosing liquid into the ligaments of the lower back in reducing pain and disability of patients with chronic back pain. The injections expose patients to potential complications.

CONCLUSION

This review is based on critical appraisal of only controlled clinical trials evaluating the efficacy of 17 different treatment modalities for acute low back pain without significant spinal pathology (i.e., acute disc herniation, cauda equina syndrome, etc.) (Table 5-6).

Of these 17 treatments, only 5 (up to 2 days bed rest, NSAIDs, muscle relaxants, manipulation, and mobilization exercise) have demonstrated level 1 evidence for efficacy. Considering that a large majority of acute low back pain patients without significant identifiable spinal pathology will have sponta-

Table 5-6. Summary of Controlled Trials of

Intervention	Control	Sample Size	No. of Trials	Statistical Significance
Bed rest				
Bed rest for 14 days	Restricted activity	80	1	Yes
Bed rest for 4 days	Analgesic	252	1	Yes
Bed rest for 2 days	Bed rest 7 days	203	1	Yes
Bed rest for 2 days	No bed rest	186	1	Yes
NSAIDs				
NSAID	Placebo	287 168	2	Yes
NSAID & muscle relaxant	Placebo	175	1	Yes
Muscle relaxants	Placebo	43 60 80 117 200 20 50	7	Yes
Manipulation				
Manipulation	Mobilization	54 95	2	Yes
Manipulation	Sham manipulation other conservative treatment		Meta-analysis of 7 trials	Yes
Exercise				
Pelvic traction and isometric exercise	Rest and hot packs	62	1	Yes
McKenzie extension exercise	Mini-back school	100	1	Yes
Graded exercise (operant conditioning) and back school	Rest Analgesics and physiotherapy	103	1	Yes
Supervised aerobic exercise	No intervention	60	1	Yes
Supervised aerobic	No exercise	60	1	Yes

Efficacious Interventions for Acute Back Pain

Result	Criticism	Level of Evidence	Grade of Recommendation	Reference
Bed rest Efficacious	Outcome assessment not blinded Validity of outcome measure	I	B	Weisel et al.[4] (1980)
Bedrest does more harm than good	Poor compliance with bed rest	I	A	Gilbert et al.[5] (1985)
Equally effective 2 days bed rest Less time off work	? generalization Poor compliance and wide variations in bed rest duration	I	A	Deyo et al.[6] (1986)
No bed rest group better	Outcome assessment not blinded	I	A	Malmivaara et al.[7] (1995)
NSAID better than placebo	Outcome assessment not blinded[9]	I	A	Amlie et al.[8] (1987) Postacchini et al.[9] (1988)
NSAID and muscle relaxant better than single drug or placebo		I	A	Basmajian[10] (1989)
Muscle relaxants better tthan placebo		I	A	Hindle[15] (1972) Gold[16] (1978) Klinger et al.[17] (1988) Baratta[18] (1982) Dapas[19] (1985) Casale[20] (1988) Arbus[21] et al. (1990)
Manipulation better in patients with pain duration of 2–4 weeks		I	A	Hadler et al.[33] (1987) MacDonald et al.[34] (1990)
Manipulation improves recovery at 2–3 weeks after start of treatment	Some patients with chronic back pain	I	A	Anderson et al.[32] (1992)
Better improvement with sometric exercise and traction		I	A	Lindstorm et al.[35] (1970)
Exercise group better on all outcome measures		I	A	Stankovic et al.[38] (1990)
Return to work faster and less sick leave in graded exercise groups		I	A	Lindstorm et al.[39] (1992)
Lower incidence of back pain and fewer days off work		I	A	Gundewall et al.[41] (1993)
Lower incidence of back pain and lost time from work in exercise groups		I	A	Kellett et al.[42] (1991)

Table 5-7. Low Back Pain Red Flags

Cancer or infection
Age > 50 (also consider abdominal aortic aneurysm) or < 20
History of cancer
Unexplained weight loss
Failure to improve with 4–6 weeks of conservative therapy
Unrelenting night pain
Intravenous drug use
Fever > 38°C
Immune suppression
Recent bacterial infection

Cauda equina syndrome or rapidly progressing neurologic deficit

Loss of bowel or bladder function
Saddle anesthesia
Leg weakness
Progressive neurologic deficit in lower extremity

History of recent trauma (i.e., motor vehicle accident or fall)

neous recovery within the first 2 weeks of onset, minimal intervention is a prudent approach during this period. The primary goal at the time of acute onset of pain is to rule out the presence of potentially life-threatening or debilitating spinal pathology (so-called Red Flags; see Table 5-7) and advise the patient on restriction of activity that produces discomfort and prescription of NSAIDs; muscle relaxants, or non-narcotic analgesics. If there is no improvement of symptoms in 2 weeks, then re-evaluation and appropriate physical therapy program should be considered. See Appendices 5-1 to 5-4.

REFERENCES

1. Anderson GBJ: The epidemiology of spinal disorders. p. 107. In Frymoyer JW (ed): The Adult Spine: Principles and Practice. Raven Press, Philadelphia, 1991
2. Spitzer WO et al: Scientific Approach to the Assessment and Management of Activity Related Spinal Disorders, A Monograph for Clinicians. Report of the Quebec Task Force on Spinal Disorders. Spine 12:7S, 1987
3. Agency for Health Care Policy and Research: Clinical Practice Guidelines 14. Acute Low Back Problems in Adults. U.S. Department of Health and Human Services. AHCPR Publication 95-0642, 1994
4. Wiesel SW, Cuckler JM, Deluca F et al: Acute low back pain. An objective analysis of conservative therapy. Spine 5:324, 1980
5. Gilbert JR, Taylor DW, Hildebrand A et al: Clinical trial of common treatments for low back pain in family practice. BMJ 291:791, 1985
6. Deyo R, Diehl AK, Rosenthal M et al: How many days for acute low back pain? A randomized clinical trial. N Engl J Med 315:1064, 1986
7. Malmivaara A, Hakkinen U, Aro T et al: The treatment of acute low back pain—bed rest, exercise or ordinary activity. N Engl J Med 332:351, 1995
8. Amlie E, Weber H, Holme I et al: Treatment of acute low back pain with piroxicam: results of a double blind placebo controlled trial. Spine 12:473, 1987
9. Postacchini F, Faccnini M, Palieri P et al: Efficacy of various forms of conservative treatment of low back pain. A comparative study. Neuroorthopedics 6:28, 1988
10. Basmajian JV: Acute back pain and spasm, a controlled multicentre trial of combined analgesic and antispasm agents. Spine 14:438, 1989
11. Gall EP, Caperton EM, McComb JE et al: Clinical comparison of ibuprofen, fenoprofen Ca, naproxen and tolmetin Na in rheumatoid arthritis. J Rheumatol 9:402, 1982
12. Brooks PM, Dau RO: Nonsteroidal anti-inflammatory drugs—differences and similarities. N Engl J Med 324:1716, 1991
13. Hingorani K: Diazepam in backache. A double blind controlled trial. Ann Phys Med 8:302, 1965
14. Boyles WF, Glassman JM, Soyka JP et al: Management of acute musculoskeletal conditions: thoracolumbar strain or sprain. A double blind evaluation comparing the efficacy and safety of carisoprodol with diazepam. Today's Ther Trends 1:1, 1983
15. Hindle TH: Comparison of carisoprodol, butabarbital and placebo in treatment of low back pain syndrome. California Med West J Med 117:7, 1972
16. Gold RH: Orphenadrine citrate—sedative or muscle relaxant? Clin Ther 1:451, 1978
17. Klinger NM, Wilson RR, Kanniainen CM et al: Intravenous orphenadrine for the treatment of lumbar paravertebral muscle strain. Curr Ther Res 43:247, 1988
18. Baratta RR: A double blind study of cyclobenzaprine and placebo in the treatment of acute musculoskeletal conditions of low back. Curr Ther Res 32:646, 1982
19. Dapas F, Hartman SF, Martinez L et al: Baclofen for the treatment of acute low back syndrome. A double blind comparison with placebo. Spine 10:345, 1985
20. Casale R: Acute low back pain—symptomatic treatment with a muscle relaxant drug. Clin J Pain 4:81, 1988
21. Arbus L, Fajadet B, Aubert D et al: Activity of tetrazepam (Myolastan) in low back pain. A double blind trial versus placebo. Clin Trials J 27:258, 1990

22. Brown FL, Bodison S, Dixon J et al: Comparison of diflunisal and acetaminophen with codeine in the treatment of initial or recurrent acute low back strain. Clin Ther, suppl. C, 9:52, 1986

23. Muncie HL, Jr., King DE, DeForge B et al: Treatment of mild to moderate pain of acute soft tissue injury: diflunisal versus acetaminophen with codeine. J Fam Pract 23:125, 1986

24. Haimovic I, Beresford HR: Dexamethasone is not superior to placebo for treating lumbosacral radicular pain. Neurology 36:1593, 1986

25. Mathews JA, Hickling J: Lumbar traction: a double blind controlled study for sciatica. Rheumatol Rehabil 14:222, 1975

26. Larsson U, Choler U, Lindstrom A et al: Auto traction for treatment of lumbago sciatica. Acta Orthop Scand 51:791, 1980

27. Weber H, Ljunggren, Walker L et al: Traction therapy in patients with herniated lumbar intervertebral discs. J Oslo City Hosp 34:61, 1984

28. Pal B, Mangion P, Hossain MA et al: A controlled trial of continuous lumbar traction in the treatment of back pain and sciatica. Br J Rheumatol 25:181, 1986

29. Coxhead CE, Meade TW, Inskip H et al: Multicentre trial of physiotherapy in the management of sciatic symptoms. Lancet 8229:1065, 1981

30. Van den Heijden GJ, Buerskens AJ, Koes BW et al: The efficacy of traction for back and neck pain: a systematic, blinded review of randomized clinical trial methods. Phys Ther 75:93, 1995

31. Shekelle PG, Adams AH, Chassin MR et al: Spinal manipulation for low back pain. Ann Intern Med 117:590, 1992

32. Anderson R, Meecker WC, Wirick BE et al: A meta analysis of clinical trials of spinal manipulation. J Manipulation Physiol Ther 15:3, 181, 1992

33. Hadler NM, Curtis P, Gillings DB et al: A benefit of spinal manipulation as adjunctive therapy for acute low back pain: a stratified controlled trial. Spine 12:703, 1987

34. MacDonald RS, Bell CM: An open controlled assessment of osteopathic manipulation in nonspecific low back pain. Spine 15:364, 1990

35. Lindstrom A, Zachrisson M: Physical therapy on low back pain and sciatica. An attempt at evaluation. Scand J Rehabil Med 2:37, 1970

36. Davies JE, Gibson T, Tester L: The value of exercises in the treatment of low back pain. Rheumatol Rehabil 18:243, 1979

37. Evans C: A randomized controlled trial of flexion exercises, education and bed rest for patients with acute low back pain. Physiother Can 39:96, 1987

38. Stankovic R, Johnell D: Conservative treatment of acute low back pain. A prospective randomized trial: McKenzie method of treatment versus patient education in "mini back school." Spine 15:120, 1990

39. Lindstorm I, Ohlund C, Eek C: The effect of graded activity on patients with subacute low back pain: a randomized prospective clinical study with an operant conditioning behavioral approach. Phys Ther 72:279, 1992

40. Faas A, Chavannes AW, Van Eijk JT et al: A randomized placebo controlled trial of exercise therapy in patients with acute low back pain. Spine 18:1388, 1993

41. Gundewall B, Lilijearrist M, Hansson T et al: Primary prevention of back symptoms and absence from work. A prospective randomized study among hospital employees. Spine 18:587, 1993

42. Kellett KM, Rellet DA, Nordholm LA: Effects of an exercise program on sick leave due to back pain. Phys Ther 71:283, 1991

43. Waterworth RF, Hunter IA: An open study of diflunisal, conservative and manipulative therapy in the management of acute mechanical low back pain. N Z Med J 98:372, 1985

44. Gibson T, Grahame R, Harkness J et al: Controlled comparison of shortwave diathermy treatments with osteopathic treatment in nonspecific low back pain. Lancet 1:1258, 1985

45. Fox EJ, Melzack R: Transcutaneous electrical stimulation and acupuncture: comparison of treatment for low back pain. Pain 2:141, 1976

46. Lehman TR, Russell DW, Spratt KR et al: Efficacy of electro-acupuncture and TENS in rehabilitation of chronic low back pain patients. Pain 26:277, 1986

47. Deyo RA, Walsh NE, Martin DC et al: A controlled trial of transcutaneous electrical stimulation (TENS) and exercise for chronic low back pain. N Engl J Med 322:1627, 1990

48. Hackett GI, Seddon D, Karminski D: Electro-acupuncture compared with paracetamol for acute low back pain. Practitioner 22:163, 1985

49. Herman E, Williams R, Stratford P et al: A randomized trial of transcutaneous electrical nerve stimulation (Codetron) to determine its benefits in a rehabilitation program for acute occupational low back pain. Spine 19:561, 1994

50. Coan RM, Wong G, Ku SL et al: The acupuncture treatment of low back pain: a randomized controlled study. Am J Chin Med 8:181, 1980

51. Mendelson G, Selwood TS, Kranz H et al: Acupuncture treatment of chronic low back pain. A double blind placebo controlled trial. Am J Med 74:49, 1983

52. TerRiet G, Kleijnen J, Knipschild P: Acupuncture and chronic pain: a criteria based meta-analysis. J Clin Epidemiol 43:1191, 1990

53. Nachemson A, Schultz A, Andersson G: Mechanical effectiveness studies of lumbar spine orthosis. Scand J Rehabil Med 9:139, 1983

54. Million R, Haavik NK, Jayson MIV et al: Evaluation of low back pain and assessment of lumbar corsets with and without back supports. Ann Rheumatol Dis 40:494, 1981

55. Walsh NE, Schwartz RK: The influence of prophylactic orthosis on abdominal strength and low back injury in the work place. Am J Phys Med Rehabil 69:245, 1990

56. Reddell CR, Congleton JJ, Huchingson RD et al: An evaluation of a weight lifting belt and back injury prevention training class for airline baggage handlers. Appl Ergonomics 23:319, 1992

57. Bergquist-Ullman M, Larsson U: Acute low back pain in industry. A controlled prospective study with special reference to therapy and confounding factors. Acta Orthop Scand 170S:1, 1977

58. Lindequist S, Lungberg B, Wikmark R et al: Information and regime at low back pain. Scand J Rehabil Med 16:113, 1984

59. Linton SJ, Jamwendo K: Low back school. A critical review. Phys Ther 67:1375, 1987

60. Kiejsers JFEM, Bonter LM, Meertens RM: Validity and comparability of studies on the effects of back schools. Physiother Theory Pract 7:177, 1991

61. Bush C, Ditto B, Fenerstein M: A controlled evaluation of paraspinal EMG feedback in the treatment of chronic low back pain. Health Psychol 4:307, 1985

62. Asfour SS, Khalil TM, Walys M: Biofeedback in back muscle strengthening. Spine 15:510, 1990

63. Flor H, Haag G, Turk DC: Efficacy of EMG biofeedback, pseudotherapy and conventional medical treatment for chronic rheumatic back pain. Pain 17:21, 1983

64. Nouwen A: EMG biofeedback used to reduce standing levels of paraspinal muscle tension in chronic low back pain. Pain 17:353, 1983

65. Dilke TFW, Burry He, Grahame R et al: Extradural corticosteroid injection in management of lumbar root compression. BMJ 16:635, 1973

66. Sonek W, Weber H, Jorgensen: Double blind evaluation of extradural predisolone for herniated lumbar disc. Acta Orthop Scand 48:635, 1977

67. Cuckler JM, Bernini PA, Wiesel SW et al: The use of epidural steroids in the treatment of lumbar radicular pain. J Bone Joint Surg [Am] 67:63, 1985

68. Ridley MG, Kingley GH, Gibson T et al: Outpatient lumbar epidural cortico steroid injection in the management of sciatica. Br J Rheumatol 27:295, 1988

69. Bush K, Hillier S: Controlled study of caudal epidural injections of triamcinolone plus procaine for the management of intractable sciatica. Spine 16:527, 1991

70. Jackson RP: The facet syndrome—myth or reality? Clin Orthop 279:110, 1992

71. Lilius G, Laasonen EM, Myelynen P et al: Lumbar facet joint syndrome. J Bone Joint Surg [Br] 71:681, 1989

72. Carette S, Marcoux S, Truchon R et al: A controlled trial of corticosteroid injections into facet joints for chronic low back pain. N Engl J Med 325:1002, 1991

73. Nash TP: Facet joints—intra articular steroids or nerve blocks. Pain Clin 3:77, 1990

74. Frost FA, Jessen B, Siggaard–Anderson J: A control double blind comparison of mepivacaine injection versus saline injection for myofascial pain. Lancet 8:499, 1980

75. Garvey T, Marks MR, Wiesel SW: A prospective, randomized double blind evaluation of trigger point injection therapy for low back pain. Spine 14:962, 1989

76. Collee G, Diykmans BAC, Vanden Brochuke JP: Iliac crest pain syndrome in low back pain. A double blind randomized study of local injection therapy. J Rheumatol 18:1060, 1991

77. Ongley M, Klein RG, Dorman TA et al: A new approach to the treatment of chronic low back pain. Lancet 18:143, 1987

Appendix 5-1
Acute Low Back Pain Pathway

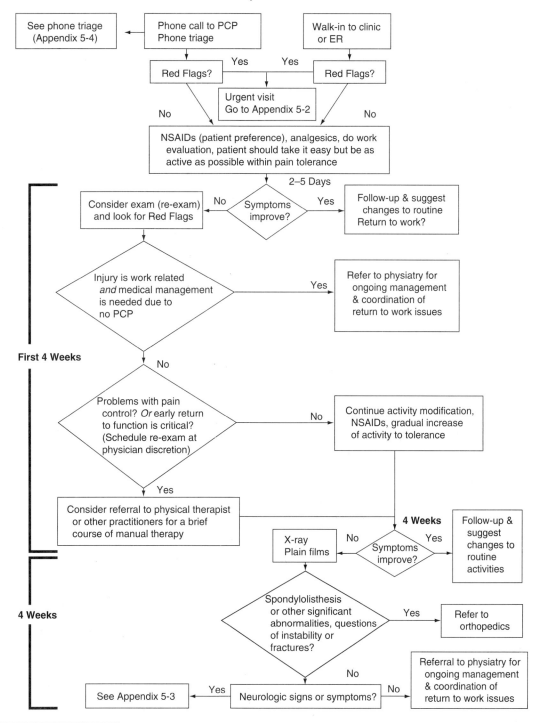

Abbreviations: PCP, primary care physician; ER, emergency room; NSAIDs, nonsteroidal anti-inflammatory drugs. (Adapted from Clinical Practice Guide #14 and Dartmouth-Hitchcock Low Back Pain Algorithm.)

Appendix 5-2
Initial Evaluation of Acute Low Back Pain

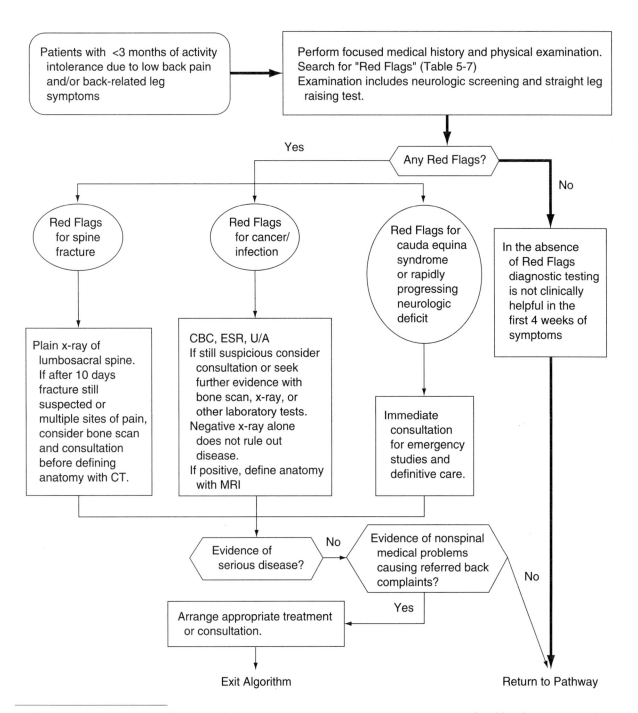

Patients with <3 months of activity intolerance due to low back pain and/or back-related leg symptoms

Perform focused medical history and physical examination. Search for "Red Flags" (Table 5-7) Examination includes neurologic screening and straight leg raising test.

Any Red Flags?

Yes

No

Red Flags for spine fracture

Red Flags for cancer/ infection

Red Flags for cauda equina syndrome or rapidly progressing neurologic deficit

In the absence of Red Flags diagnostic testing is not clinically helpful in the first 4 weeks of symptoms

Plain x-ray of lumbosacral spine. If after 10 days fracture still suspected or multiple sites of pain, consider bone scan and consultation before defining anatomy with CT.

CBC, ESR, U/A If still suspicious consider consultation or seek further evidence with bone scan, x-ray, or other laboratory tests. Negative x-ray alone does not rule out disease. If positive, define anatomy with MRI

Immediate consultation for emergency studies and definitive care.

Evidence of serious disease?

No

Evidence of nonspinal medical problems causing referred back complaints?

No

Arrange appropriate treatment or consultation.

Yes

Exit Algorithm

Return to Pathway

Abbreviations: CT, computed tomography; MRI, magnetic resonance imaging; CBC, complete blood count; ESR, electro skin resistance; U/A, urinalysis.

(Adapted from Clinical Practice Guide #14 and Dartmouth-Hitchcock Low Back Pain Algorithm.)

Appendix 5-3
Management Protocol for Neurologic Signs
or Symptoms Still Evident After 4 Weeks

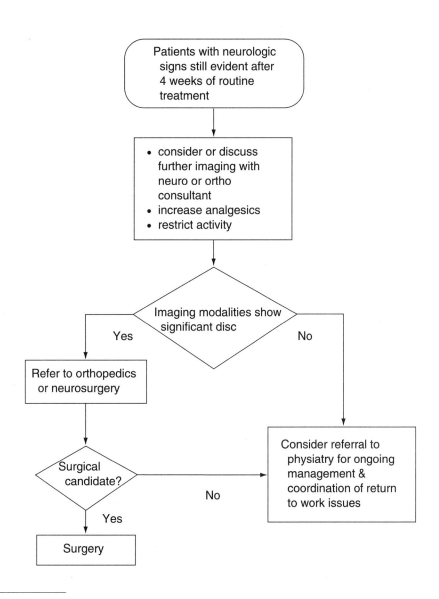

(Adapted from Clinical Practice Guide #14 and Dartmouth-Hitchcock Low Back Pain Algorithm.)

Appendix 5-4
Phone Triage

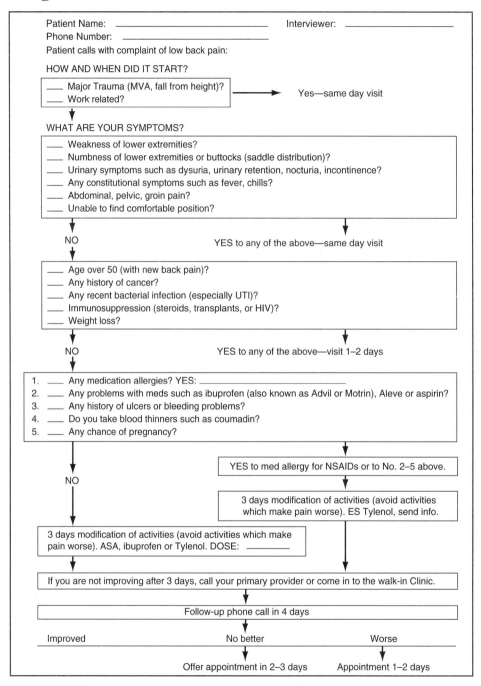

Patient Name: _____   Interviewer: _____

Phone Number: _____

Patient calls with complaint of low back pain:

HOW AND WHEN DID IT START?

| ____ Major Trauma (MVA, fall from height)? |
| ____ Work related? |

→ Yes—same day visit

WHAT ARE YOUR SYMPTOMS?

____ Weakness of lower extremities?
____ Numbness of lower extremities or buttocks (saddle distribution)?
____ Urinary symptoms such as dysuria, urinary retention, nocturia, incontinence?
____ Any constitutional symptoms such as fever, chills?
____ Abdominal, pelvic, groin pain?
____ Unable to find comfortable position?

NO   YES to any of the above—same day visit

____ Age over 50 (with new back pain)?
____ Any history of cancer?
____ Any recent bacterial infection (especially UTI)?
____ Immunosuppression (steroids, transplants, or HIV)?
____ Weight loss?

NO   YES to any of the above—visit 1–2 days

1. ____ Any medication allergies? YES: _____
2. ____ Any problems with meds such as ibuprofen (also known as Advil or Motrin), Aleve or aspirin?
3. ____ Any history of ulcers or bleeding problems?
4. ____ Do you take blood thinners such as coumadin?
5. ____ Any chance of pregnancy?

YES to med allergy for NSAIDs or to No. 2–5 above.

3 days modification of activities (avoid activities which make pain worse). ES Tylenol, send info.

NO

3 days modification of activities (avoid activities which make pain worse). ASA, ibuprofen or Tylenol. DOSE: _____

If you are not improving after 3 days, call your primary provider or come in to the walk-in Clinic.

Follow-up phone call in 4 days

Improved   No better   Worse

Offer appointment in 2–3 days   Appointment 1–2 days

Abbreviations: MVA, motor vehicle accident, UTI, urinary tract infection; HIV, human immunodeficiency virus; NSAIDs, nonsteroidal anti-inflammatory drugs; ASA, acetylsalicylic acid.

(Adapted from Dartmouth Hitchcock Low Back Pain Algorithm.)

6

Persistent Pain

Eldon Tunks
Joan Crook

Although the randomized controlled trial (RCT) is the gold standard in studies of treatment efficacy, few have been conducted in the area of persistent pain. Obstacles to research include the diagnostic diversity of persistent pain problems, the diversity of behavioral treatments, the theoretical and practical problems in outcome measurement, and the fact that many behavioral treatment programs are multimodal and admit persistent pain sufferers with nonuniform medical diagnoses. These factors make it difficult to compare studies, to create appropriate control groups, and to accomplish follow-up studies of sufficient length. On the other hand, there are enough adequate studies and enough clinical experience to provide support for the guidelines presented here as an algorithm.

In clinics dealing with persistent pain, the majority of patients fall into the categories of persistent soft tissue pains, persistent headaches, postinjury persistent back and neck pains with disability, and persistent pain with emotional disorder or somatization. This chapter discusses these categories of persistent pain, which represent the more usual pain clinic practice, and which are the main focus of behavioral management. Other pain problems, such as intractable pain of malignancy, neuralgias, reflex sympathetic dystrophies, central pain syndromes, persistent chest or gut pains, and pain in children are not described in this chapter.

BEHAVIORAL INTERVENTIONS

There is no unique chronic pain syndrome—biomedical and psychological variables differ greatly among patients.[1] A minority of pain sufferers are responsible for most health care use. Typically, they have a chronic or prolonged clinical course, are more disabled, appear to be more refractory to treatment, and demonstrate involvement of more psychosocial factors.[2–4] Although the risk of reinjury is a factor in many cases,[4,5] psychological factors are also important.[2,6] For this broad cross-section of patients, behavioral interventions have demonstrable efficacy in addressing the subjective and functional aspects of the problem at post-treatment and at follow-up.[7,8]

MULTIMODAL PAIN PROGRAMS

Most behaviorally oriented chronic pain management programs combine a cognitive-behavioral treatment focus, which is guided by progressive quotas of functional goals; withdrawal of excessive analgesics and sedatives; relaxation and coping skills training; nonpharmacologic treatments such as aerobic exercise, pacing, and problem-solving techniques; improvement of body mechanics and ergonomics; patient education; and often family and social system intervention.

Trials Using an Untreated Control Group

To address the difficult question of control group, a frequent strategy has been to use an untreated control group derived from patients accepted for treatment but not authorized by insurers. Although this strategy introduces the possibility of group differences associated with the factor of nonauthorization, it has been used several times with consistent results.

Guck et al.[9] studied chronic pain patients with mixed diagnoses. They identified 20 patients who qualified for the chronic pain management program and who wanted to participate, but were denied financial coverage. These patients were the control group. Of the 96 patients who completed the 4-week pain management program, 20 were randomly selected and stratified to match the elapsed times since evaluation. These patients were the treated group. The groups appeared well matched at pretreatment except that the mean pain history of the treated group was 49, versus 69 months for the untreated group, a statistically nonsignificant difference, but perhaps a clinically important difference. The control group had a greater proportion of subjects with back and/or leg pain. Both of these pretreatment differences might systematically bias the outcome toward the treatment group.

At the 1- to 5-year reanalysis, 60 percent of the treated patients met all the criteria of success of employment or equivalent, no compensation for pain problems, no pain-related hospitalization or surgery since treatment, and no prescription narcotic or psychotropic medication. None of the controls met these criteria. The treated patients were significantly better with respect to pain, pain-related hospitalizations, uptime, and depression variables. The untreated patients had significantly more pain interference with common activities and less employment.

Mayer et al.[10] used a similar strategy to compare 66 treated low back pain patients with 38 untreated low back pain patients. The program (PRIDE) was a particularly vigorous multimodal program running 57 hours a week for 3 weeks, followed by daily outpatient visits until maximum benefit or return to work was achieved, at an average of 5 weeks. The elements of the program included fitness and endurance training with use of objective physical performance measures; relaxation and cognitive-behavioral training; and family, individual, and group therapy. At 3- and 6-month follow-up periods, functional and psychological measures showed significant improvement when compared to admission in the treatment group. At 1-year follow-up, 86 percent of the treatment group was employed versus 45

percent of the control group and 20 percent of the dropout group.

Treatment of Persistent Pain

Deardorff et al.[11] studied 42 treated and 15 untreated patients with mixed diagnoses. The study weaknesses included the small number of control subjects, greater pain intensity and interference ratings at preassessment of the treated patients compared to controls, and an older treated group. One might expect that these factors might bias the favorable outcome toward the control group, but, in fact, the treatment group did better. Both groups reported reduced pain levels after 11 months average follow-up. The treated group showed a return to work rate of 48 percent, with an additional 28 percent in vocational rehabilitation. None of the untreated group returned to work or vocational rehabilitation.

Randomized Controlled Trials

Several RCT studies have compared multimodal therapies with control conditions in pain management.

Mixed Chronic Pain Diagnoses

Linton et al.[12] randomly assigned chronic pain patients with mixed diagnoses to three outpatient conditions: waiting list control, regular rehabilitation clinic treatment, or regular treatment plus operant behavior therapy and relaxation training. The regular treatment patients received more therapeutic contact than patients in the behavioral condition. Only the patients in the behavioral condition showed a significant reduction in pain intensity. The behavioral treatment group achieved significantly superior control in daily activity compared to the waiting list. The behavioral treatment condition was superior to the other conditions in the categories of reduced medication intake, improved sleep, and depression.

Peters and Large[13] attempted to randomize 85 chronic pain patients with mixed diagnoses: 33 were assigned to inpatient multimodal therapy, 29 to outpatient multimodal therapy, and 23 to a no-treatment control condition. Of these, 29 inpatients, 23 outpatients, and 16 controls participated enough to be studied. The characteristics of the noncompleters was not reported. The inpatient group had a higher proportion of women and were more depressed and psychologically distressed at pretreatment. This inequality might bias the inpatient group toward a worse prognosis or toward greater regression toward the mean on some measures. Patients in both treatment groups improved with respect to psychological distress, pain behavior, disability, and pain after exercise when compared with the control group. The outpatients, who were similar to the control group, improved more with respect to pain complaint.

Chronic Low Back Pain Diagnosis

Talo et al.[14] conducted an RCT on 173 patients with chronic low back pain and the following characteristics: duration at least 6 months, age 30 to 47 years, no compensation/pension claim, no more than one back surgery, and no contraindication for heavy exercise. Patients were stratified by age (less than 40 and greater than 40) and gender and randomized to three groups. The functional activation program was based on the PRIDE model. A spa resort-type program was about half the intensity and hours of treatment, had more passive modalities, and lacked stress management. Those unfit for functional activation were also randomized to the spa resort or to some other type of care. Thus, two equally fit groups were randomized into the activation and spa programs, and a fit and unfit group were assigned to the spa program.

At 12 months, the activation and spa patients had improvement in measures of coping, psychological distress, and pain variables, but the unfit spa subjects had little change in status. Patients who on pretreatment measures were good copers did equally well in either program. The mental health of interpersonally distressed or adaptive copers improved more in the activation program; in dysfunctional patients, mental health improved more in the spa program. In the spa program, fit patients achieved more psychosocial adjustment and reduced medication and depression; unfit patients increased in psychological distress and dysfunction.

Alaranta et al.[15] studied chronic low-back pain patients using the same inclusion criteria as Talo et al.[14] Patients were randomized to two groups: 152

received in-house functional activation (based on the PRIDE model), and 141 received a less strenuous in-house program, with lighter and unspecific exercise, including many passive modalities, and excluding stress management, for about half the number of hours compared to the experimental program. At pretreatment, the groups were similar in measures of employment and in sick leave during the preceding 12 months.

The findings were of greater mean improvements in outcome measures in males than in females, and the male/female differential of improvement was more evident during longer follow-up. At 3 and 6 months, men and women in the functional activation group had a lower self-rating of pain disability. At 3 months, men and women in the functional activation program improved more in measures of flexibility and strength, had less pain on activity, and better ability to do strenuous leisure activities. At 12 months, men but not women in the functional activation group did better in these measures.

At 12 months only, men in the functional activation group were better on the World Health Organization (WHO) Occupational Handicap measure; however, using this measure, 70 percent of both treatment groups had no or very mild problems in work and ordinary activities. The functional activation group and reference group were not significantly different during follow-up on measures of use of health care services, sick leaves, retirements, and psychological measures.

Turner et al.[16] randomly assigned 96 low back pain patients to one of four groups: outpatient group behavioral therapy, aerobic exercise, behavior and exercise therapies, or waiting-list control. Patients were followed at post-treatment and at 6 and 12 months after treatment. At post-treatment, the combined exercise-behavioral treatment group was significantly more improved than the control patients, but at the follow-ups, all three treatment conditions were significantly improved from pretreatment, with no differences among the treatment groups.

Heinrich et al.[17] studied chronic back pain patients (pain longer than in most other studies). Fifty-one met the screening criteria and were assigned alternately to either the behavior therapy or the physical therapy groups. The only pretreatment group differences was pain duration, which was 22 years in the behavior therapy group and 14 years in the physical therapy group. The behavior therapy condition included patient education, communication and assertiveness skills, coping skills training, relaxation, goal setting, and group treatment. The physical therapy condition included back school and other education, relaxation and self-help techniques, problem solving, ergonomics, and group treatment. Five patients dropped out of the behavior therapy and 13 dropped out of the physical therapy, leaving 18 behavior therapy patients and 15 physical therapy patients who completed the postevaluation.

At 6 months, 16 behavior therapy and 9 physical therapy patients completed follow-up. When the 26 dropouts were compared to the 25 completers, the dropouts were younger (41 versus 48 years), had shorter pain histories (8 versus 18 years), were more often divorced or separated, and were more likely to use alcohol. The effect of the dropouts on the demographic data of the remaining treatment groups was not described. On follow-up, there was no difference in reported activity level or physical limitations between the treatment groups, although measures of back care appeared to improve more in the physical therapy group than in the behavior therapy group. Both treatment groups were less depressed and less painful at post-evaluation and 6-month follow-up.

Nicholas et al.[18] randomly allocated 60 chronic low back patients to six groups; after the pretest, results were available on 58. All six groups received physiotherapy with exercise and back education. Two groups had cognitive therapy with or without relaxation, two groups had operant behavioral therapy with or without relaxation, and two control groups had either nondirective discussion sessions or no discussion sessions. Thirty-nine subjects were available at the 6- and 12-month follow-ups. Because of the number of dropouts, the four psychological treatment groups were combined, and the two physiotherapy-alone groups were combined for analysis, and Bonferroni correction was used to adjust for the large number of variables. No information was given on the pretest characteristics of dropouts. The relaxation condition included audiotapes. The behavior therapy condition allowed therapist praise for completed tasks, but the cognitive therapy condition did not. Although all groups improved on variables of pain, function, coping, and medication use, the improvement was greater at post-treatment with the psychological interventions plus physiotherapy than it was with the control plus physiotherapy groups. These differences were only weakly maintained at 6- and 12-month follow-ups. Relaxation therapy had little effect on the effectiveness of either cognitive or operant behavior treatments. Considering the sample size problems and the constrictions in the application of the experimental conditions, it is unlikely that significant differences could have been detected.

Nicholas et al.[19] also studied 20 chronic low back pain patients with a greater than 6-month history of pain and who were not candidates for invasive procedures. Age ranged between 20 and 60 years. These patients were not due for insurance compensation settlement within 12 months. The mean duration of low back pain was 5.5 years, with a range of 6 months to 20 years. Patients were randomized to two groups. (No information was given regarding compatibility of the groups with respect to age or pain durations.)

Both groups received back care classes 2 hours a week. One group received 1.5 hours a week of cognitive-behavioral and relaxation therapy; the other received an equal amount of time in nondirective group discussions about their experiences with back pain. In the post-treatment assessment, the cognitive-behavioral group did better than the nondirective treatment with respect to sickness impact, coping skills, self-efficacy, and medication use. (Measures of pain and depression did not show significant change.) At 6-month follow-up, the trends were still present, but the outcomes of the two groups were more similar. (The trends in favor of the treatment group might have been more significant with a larger sample size.)

Long-term Outcome

McArthur et al.[20] studied 702 consecutive admissions to a multimodal chronic pain clinic on a variety of measures including physical performance, psychological measures, pain self-report, and pain-related performance; data were available on 360 patients. Both program completers and noncompleters were evaluated for change on these measures. The noncompleters had somewhat worse function at admission.

There was significant improvement in most of the completers, but not in the noncompleters. The authors then reported a yearly follow-up for 5 years of patients who had completed the program.[21] In the first 4 years, there was little change in pain status, and for the first 3 years little change in reports of the degree to which pain interfered with activity. There was a steady increase in return to work, beginning at 33 percent at 6 months. There was a steady decrease in use of medications and in litigation.

Crook et al.[22] found in a follow-up of an epidemiologic survey that after 2 years, family practice clinic patients with persistent pain had a 35 percent probability of no longer suffering persistent pain, compared to 15 percent of patients referred to a chronic pain clinic.

Maruta et al.[23] carried out a 3-year follow-up of a cohort of 239 patients with chronic pain who had completed a chronic pain program. Mean pain duration was 6.7 years, average previous surgeries was two, and mean absence from full-time work was 2 years. Forty-three percent received disability compensation. At least 39 percent had maintained moderate to marked improvement in attitude modification, medication reduction, and functioning; and 36 percent were partially improved. Although this was not a controlled study, the outcomes suggest good improvement with multimodal treatment.

Härkäpää et al.[24] randomly assigned 476 chronic back pain sufferers to inpatient or outpatient treatment, or no-treatment control. All had back pain for at least 2 years, all had strenuous jobs, and pain interfered with working capacity. Inpatient treatment was 3 weeks and outpatient treatment was 15 weeks. Both included back school, exercise, relaxation, heat or electrotherapy, and coping skills classes. A refresher program 1.5 years later was 2 weeks for inpatients and 8 sessions for outpatients.

Low back pain decreased more in both treatment groups at 3 months, and in the inpatient group only at 1.5 years and 22 months. At 2.5 years, there were no differences between groups. At 2.5 years, 25 percent of inpatients, 14 percent of outpatients, and 10 percent of controls showed clear gains in low back pain disability index. Inpatients had the best long-term (2.5 years) compliance with prescribed exer-cise. Sick time increased in all during follow-up, but increased less in inpatients than in controls at 2.5 years, whereas outpatients' sick time was between control and inpatient means.

As part of the same study, Mellin et al.[25] noted more consistent improvement on an index derived from combined physical measures in the inpatients.[25] Between-group comparisons showed that inpatients were doing better than outpatients or controls at 2.5 years. In women, improvements in the index were seen up to 2.5 year follow-up for both treatment groups.

Lindstrom et al.[26] studied low back pain patients who had been sicklisted 8 weeks, but who had been without back pain in the 12 weeks before the latest sicklisting. They were randomized—51 to an activity group with return-to-work expectation, functional capacity measures, individualized submaximal graded exercise with operant behavioral approach, work place visit, and back school and 52 to a control group with traditional care from their regular physician.

Men in the activity group returned to work earlier, but at 1 year, the rate of return to work was similar in the activity and control conditions. At 2 years, average durations of sicklistings for back pain, and total durations of sicklistings, were still less in the activity group, which also had a greater number of patients with no pain recurrences. Between-group comparisons showed no significant difference with respect to rate of return to work or sick leave at 2 years for women.

Prognostic Factors

Chronic physical and psychosocial maladies coexist in specialty clinics.[27,28] The unique characteristics of the study samples of pain clinic patients must be considered in any review.[2] Potential prognostic demographic factors (e.g., age, employment status on program entry) were often not controlled, particularly in the early studies.[11] In many studies, heterogeneous pain diagnoses often have been considered together, so that prognostically different subgroups have not been identified (e.g., migraine, or musculoskeletal pain). Patients from important diagnostic subgroups may respond to different treatment factors and may be selected differently by program entry criteria. As a result, recruitment methods may influence outcome regardless of potential treatment efficacy.[23,29,30]

Psychological variables are responsible for a substantial proportion of the variance in outcome scores, even after disease activity has been considered. Psychological factors influence how patients respond to treatment of low back pain, whether by physiotherapy,[31] rehabilitation,[32] or surgery.[33] Emotional patterns, primarily involving levels of depression,[32] mood,[34,35] and emotional distress,[36] for example, were cited as influencing the course of treatment.

Different sets of predictors may be identified for subgroups of patients. For example, Dworkin et al.[32] examined the hypothesis that treatment responses in chronic pain patients with and without depression would be predicted by different patterns of variables in short-term outcome of pain clinic treatment. Employment status,[37] pretreatment compensation,[38] and length of time between onset and treatment,[39] have been seen as closely related to treatment outcome. Being unemployed at the beginning of treatment, receiving compensation before treatment, and increasing length of time between onset and treatment were all related to poor treatment outcomes. When employment and compensation were used jointly to predict long- and short-term outcome in multiple regression analysis, however, only employment was significant.[37]

The time that multimodal pain clinic treatment is initiated during the clinical course of the disorder is important. Randomized controlled clinical trials are needed to address not only whether specialized pain treatment is effective, but more specifically, at what time during the course of the impairment the treatment is most successful, at what cost, and for what group of patients.

Chronic Pain Prevention

Philips et al.[40] conducted an RCT in 117 cases of acute back pain, who were referred from general practitioners and emergency departments. The initial visit occurred an average of 7 days after onset, the second visit at 3 months, and the third at 6 months after onset. Patients were randomized to treatment groups of (1) exercise with "letting pain guide" and

behavioral counseling, (2) graded and gradual reactivation approach and behavioral counseling, and (3) graded and gradual reactivation and control nonbehavioral counseling.

The group with the graded reactivation treatment was not different from the "pain as guide" group in development of chronic pain at 6 months. However, the groups receiving behavioral counseling had a somewhat greater percentage of patients reporting "no pain" at 6 months, but the behavioral changes noted did not prevent chronic pain from developing.

Fordyce et al.[41] conducted an RCT comparing outpatient operant behavioral therapy and traditional management for acute back pain. After random assignment and attrition, there were 29 men and 21 women in the behavioral group, in which the use of analgesics, exercises, and activity limits were all based on quotas leading to restoration of normal activity. There were 36 men and 21 women in the traditional condition, in which use of these treatments was based on symptoms. No significant group differences at admission or at 6 weeks were found with respect to demographic, employment, sickness, medication, or back examination findings. At follow-up (9 to 12 months) the behaviorally treated group fared significantly better on the health care utilization, "claimed impairment" and pain drawings, whereas the traditionally treated group had worsened on the "claimed impairment" variable.

Linton and Bradley[42] conducted a prospective cohort study of hospital employees with a prior history of sicklisting for back pain. These subjects attended a course including back education, stress control, fitness training, goal setting, problem-solving, and focus on life-style. After 18 months follow-up, subjects had less pain, used less medication, and were more active. In addition, a trend toward increasing sicklistings was reversed.

In a similar study by Kellett et al.[43] subjects with short-term back pain were randomly assigned to active exercise (n = 58) or to a control condition (n = 53). The 1.5 years before and after intervention were compared. The episodes of back pain and sick days from back pain decreased by 50 percent in the active exercise group but increased in the control group.

Summary

Multimodal therapy for chronic pain is more effective than comparison treatments or no treatment. This efficacy is particularly demonstrable 6 months after treatment. Benefits are found in measures including psychological distress, function, return to work, and pain. When there is goal-oriented multifocused treatment, the addition of single modalities such as relaxation may not improve the overall efficacy, suggesting that individual modalities may have nonspecific effects on outcomes. Functional measures, such as goal setting and graded systematic exercise with monitoring, improve the outcomes in terms of psychological and functional measures.

Gender-specific outcomes have received some attention. Women and men both improve in vigorous multimodal programs. However, on longer term follow-up—greater than 6 months—the outcomes of women treated in multimodal and comparison programs become more alike. The women treated in multimodal programs, however, seem for the most part to maintain their improvement. On longer follow-up, men treated in multimodal programs continue to show greater benefits than men treated in comparison programs. Hansen et al.,[44] however, found that there may be greater relative benefit of a physically vigorous program for patients who are initially unfit, or for women.

Several hypotheses need to be tested. A factor influencing successful reintegration whether the physical fitness is adequate for the work, especially for male laborers.[10] On the other hand, success for women may depend partly on physical fitness, but also on overcoming barriers of a psychosocial character, which might be addressed in other types of treatment programs, as well as in multimodal programs.

In several studies, the interaction of the natural progression/regression of chronic pain conditions has apparently interacted with the effects of treatment, so that the short-term effects are more related to the treatment, but long-term effects were influenced by nontreatment factors. The epidemiologic studies of the long-term follow-up of chronic pain should be considered when interpreting long-term follow-up of multimodal (and other) treatment programs. The prevention of chronic pain has not yet been shown to be possible, although a modest reduction of trend toward sicklisting or chronic pain has been demonstrated in some studies of multimodal programs. In terms of weighting the significance of short-term versus long-term outcomes, the greater clinical efficacy should be demonstrable in short-term improvement of function and return to work, and interruption of the pattern of evolution toward chronic pain.

Several factors influencing efficacy have been examined. Factors such as length of treatment, age, illness duration, or litigation were not correlated with the effect sizes in one meta-analysis. This lack of correlations has implications for the practice of excluding patients from treatment on the grounds of compensation or litigation. If duration of treatment is not associated with effect size, more economical treatment may be possible. These factors need more prospective testing.

UNIMODAL THERAPIES FOR CHRONIC PAIN

Behavioral or Psychological Treatment

Kerns et al.[45] studied 28 patients with chronic pain of mixed diagnoses. They were randomized—10 to operant behavioral therapy, 10 to cognitive-behavioral therapy with coping skills training, and 8 to a waiting-list control group. Patients were followed up at 3 and 6 months post-treatment. Of the 10 patients in the behavioral group, 6 were lost to follow-up. At post-treatment, both treatment groups improved in goal attainment. The cognitive behavioral group showed pain improvement at post-treatment, and at 3 months, but less significantly at 6 months. (The study is weak because of small sample size, short follow-up, and high percentage of dropouts.)

Dolce et al.[46] studied 14 chronic pain patients in a within-subjects, repeated-measures design. Patients were treated in a multimodal program. As specific quotas were set, exercise tolerance increased steadily. Self-efficacy expectancies improved for 82 percent and worries decreased for 71 percent of patients. In a study of experimental cold-pressor pain in 64 college volunteers, Dolce et al.[47] showed that setting quotas significantly improved pain tolerance performance. Financial incentives did not improve tolerance more than quotas alone, and giving an inactive placebo apparently worsened performance, perhaps by undermining the subjects' belief in their ability to cope with the stressor.

Altmaier et al.[48] conducted an RCT in which 33 chronic low back pain patients were randomized to one of two 3-week inpatient conditions. Each included a multimodal back education and physical conditioning program, and one also included a cognitive-behavioral program. Patients were work disabled from 3 to 30 months and were not surgical candidates, were not involved with compensation, and did not demonstrate significant depression or anger. By the 6-month follow-up, 81 percent of patients had either returned to work or had attempted to return to work. Measures of pain, interference, disability, and physical measures were not significantly different between groups, suggesting that if a program is functioning effectively, with a clear focus on improving function and return to work, it is unlikely that adding other psychological elements will improve the results.

Pilowsky and Barrow[49] studied 102 patients with chronic pain (21 percent less than 1 year and 46 percent 2 to 5 years) who had functional impairment and lesions that were not commensurate to their pain. Patients were randomly assigned to four groups: amitriptyline plus 12 weekly sessions of psychotherapy, amitriptyline plus six 15-minute supportive therapy sessions, placebo plus 12 weekly sessions of psychotherapy, or placebo plus six 15-minute supportive therapy sessions. Amitriptyline serum levels tended to be below the usual antidepressant level. Patients were followed for up to 1 year, but the report concerned only the 12-week post-treatment findings.

Amitriptyline was associated with a greater increase in productivity and reduction of time in pain. Psychotherapy was associated with an increase in pain, but also an increase in productivity. (The selection criteria were likely to include a majority of patients with somatoform disorders who may be unlikely to respond either to psychotropic drugs or psychotherapy. The modest results of the study should be interpreted cautiously.)

Pilowsky et al.[50] reported a study of 64 chronic pain patients who probably had somatoform disorders. They were randomized to treatment with amitriptyline and cognitive behavioral therapy, or to amitriptyline and supportive therapy. In this initial group, baseline scores did not differ between the completers (40) and dropouts (18). At the end of 8 weeks, the completers were assigned to follow-up: 19 to treatment group and 21 to comparison group. Control (supportive therapy) patients were allowed to change to cognitive behavioral therapy if they wished—eight of original controls proceeded to cognitive behavioral therapy. At this point, the treatment group was older than the control group (47 and 40 years, respectively) and the treatment group reported more "superficial pain" than the control group. The cognitive behavioral therapy and amitriptyline treatment group experienced less time in pain and less average intensity of pain at 3 and 6 months, and no difference at these follow-up times in productivity. Sample size may have been too small to show statistically significant changes.

Holroyd et al.[51] randomly assigned 41 recurrent tension headache patients to home-based cognitive therapy or to amitriptyline therapy at doses individualized from 25 to 75 mg/day. With either patient-rated daily headache recordings or neurologist-rated improvement, both treatments produced clinically significant improvements, with cognitive therapy yielding somewhat more favorable outcomes than amitriptyline.

Relaxation

In controlled studies and in clinical practice, relaxation therapy has proved efficacious. It is an important ingredient in other procedures such as biofeedback, desensitization and assertiveness training, and some kinds of cognitive-behavioral therapy. Relaxation compares favorably with other psychological treatment methods and with biofeedback.[52–56] Operant behavioral therapy may be effective in reducing medication intake, reducing verbal and nonverbal expressions of pain, and increasing activity, and relaxation therapy may be somewhat more effective in reducing the subjective experience of pain and emotional distress.[57,58] On the other hand, relaxation therapy may be nonspecific in its effect, but efficacious.[18,52]

Sorbi and Tellegen[59] randomly assigned migraine patients to relaxation or to "stress-coping training." Both groups improved significantly, but the relaxation patients perceived significantly better training effects in migraine duration, drug consumption, and awareness of stress, whereas the stress-coping patients more often believed that they had acquired control over stressful events. These group differences faded during 8 months of follow-up.

Attanasio et al.[60] randomly assigned 25 tension headache sufferers to three conditions: combined treatment in the therapist's office using relaxation and cognitive therapy with instructions for home practice, home-based treatment using relaxation and cognitive treatment, or home-based relaxation only. All three groups improved: 71 percent of subjects in the combined office-based treatment, 62 percent of those in the combined home-based treatment, and 50 percent of those in the home-based relaxation group showed meaningful improvement in headache. (Sample size was small and the differences were not statistically significant.)

Biofeedback Training

The main application of biofeedback training has been in the area of headache management; it also has been applied successfully to other pain and rehabilitation problems.

Several reviews have concluded that in most cases, biofeedback training is about as effective as relaxation, and both are better than placebo or no-treatment conditions.[52-56,62-68] The physiologic function that is monitored may show a training effect in the desired direction, but this effect is often small, and it may be difficult to establish a clear relationship between the symptomatic improvement and the biofeedback training-monitored physiologic change. Relaxation or cognitive coping skills also may be active ingredients in the therapeutic effect of biofeedback training.

Bell et al.[69] randomly assigned 24 tension headache sufferers to four groups. The biofeedback group was combined with lessons in the use of imagery, awareness of inner states, a brief relaxation technique, home practice, and methods for applying the coping skills. The psychotherapy group consisted in the same number of hours of treatment devoted to discussion of stressors, headache triggers, coping, dealing with unpleasant affect, and some psychodynamic issues, and use of imagery to deal with pain. The combined group included both treat-

ments. There was also a waiting-list control group. All three treatment groups improved significantly with respect to controls on the variables of headache symptoms, psychological improvement, medication use, and decline in muscle spasms. Improvement was superior in degree for all biofeedback patients for ability to relax, need for medication, psychological distress variables, and total complaints. Psychotherapy combined with biofeedback training was no more effective than biofeedback training alone. (With such a small sample size, however, detection of significant differences would be unlikely.)

Lacroix et al.[70] assigned 55 inpatients with back and neck pain and tension headache to frontalis electromyographic (EMG) biofeedback, relaxation, combined relaxation-biofeedback, or no-treatment control. Patients also participated in active rehabilitation. A small but significant improvement was found for all three treatment groups, whereas the control group steadily worsened with regard to headache frequency. Patients who received the relaxation training reported more improvement in all aspects of headache symptoms at the 6-month follow-up.

The beneficial effects of biofeedback training are stable over time. Flor et al.[71] followed back pain patients for 2.5 years. Patients had been subjects in one of three groups: all three groups had conventional treatment, and the experimental groups had either EMG biofeedback or pseudofeedback. On follow-up, pain improved 68 percent in the biofeedback group and 14 percent in the other groups. Biofeedback patients reported significant improvement in pain interference, medication use, pain-related behaviors, pain on activity, and recourse to other treatment. They also used more psychological strategies for coping.

META-ANALYSES OF NONMEDICAL TREATMENTS

Malone and Strube[35] identified 109 studies of which 48 provided sufficient information to calculate effect sizes. Autogenic, biofeedback, cognitive, hypnosis, operant, multimodal treatment packages, pill placebo, relaxation, and transcutaneous electrical nerve stimulation (TENS) studies were included. Treatment types associated with the largest effect sizes were autogenic (2 studies), hypnosis (1 study), placebo (3 studies), multimodal package (11 studies), biofeedback (24 studies), and relaxation (7 studies).

Outcome measures associated with the least variability in effect sizes (reflecting consistency) were subjective symptoms, EMG or temperature recordings, and mood; these measures consistently showed improvement. In a comparison of "percentage of patients improved and treatment type," improvement occurred in 77 percent of the no treatment group, 84 percent of the biofeedback group, and 95 percent of the relaxation group. All other treatments were associated with patient improvement rates of less than 77 percent. (Although the comparison is crude because of marked variability in study type, the results do not provide evidence of greater efficacy than control condition for many methods.) The "percentage of improved patients as a function of outcome measure" was also calculated. Mood was 100 percent; and only "intensity," "duration," and "frequency" were above the 75 percent levels.

Holroyd and Penzien[72] restricted their search to studies of propranolol, relaxation and thermal biofeedback together, placebo, and no-treatment controls for recurrent migraine. They identified 73 applicable studies. The average percentage of improvement was calculated as a function of treatment type; the average group improvement was 55.1 percent for relaxation/biofeedback training, 55.1 percent for propranolol, 12.2 percent for placebo, and 1.1 percent for the untreated condition. There was a significant difference between the mean improvements for the drug or relax/biofeedback training conditions and the control conditions. Using the more conservative measure of daily headache recording, the same significant differences were still obtained.

Flor et al.[73] conducted a meta-analysis of studies from 1960 to 1990. Of these, 65 met the study criteria. Most of these were multimodal studies and most involved chronic low back pain, with high rates of unemployment, medication use, surgeries, compensation, and litigation. Effect sizes for control groups were close to zero at short-term (mean, 5 weeks) and long-term follow-up (mean, 95 weeks). Treatment groups showed effect sizes of 1.51 and 1.31 at short- and long-term follow-up, respectively. Comparing the between-group (treatment vs control)

effect sizes, the short-term effect size was 0.62, and the long-term effect size was 0.81.

These results showed substantial gains of treated groups over control groups at short- and long-term follow-up. Multimodal programs demonstrated superior results in comparison to unimodal nonmedical or unimodal medical treatments. Outcome measures demonstrating the largest change were psychophysiologic measures, followed by mood, pain, and behavioral measures. Similarly, specific behavioral change levels also showed high effect sizes, including work, medication, and activity. Treated patients showed a 43 percent increase in returning to work, compared to a 25 percent increase in the untreated groups. Thus, improvements are far-reaching, including psychological, subjective, economic, and functional dimensions. There were virtually no significant correlations between effect sizes and the variables of age, pain duration, litigation, compensation, or durations of treatment.

Bigos et al.[74] conducted an extensive and scholarly review of RCTs and meta-analyses of the assessment and treatment of acute low back pain. Treatment recommendations were based on more than 180 controlled studies. About half were of samples of either chronic patients or combined acute and chronic patients. Where possible, the authors performed meta-analytic analyses. Conclusions and recommendations were based on the quality and consensus of high-quality scientific studies. Although the emphasis of the monograph is on acute low back pain, there is considerable relevance for chronic patients. Extrapolating from their findings, particularly where they depended on studies of chronic low back patients, they concluded the following:

Provision of accurate information regarding the usually benign natural history of low back pain, regarding the means of limiting symptoms and disability, and regarding investigation and treatment options tend to speed recovery.

Controlled studies did not show that antidepressants were more effective than placebo in reducing the subjective distress or impairment associated with chronic low back pain.

Controlled studies of manipulation show at least short-term effect in reducing recovery time in low back sufferers.

Various common physical treatments (passive therapies) do not appear to be clearly better than no treatment in samples that include chronic low back sufferers. Biofeedback for chronic low back pain yields unimpressive and contradictory clinical results.

Controlled studies of facet joint injections using steroid, local anesthetic, or saline did not show significant advantages at 3 months or advantages at 6 months in terms of the percentage of patients with sustained improvement. Studies of epidural steroid injections show short-term benefits within the month after treatment, but not on longer-term follow-up.

Although a few studies of acupuncture in chronic low back pain demonstrated greater benefit in patients receiving "needling" than in those receiving "no needling," studies were not able to demonstrate specificity for traditional acupuncture points, and most studies were performed too poorly to allow conclusions.

Active exercise is almost universally used in chronic pain management programs. Exercise regimens vary considerably in components and intensity and are usually combined with other components such as patient education and behavior modification techniques. There is generally a consensus that such active exercise programs are more beneficial than programs lacking active exercise.

Several studies also demonstrate a "secondary prevention" of recurrent back pain episodes or sicklistings in patients who participate in programs including active exercise.

Summary of Behavioral Treatments

It appears that unimodal psychological/behavioral programs are efficacious, although perhaps not as efficacious as multimodal therapies. The importance of structured objective behavioral goals is noted. Alternatives to behavioral treatment include biofeedback, relaxation, and cognitive treatments. Evidence for the short-term specificity of treatment effect for some of these treatments is present, but after a few months, the outcomes of these various alternatives become more similar.

PHYSICAL THERAPY, BED REST, AND EXERCISE

Chronic low back pain responds poorly to most single passive therapies or to prolonged bed rest.[4,75,76]

In a review of good-quality, randomized controlled studies, Nachemson[76] concluded that there was strong to conclusive evidence of effectiveness of physical treatments in certain circumstances. For low back pain without radiation below the knee, bed rest of not more than 2 days was considered effective for pain in the first 6 weeks, whereas bed rest of more than 7 days was considered not effective. Paracetamol and nonsteroidal antiinflammatory drugs (NSAIDs) were considered effective only during the first 3 months. Manipulation and back school were both considered effective during the period of weeks 1 through 6. Supervised fitness programs were considered effective for back pain from 7 weeks to 3 months. For back pain with sciatica radiating below the knee and possibly with neurologic signs, 1 week, but not 2 weeks, of bed rest was considered effective during the first 3 months, and surgery was considered effective in the periods of 5 weeks to 3 months with pain lasting longer than 3 months.

In the meta-analysis by Flor et al.,[73] effect sizes demonstrated that conventional physical therapy was better than medical treatment or no treatment, but was inferior to multidisciplinary approaches. Greater success is demonstrated with active exercise aimed at promoting fitness, improving body mechanics, and improving confidence.

In the review and meta-analysis by Bigos et al.,[74] little or no significant benefit could be demonstrated in chronic back pain sufferers using antidepressants, passive physical therapies, biofeedback, and "trigger point" and facet joint injections. There was some equivocal benefit for chronic back pain sufferers with acupuncture. Possible short-term benefits were demonstrated using manipulation and epidural steroid injections. Of all single modalities, those with the greatest apparent efficacy were patient education and active exercise programs.[74] Bridging the gap between the clinic and the work setting and using functional measures relevant to the patient's work activity have produced remarkable results.[10]

Malmivaara et al.[77] conducted an RCT in patients with acute or recurrent low back pain of less than 3 weeks' duration. After randomization, 67 patients were assigned to 2 days bed rest, 52 patients to exercise and normal activity as tolerated, and 67 patients to normal activity as tolerated. Eighty-seven percent of patients completed the 12-week assessment; the dropouts were not significantly different from completers in baseline variables.

At 3 weeks, the activity-as-tolerated group fared better than the other treatment groups with respect to number of sick days, pain duration, pain intensity, ability to work, and the Oswestry Back Disability Index. At 12 weeks, patients assigned to bed rest recovered significantly more slowly than activity-as-tolerated group with respect to sick days, pain, ability to work, lumbar flexion, and the Oswestry index. The exercise group recovered more slowly than the activity-as-tolerated group with respect to sick days and lumbar flexion. Costs and use of health care services were lowest in the activity-as-tolerated group. A possible interpretation would be that an immediate focus on normality rather than on symptoms and treatment is likely to have a more beneficial effect in episodes of acute or subacute back pain.

Mitchell et al.[78] conducted a multicenter study of clinics providing intensive exercises, work conditioning, return-to-work expectations, and patient education. Average duration of injury to treatment was 41 days. Two-thirds of the patients had low back pain. Seven hundred three patients were matched by age and sex to another group of 703 who were treated by their own practitioners.

The clinic patients returned to work significantly earlier, with substantial savings in indemnities, health care costs, and wages. With several months of follow-up, the proportion of those returned to work became more similar in the clinic and control patients, but the accumulated savings remained significantly greater for the clinic group.

Manniche et al.[78] conducted an RCT of 105 patients between the ages of 20 and 70 who had at least 0.5 years of low back pain and recurrent acute back pain within the previous year. They were randomly assigned to a 3-month intensive treatment group, a light treatment group that performed about one-fifth of the intensive treatment group's exercise, and a passive treatment group that received thermotherapy, massage, and mild exercise. At post-treatment and 3-month follow-up, the intensive training group had improved more than the other groups based on a scale measuring back pain and function. The improvement in the light exercise group was less pronounced. At 3- and 6-month follow-up, the intensive group had greater isometric endurance. Those who continued exercise once a week still maintained a favorable result in pain and function measures at 1 year. In this study, the same favorable results were seen with subgroups composed of women, those with greater pain severity, those with longer pain durations, older age, those with sciatica, or those with spinal radiographic findings.

Hansen et al.[44] randomized 150 patients with chronic or recurrent low back pain to three groups: intensive back muscle exercises, conventional physiotherapy with isometric exercises for trunk and leg muscles, or placebo treatment using semihot packs and light traction. Biweekly treatment was continued for 4 weeks, with follow-up at program completion, and 1, 6, and 12 months after program completion. On variables of pain and treatment effect, intensive back exercise appeared to be most effective for women or for those with sedentary or light jobs. Men or those with more strenuous jobs fared better with physiotherapy.

MANIPULATIVE THERAPY

Meade et al.[80] conducted a multicentered RCT of chiropractic manipulation or outpatient hospital treatment for chronic low back pain. Seven hundred forty-one patients between the ages of 18 and 65 were treated according to discretion of the respective clinicians and followed for 2 years. Outcomes included a disability questionnaire and mobility measures. Chiropractic treatment was more effective for patients with more severe or chronic back pain.

Koes et al.[81] conducted an RCT with 256 patients with nonspecific back and neck pain of at least 6 weeks duration, who had received no manual or physiotherapy in the last 2 years. The physiotherapy condition included exercise, massage, heat, electrotherapy, ultrasound, and short-wave diathermy. Manual therapy included manipulation and mobilization of the spine. General practitioner treatment included medication, advice, home exercise, and bed rest. The placebo condition involved nonfunctioning diathermy and ultrasound devices. In patients with pain complaints of a year or greater, and in those younger than 40, pain improvement and physical functioning were greatest with manual therapy, followed by physiotherapy. Global perceived improvement was greater with these treatments than with general practitioner or placebo treatment.

Anderson et al.[82] conducted a meta-analysis of 23 RCTs that compared spinal manipulation therapy to nonmanipulative or sham therapies for low back pain. Of the 44 effect sizes, 38 indicated that spinal manipulation was better than the comparison therapy. Higher effect sizes were found in younger patients and in those who had experienced back pain for 6 or fewer weeks. Some of the overall effect sizes were pain, 0.38; global clinician rating, 0.38; global patient rating, 0.18; flexion, 0.34; work, 0.40; and daily activities, 0.30.

Gross et al.[83] conducted a meta-analysis about conservative management of mechanical neck disorders. From a large number of reports, 24 RCTs and eight before-after trials met selection criteria. Eight of these were adequately strong in terms of methodologic quality. In two controlled trials and two RCTs comparing manual therapy alone to another condition, no differences between groups could be demonstrated. Six studies involved manual therapy combined with other forms of physical medicine, drug, or education treatments. The study population's diagnoses varied from acute to chronic.

The pooled effect sizes of five similar trials yielded an effect size of –0.6 at 1 to 4 weeks, which is consistent with moderate to large pain reduction, and an effect size of –0.5 at 6 to 8 weeks treatment, which is consistent with moderate pain improvement. Two combined trials using EMG therapy showed significantly reduced pain. Two combined trials using laser therapy failed to show significant effect. Single studies involving spray-and-stretch, infrared light, and exercise with drug therapy and advice lacked sufficient evidence to independently confirm a significant effect. Two acupuncture RCTs and three traction RCTs provided insufficient extractable data to confirm significant effect. A controlled trial of TENS showed no significant difference between TENS and comparison groups.

Although trials using muscle relaxants and anti-inflammatory drugs were reported as showing significant improvements, data or methodologic problems prevented the authors from drawing conclusions from studies of analgesics, relaxants, or anti-inflammatory drugs. On one trial, short-term pain reduction was attributed to patient education, relaxation, and exercise (benefits were not evident after 8 weeks). In the 8 studies involving education along with other components, however, the design or data would not allow for confirmation of the effects of education.

Summary

Evidence suggests that manipulation and physical therapy may be better than medical or no treatment. In some studies, manipulation or mobilization appears to be more efficacious than physical therapy, but it is likely that physical therapy for subacute or chronic pain is less efficacious than exercise and activation. Comparative studies have not yet been performed between manipulative therapies and multimodal or behavioral therapies. There is some contradictory evidence regarding whether manipulation or mobilization are effective in pain of longer duration.[76,80,82]

PHARMACOLOGIC TREATMENT

The pharmacologic treatment of chronic pain can involve the use of medications for the treatment of the pain intensity itself or the use of medications to treat conditions (especially depression or anxiety) associated with the chronic pain.

Antidepressants

Antidepressants, particularly the tricyclic antidepressants (TCAs), are useful in management of neuralgias and prevention of headaches. In "mixed" categories of chronic pain sufferers, tricyclic antidepressants such as doxepin also may be of some benefit.[84,85] Not all chronic pain sufferers respond to antidepressants, and analgesic effects may not be demonstrable after a few months.[49,74,86] The analgesic effects from antidepressants are sometimes linked to the coexistence of a treatable depression,[84,85,87] and often the analgesic effect is independent of depression.[88–91]

There are a few studies of monoamine oxidase inhibitors (MAOIs)[92,93] and of the newer selective serotonin reuptake inhibitors (SSRIs)[94,95] for pain conditions. There are no studies of combination treatments for pain with depression, such as combining TCAs with some SSRIs.

A meta-analytic study demonstrated the greatest effect sizes with TCAs and lesser effect associated with heterocyclic agents.[96] Larger effect sizes appeared to be linked more with mixed effects than to serotonergic or adrenergic reuptake inhibition. The disorders associated with larger effect sizes were headaches and neuralgias. In that study, effect sizes were not associated with organic or psychic diagnoses, the coexistence of depression, or the antidepressant effect of the drug.[96]

Summary of Antidepressant Use

The old debate as to whether pain causes depression or depression causes pain can be resolved with the recognition that each predicts the other; that is, there is a complex biopsychosocial causality. One should recognize the importance of affective disturbance. Whether or not antidepressants are attempted for pain treatment, antidepressants should be considered in the presence of psychological indicators of a treatable affective condition.

At least a temporary analgesic effect has been found for some antidepressants in some pain conditions. There is still no theory to adequately predict or explain this analgesic effect, which in many cases is independent of antidepressant effect. When it occurs, the effect is often mild and temporary.

Pharmacologic Agents as Analgesics in Musculoskeletal Pain

Back Pain

Although acute back pain benefits from short-term use of nonsteroidal analgesics, the efficacy of medications in chronic low back pain has not been proven.[4,74] In fact, patients with chronic back pain referred to pain clinics often present with dependencies, abuse, or addiction to analgesics and sedatives.

Withdrawal of these drugs is usually a component of treatment in chronic pain management programs.

Zitman et al.[97] conducted a double-blind RCT comparing amitriptyline to placebo. Pain diagnoses were mixed, with mean duration of 5.1 years, and mean number of surgical operations at 1.3. Severe psychiatric disorders were excluded, but 20 patients had Axis I psychiatric disorders. At the baseline, the placebo group had higher pain levels.

By 12 weeks, the pain levels in placebo and amitriptyline groups were no longer significantly different. The only apparent significant difference was a transient improvement in hours slept, at 2 weeks, in the amitriptyline group. As with the Pilowsky et al. study,[49] the lack of clear evidence of effect also should be considered in the light of the patient population, which included a high percentage of psychogenic pain diagnoses in very chronic pain patients who did not exhibit major depression. These patients would have a low likelihood of responding to antidepressants and would not be the patients normally chosen for such treatment.

Hameroff et al.[85] conducted a double-blind RCT comparing doxepin and placebo, in 30 patients suffering chronic low back and/or neck pain with depression. Presumably, they were quite chronic—the mean number of surgeries was 1.4 with a range of 0 to 15. Doses used were consistent with antidepressant effect. Doxepin was significantly better than placebo in relieving depression and psychological distress, sleep disturbance, and incidence of pain.

Pheasant et al.[98] conducted a randomized double-blind crossover study of amitriptyline in low back pain. The active drug was significantly associated with greater reduction in analgesic use and improved mood, but not activity level.

Chronic Fibromyalgia

Quimby et al.[99] reported a double-blind RCT comparing cyclobenzaprine and placebo for chronic fibromyalgia. Some but not all patients improved with cyclobenzaprine; more improved with cyclobenzapine than with placebo.

Carette et al.[86] compared amitriptyline, cyclobenzaprine, and placebo, in a double-blind RCT in 208 patients with chronic fibromyalgia. At 1 month, clinical improvement was found in 21% and 12% of amitriptyline and cyclobenzaprine patients, respectively, and in no patients treated with placebo. At 6 months, improvement was found in 36% and 33% of amitriptyline and cyclobenzaprine patients, respectively, and in 19% of the placebo group. Thus, the short-term analgesic effect of the active drug was significantly better than placebo, but could not be demonstrated on long-term follow-up.

In a small RCT (only nine patients with fibromyalgia completed the study) comparing cyclobenzaprine with placebo, Reynolds et al.[100] found that pain, tenderness, sleep, and mood were unchanged by cyclobenzaprine. With such a small sample size, a significant difference could easily be undetected.

Jaeschke et al.[101] conducted 23 double-blind multiple cross-over N-of-1 RCTs using amitriptyline for the treatment of fibromyalgia. Symptoms and tender points were assessed. By symptom questionnaires, 18 of 23 trials favored amitriptyline, but only seven of these trials reached statistical significance. Five of 23 trials favored placebo. By tender point count, 15 favored amitriptyline, but only four reached statistical significance, and seven trials favored placebo. The variables associated with the greatest statistical significance were combined symptoms questionnaire and tender point counts. Symptoms significantly associated with improvement included energy, aches and pains, sleep, headache, tiredness, stiffness, and bowel problems. Generally, when benefit was noted with amitriptyline, it occurred immediately or within the first 2 weeks.

CHRONIC HEADACHE

This category of persistent pain is commonly seen in chronic pain clinics as the main presenting problem, or in association with other chronic pain problems. Although RCT literature regarding this problem is sparse, there is a good level of consensus regarding its significance and management.

About three-fourths of these cases represent transformed migraine. In these headaches, migraine symptoms have gradually increased in frequency along with unsuccessful and escalating use of abortive medications, until the pattern is of a daily or near-daily headache with mixed picture of ten-sion headache alternating with more severe vascular features. About one-fourth of these cases begin with tension-type headaches or sudden-onset chronic headache, or the chronic pattern has been precipitated by an accident.[102]

Excessive and prolonged use of combinations of abortive medication appears to be etiologic in many of these cases. Medications responsible include acetaminophen or acetylsalicylic acid, usually in combination drugs, ergotamine, caffeine, and opiates.[102,103]

Detoxification

About 75 percent of patients who cease their excessive daily use of these substances improve significantly—that 25 percent do not, demonstrates that other factors are also at work in the etiology of this problem.

Those who do not improve usually do not become worse when they stop taking their daily abortive medications.[103–105] The chronic headache, however, may be difficult to treat because of poor compliance with the detoxification regimen. If patients continue to abuse mixed analgesics and ergotamine, the headache is less likely to respond to appropriate prophylactic drugs. In these cases, one option is to admit the patient to an environment in which medical and psychological support can be given, and compliance monitored.

On an inpatient basis it is possible to use intravenous dihydroergotamine or intravenous hydrocortisone to break the headache cycle.[102,106] Intravenous dihydroergotamine also has been used on an outpatient basis.[107] Such regimens have good efficacy when measured at short-[64] and long-term follow-up.[108]

A controlled clinical trial has shown good efficacy of dihydroergotamine at 2 days, and two-thirds of patients sustained benefit at a mean of 15 months. A comparison group of diazepam-treated patients had a significantly worse short- and long-term outcome.[106]

The challenge is to convince patients to accept detoxification. This goal is difficult to achieve because (1) the pain is often severe, (2) patients tend to panic when their headache worsens, (3) many abortive medications are available without prescription, and (4) patients often observe that there is short-term partial pain relief when they take their analgesics and a sudden aggravation of the chronic headache when they miss a dose. Most chronic headache sufferers experience psychological disturbance, especially depression and anxiety, which may require treatment with antidepressants.

Offending medications often can be withdrawn on an outpatient basis with education and support.[105] For the most part, it is necessary to institute prophylactic medications, singly or in combination, to reduce the frequency of headaches. These medications include β-adrenergic blockers, TCAs, calcium channel blockers, and methysergide. Patients must be informed that most prophylactic medications do not work well if the abused drugs are still being used, and that the beneficial effects of detoxification may not appear for 1 to several weeks.

Prophylaxis

Although controlled studies have shown that β-adrenergic blockers such as propranolol or metoprolol, calcium channel blockers such as verapamil or flunarizine, and TCAs such as amitriptyline or pizotyline are effective in chronic headache prophylaxis,[109–115] behavioral treatments are at least as effective.[51] SSRIs have shown promise in a few controlled studies,[94,95] but their relative effects on the variables of pain and depression need to be clarified. Few controlled studies involving MAOIs for headache have been published.[92,93]

Supportive Therapies

Physical Therapies

Relevant therapies include active exercise, diets to minimize headache triggers, reduced smoking, improved sleeping habits, and instruction in good posture and body mechanics.[102,116] Uncontrolled studies of treatments using spray-and-stretch and massage for myofascial features and splint therapy or occlusal correction have been published.[117] One controlled study casts doubt on the efficacy of splint therapy.[118]

Psychological Treatment

In the context of patient education and detoxification from medications of abuse, other treatments have included biofeedback,[72] imagery, self-hypnosis, and relaxation therapies.[119,120] Multimodal therapies also have been used.[102]

PAIN WITH DEPRESSION

Patients who are referred to pain clinics have a much higher prevalence of psychological distress than those who are not referred.[2] A purely behavioral approach to persistent pain management is probably effective and appropriate in many but not all cases, because many patients demonstrate comorbidity of chronic pain and serious depression and other serious psychiatric symptoms.[121–124] Some studies suggest that psychological disturbances such as depression cause pain.[92,125–127] Other studies suggest that depression is a result of persistent pain,[122,123] rather than a function of preexisting psychodynamic factors.[128] One study suggests that persistent pain predicts depression, and almost equally depression predicts pain.[121] Patients who are both depressed and in pain show greater pain intensity and impairment and greater pain behavior.[129] The best care will probably be provided if judicious and selective use of antidepressants is a cotreatment of associated psychiatric disorders, especially depression and anxiety.

Pharmacologic Treatment

In terms of pharmacologic treatment of depression associated with chronic pain the following recommendations are made:

1. If the depression is (a) persistent for several months, (b) significantly interfering with function or treatment, (c) causing moderate to severe distress, (d) associated with a clinically significant degree of psychological distress such as anxiety, anger, or suicidal thoughts, (e) has diagnostic characteristics of major depression, (f) occurs in a patient with a previous history or significant family history of major depression, it requires independent treatment.
2. If antidepressants have been used previously but have not been effective, one should determine if

adequate doses were taken for sufficient time, or if there were limiting side effects.

3. Drug classes that were taken adequately but without adequate result would not be the drugs of first choice.

4. In general, if insomnia is a problem, the more sedating TCAs may be used. The less sedating antidepressants may be preferable for depressions associated with poor energy. TCAs also may be considered for their possible analgesic effects for some pain types.

5. If poorly tolerated, SSRIs may be used, with or without a modest evening dose of desipramine or amitriptyline (TCAs), which might potentiate the antidepressant effect.

6. For resistant depressions, other agents such as MAOIs, lithium, or carbamazepine (for bipolar sufferers only) or atypical antidepressants such as trazodone or venlafaxine can be used.

7. Most antidepressants will alleviate the anxiety symptoms or anxiety disorders that are commonly associated with pain and depression.

Psychotherapy

Psychological treatments are also effective in treatment of psychological distress associated with pain; but the studies of individual or group psychotherapies for pain have been few, often flawed, and consistent data are still lacking. The clinical impression is that in multimodal treatment, or in treatment of subacute or chronic pain, at least supportive psychotherapy is necessary. In selected cases, it is necessary to provide family intervention or individual psychotherapy. Many multimodal therapies depend on group treatment to facilitate support, reinforcement, patient education, and corrective emotional experience.

ALGORITHMS FOR CHRONIC PAIN MANAGEMENT

The algorithm presented here is based on evidence from controlled trials where possible and on clinical experience where good studies are not available. Scientific data come from clinical trials, follow-up studies, and epidemiologic studies dealing with chronic pain. The monograph by Bigos et al.[74] reviews the available controlled studies of acute back pain and presents algorithms for acute pain assessment and treatment.

The overall perspective presented in the algorithms is that acute pain needs to be managed expeditiously to prevent complications or impairments (Fig. 6-1). In a minority of cases, pain problems may become recurrent or persistent. At about 3 months of nonresolution or of recurrent pain episodes, the pain problem should be carefully reevaluated from a medical, rehabilitational, and psychiatric point of view. In many cases, a physical activation program with work-reentry focus is required, especially if sicklisting is an issue. Depression or psychological distress may become evident as complicating factors at the subacute or chronic stages. As pain becomes chronic, case management, functional rehabilitation, and psychological treatment are likely needed in the context of a multimodal program.

Over the span of injury, pain, and chronicity, there should be an ongoing assessment of outcomes (Fig. 6-1). Treatments effective at the acute stage may be ineffective at the subacute or chronic stage. It is necessary to increase the emphasis on restoration of function, on behavioral-psychological techniques, and multimodal intervention in the subacute and chronic stages of pain. As one reaches the subacute or chronic pain stages, one must evaluate the treatment plan in the light of demonstrated efficacy of treatment measures for that stage of pain.

Acute Pain

Acute pain can be conceptualized as pain associated with a temporary physical condition, in parallel with a process and timeline of natural healing and resolution. This process is expected to run its course in a matter of days to weeks. In the case of acute or recurrent back pain, the general principles are to promote healing, protect, palliate, and progressively restore function. These goals might be achieved by judicious use of rest and modification or restriction of activity, time-limited use of analgesic or relaxants, and maintenance of an expectation of normal recovery while progressively restoring daily activity and implementing exercise. The vast majority of acute pain episodes resolve in days to weeks. A small but

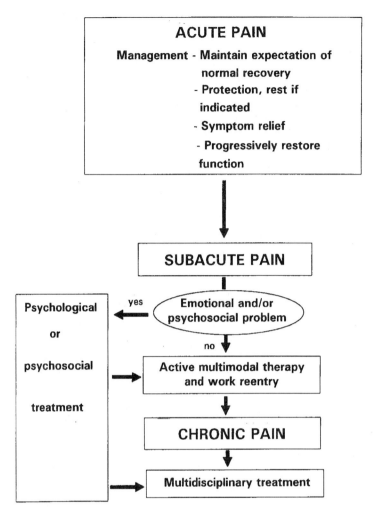

Fig. 6-1. Management of acute, subacute, and chronic pain.

important minority (about 5 to 10 percent) develop subacute or recurrent pain.

Subacute Pain

Subacute pain might be conceptualized as pain lasting more than the normal tissue healing time (usually 1 to 8 weeks), enduring 3 months or more, or being recurrent past the normal time of resolution (Fig. 6-2). Management should include patient education and counseling, with active physical treatment rather than passive modalities. Manipulative treatment may be of value as well, although the relative efficacy of manipulative therapies with respect to active exercise has not been investigated. If there is sicklisting or functional impairment in daily activity because of the pain, a multifaceted treatment program is indicated, consisting of education, counseling or back school, some form of coping skills training or relaxation training, and active exercise with progressive quotas, work hardening, and work reentry. In some settings, the program might involve referral to a specific multimodal treatment unit or early intervention unit, but there is no reason that a primary care worker cannot coordinate such a program if access to the necessary treatment elements were available. Vocational counseling and liaison with the workplace are strongly advisable.

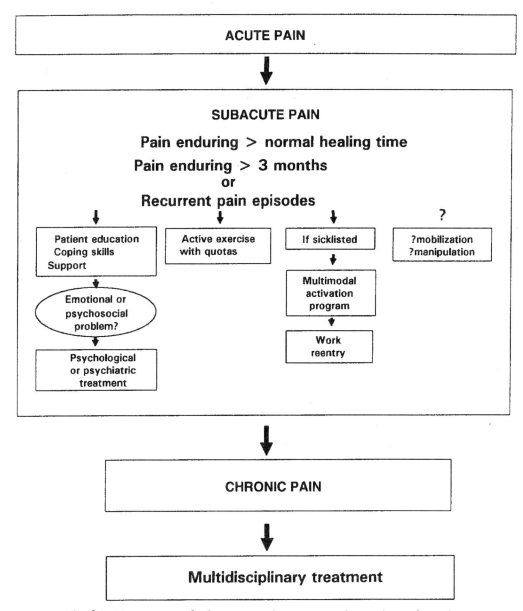

Fig. 6-2. Management of subacute pain (approximate duration) 3 to 6 months.

Persistent Pain

Barriers to recovery such as psychosocial problems or depression should be identified and psychological, psychosocial, or psychopharmacologic treatment initiated (Fig. 6-3). Untreated psychosocial problems and depressions can seriously impair function, prolong recovery, and interfere with rehabilitation.

Depression and other psychological or social problems frequently coexist with and may be triggered by persistent pain. Treatment may be pharmacologic and/or psychological. In many patients, active rehabilitation treatment, or even the knowledge that active rehabilitation is to begin, has a therapeutic effect in relieving anxiety and depression. However, more serious mood disturbance,

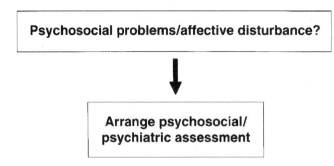

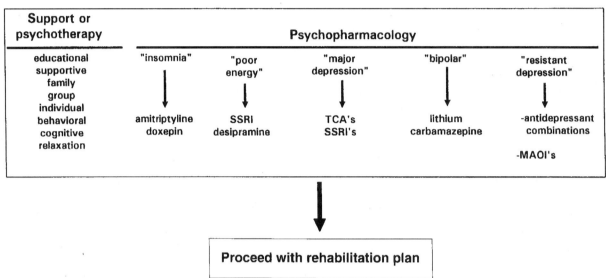

Fig. 6-3. Psychosocial intervention for subacute or chronic pain.

and in some cases major depressions, can also occur.

Pharmacologic Aids

Pharmacologic treatment may be useful in several types of situations.

1. A TCA may be indicated for a specific pain syndrome (e.g., chronic headache or neuralgia).
2. For pain associated with insomnia, sedating antidepressants may be helpful (e.g., amitriptyline, doxepin, trazodone).
3. For persistent pain associated with fatigue or poor energy, and depression with hypersomnia and fatigue, energizing antidepressants such as desipramine or SSRIs can be used.

4. For major typical and atypical bipolar depression, lithium carbonate and carbamazepine are some drugs of choice.
5. For resistant depressions and dysthymias, MAOIs and combination antidepressant regimens may be used.

Psychotherapy

Psychotherapy (supportive, individual, group, or family) should be used in the treatment of psychological complications.

1. Supportive psychotherapy is the key ingredient in any healthy and productive client-clinician relationship.
2. Supportive therapy is always necessary when treatment is multimodal, when compliance is a

problem, when morale is poor, when there is affective distress, when several agencies may fragment the therapeutic alliance, or when there is a family or social problem.

3. Supportive therapy is always necessary when psychotropic medication is being used for serious psychological distress or major depression.

4. More intensive psychotherapies are often necessary to deal with personality adjustment and family problems that are often comorbid with chronic pain.

Chronic State

If improvement has not occurred despite such active functionally oriented treatment, consideration should be given for referral to a multimodal chronic pain clinic.

If pain becomes chronic, there needs to be a broad reevaluation of the problem from a medical, psychological, functional, and social perspective (Fig. 6-4). (For this discussion 6 months is used as a marker for chronicity, although 3 to 6 months can be considered the beginning of chronicity.) A multimodal treatment program is usually required. The probability of significant psychological or social adjustment problems is about 25 to 50 percent. Such problems must be identified and treated appropriately.

Referral to a multimodal pain clinic should be considered, but whether or not a specific chronic pain service is available, a multimodal treatment approach is needed. Treatment should include an educational component dealing with acceptance of chronic pain management instead of pain cures and passive treatments, and with the distinction of hurt versus harm. Treatment should include coping skills training (or

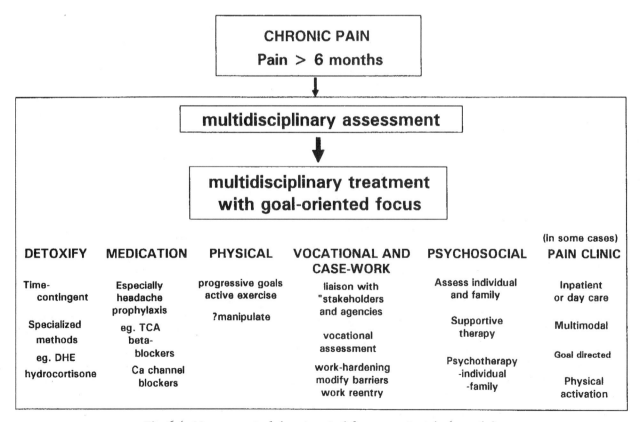

Fig. 6-4. Management of chronic pain (after approximately 6 months).

an equivalent, such as relaxation training). Personal responsibility for activity should be promoted through progressive goals of restoration of family roles, personal function, and working roles.

If abuse of analgesics and various other drugs or alcohol has become a complicating factor, detoxification is required along with behavioral techniques to promote self-help and coping skills. Exercise should be quota-based, progressive, and relevant to the work and personal life-style requirements of the individual. Vocational counseling and liaison with the workplace are strongly advisable.

Medical Treatment

Medical treatments appropriate to a multimodal chronic pain clinic include the following pharmacologic measures:

1. Abused medication may be systematically withdrawn either by masked solution or goal-setting and quotas, both using time-contingent dosing and gradual withdrawal. With some headache problems, withdrawal of abortive analgesic medication may be supported by prescription of hydrocortisone or dihydroergotamine injections, followed by prescription of prophylactic medication.
2. Certain drug regimens are effective in pain relief itself (e.g., capsaicin, TCAs, or anticonvulsants in neuralgia pain).
3. For chronic headache, a variety of medications may be used in prophylaxis (e.g., amitriptyline, some calcium-channel blockers, and β-adrenergic blockers).
4. There is some limited benefit from muscle relaxants and TCA in the treatment of chronic fibromyalgia (e.g., cyclobenzaprine or amitriptyline).

Physical Treatments

Physical treatments appropriate for chronic pain, especially chronic low back pain, include the following:

1. Active exercise, especially when there is use of patient-endorsed goals, and progressive quotas are important.

2. Manipulation or mobilization is beneficial in spinal pain of short duration and may be of some benefit for subacute or chronic low back pain and appears to be as effective as, or more effective than, passive physical therapy. Although comparison studies have not yet been carried out, active multimodal therapies will likely prove more effective than manipulation/mobilization.

REFERENCES

1. Tunks E: Is there a chronic pain syndrome? p. 257. In Lipton S, Tunks E, Zoppi M (eds): Advances in Pain Research and Therapy. Vol. 13. Raven Press, New York, 1990
2. Crook J, Tunks E, Rideout E, Browne G: Epidemiologic comparison of persistent pain sufferers in a specialty pain clinic and in the community. Arch Phys Med Rehabil 67:451, 1986
3. Spengler DM, Bigos SJ, Martin NA et al: Back injuries in industry: a retrospective study. I. Overview and cost analysis. Spine 3:241, 1986
4. Spitzer WO, Abenhaim L, Dupuis M et al: Scientific approach to the assessment and management of activity-related spinal disorders. Spine, suppl. 7, 12:S1, 1987
5. Magora A: Investigation of the relation between low back pain and occupation. Industr Med Surg 39:504, 1970
6. Magora A: Investigation of the relation between low back pain and occupation. V. Psychological Aspects. Scand J Rehabil Med 5:191, 1973
7. Roberts AH, Reinhardt L: The behavioral management of chronic pain: long-term follow-up with comparison groups. Pain 8:151, 1980
8. Aronoff GM, Evans WO, Enders PL: A review of follow-up studies of multidisciplinary pain units. Pain 16:1, 1983
9. Guck TP, Skultety FM, Meilman PW, Dowd ET: Multidisciplinary pain center follow-up study: evaluation with a no-treatment control group. Pain 21:295, 1985
10. Mayer TG, Gatchel RJ, Kishino N et al: Objective assessment of spine function following industrial injury. Spine 10:482, 1985
11. Deardorff WW, Rubin HS, Scott DW: Comprehensive multidisciplinary treatment of chronic pain: a follow-up study of treated and non-treated groups. Pain 45:35, 1991
12. Linton SJ, Melin L, Stjernlöf K: The effects of applied relaxation and operant activity training on chronic pain. Behav Psychother 13:87, 1985

13. Peters JL, Large RG: A randomised control trial evaluating in- and outpatient pain management programmes. Pain 41:283, 1990

14. Talo S, Rytökoski U, Puukka P: Patient classification, a key to evaluate pain treatment: a psychological study in chronic low back pain patients. Spine 17:998, 1992

15. Alaranta H, Rytökoski U, Rissanen A et al: Intensive physical and psychosocial training program for patients with chronic low back pain: a controlled clinical trial. Spine 19:1339, 1994

16. Turner JA, Clancy S, McQuade KJ, Cardenas DD: Effectiveness of behavioral therapy for chronic low back pain: a component analysis. J Consult Clin Psychol 58:573, 1990

17. Heinrich RL, Cohen MJ, Naliboff BO et al: Comparing physical and behavior therapy for chronic low-back pain on physical abilities, psychological distress, and patients' perception. J Behav Med 8:61, 1985

18. Nicholas MK, Wilson PH, Goyen J: Operant-behavioral and cognitive-behavioral treatment for chronic low back pain. Behav Res Ther 29:225, 1991

19. Nicholas MK, Wilson PH, Goyen J: Comparison of cognitive-behavioral group treatment and an alternative non-psychological treatment for chronic low back pain. Pain 48:339, 1992

20. McArthur DL, Cohen MJ, Gottlieb HJ et al: Treating chronic low back pain. I. Admissions to initial follow-up. Pain 29:1, 1987

21. McArthur DL, Cohen MJ, Gottlieb HJ et al: Treating chronic low back pain. II. Long-term follow-up. Pain 29:23, 1987

22. Crook J, Weir R, Tunks E: An epidemiological follow-up survey of persistent pain sufferers in a group family practice and specialty pain clinic. Pain 36:49, 1989

23. Maruta T, Swanson DW, McHardy MJ: Three year follow-up of patients with chronic pain who were treated in a multidisciplinary pain management center. Pain 41:47, 1990

24. Härkäpää K, Mellin G, Järvikoski A, Hurri H: A controlled study on the outcome of inpatient and outpatient treatment of low back pain. Scand J Rehabil Med 22:181, 1990

25. Mellin G, Härkäpää K, Hurri H, Järvikoski A: A controlled study on the outcome of inpatient and outpatient treatment of low back pain. Scand J Rehabil Med 22:189, 1990

26. Lindstrom I, Öhlund C, Eek C et al: The effect of graded activity on patients with subacute low back pain: a randomized prospective clinical study with an operant-conditioning behavioral approach. Phys Ther 72:279, 1992

27. Eastwood M: Epidemiological studies in psychosomatic medicine. p. 411. In Lipowski ZJ, Lipsitt DR, Whybrow PW (eds): Psychosomatic Medicine. Oxford University Press, New York, 1977

28. Crook J: Women in pain. p. 113. In Copp LA (ed): Recent Advances in Nursing: Perspectives on Pain. Churchill Livingstone, Edinburgh, 1984

29. Deyo RA, Bass JE, Walsh NE et al: Prognostic variability among chronic pain patients: implications for study design, interpretation, and reporting. Arch Phys Med Rehabil 69:174, 1988

30. Turk DC, Rudy TE: Neglected factors in chronic pain treatment outcome studies—referral patterns, failure to enter treatment, and attrition. Pain 43:7, 1990

31. Bergquist-Ullman M, Larsson U: Acute low back pain in industry: a controlled prospective study with special reference to therapy and confounding factors. Acta Orthop Scand, suppl. 170:1, 1977

32. Dworkin RH, Richlin DM, Handlin DS, Brand L: Predicting treatment response in depressed and nondepressed chronic pain patients. Pain 24:343, 1986

33. Doxey NC, Dzioba RB, Mitson GL, Lacroix JM: Predictors of outcome in back surgery candidates. J Clin Psychol 44:611, 1988

34. Linton SJ, Kamwendo K: Risk factors in the psychosocial work environment for neck and shoulder pain in secretaries. J Occup Med 31:609, 1989

35. Malone MD, Strube MJ: Meta-analysis of non-medical treatments for chronic pain. Pain 34:231, 1988

36. Waddell G, Main CJ, Morris E et al: Chronic low-back pain, psychologic distress, and illness behavior. Spine 9:209, 1984

37. Dworkin RH, Handlin DS, Richlin DM et al: Unravelling the effects of compensation, litigation, and employment on treatment response in chronic pain. Pain 23:49, 1985

38. Carron H, DeGood DE, Tait R: A comparison of low back pain patients in the United States and New Zealand: psychosocial and economic factors affecting severity of disability. Pain 21:77, 1985

39. Stieg RL, Williams RC: Chronic pain as a biosociocultural phenomenon: implications for treatment. Semin Neurol 3:370, 1983

40. Philips HC, Grant L, Berkowitz J: The prevention of chronic pain and disability: a preliminary investigation. Behav Res Ther 29:443, 1991

41. Fordyce WE, Brockway JA, Bergman JA, Spengler D: Acute back pain: a control-group comparison of behavioral vs traditional management methods. J Behav Med 9:127, 1986

42. Linton SJ, Bradley LA: An 18-month follow-up of a secondary prevention program for back pain: help

and hindrance factors related to outcome mainte-nance. Clin J Pain 8:227, 1992

43. Kellett KM, Kellett DA, Nordholm LA: Effects of an exercise program on sick leave due to back pain. Phys Ther 71:283, 1991

44. Hansen FR, Bendix T, Skov P et al: Intensive, dynamic back-muscle exercises, conventional physio-therapy, or placebo-control treatment of low-back pain: a randomized, observer-blind trial. Spine 18:98, 1993

45. Kerns RD, Turk DC, Holzman AD, Rudy TE: Com-parison of cognitive-behavioral and behavioral approaches to the outpatient treatment of chronic pain. Clin J Pain 1:195, 1986

46. Dolce JJ, Crocker MF, Moletteire C, Doleys DM: Exer-cise quotas, anticipatory concern and self-efficacy expectancies in chronic pain: a preliminary report. Pain 24:365, 1986

47. Dolce JJ, Doleys DM, Raczynski JM et al: The role of self-efficacy expectancies in the prediction of pain tolerance. Pain 27:261, 1986

48. Altmaier EM, Lehmann TR, Russell DW et al: The effectiveness of psychological interventions for the rehabilitation of low back pain: a randomized con-trolled trial evaluation. Pain 49:329, 1992

49. Pilowsky I, Barrow CG: A controlled study of psy-chotherapy and amitriptyline used individually and in combination in the treatment of chronic intractable, 'psychogenic' pain. Pain 40:3, 1990

50. Pilowsky I, Spence N, Rounsefell B et al: Out-patient cognitive-behavioral therapy with amitriptyline for chronic non-malignant pain: a comparative study with 6-month follow-up. Pain 60:49, 1995

51. Holroyd KA, Nash JM, Pingen JD et al: A comparison of pharmacological (amitriptyline HCL) and nonphar-macological (cognitive-behavioral) therapies for chronic tension headaches. J Consult Clin Psychol 59:387, 1991

52. Jessup BA, Neufeld RWJ, Merskey H: Biofeedback therapy for headache and other pains: an evaluative review. Pain 7:225, 1979

53. Zitman FG: Biofeedback and chronic pain. p. 795. In Bonica JJ, Lindblom U, Iggo A (eds): Advances in Pain Research and Therapy. Vol. 5. Raven Press, New York, 1983

54. Turner JA, Romano JM: Evaluating psychologic inter-ventions for chronic pain: issues and recent develop-ments. p. 257. In Benedetti C, Chapman CR, Moricca G (eds): Advances in Pain Research and Therapy. Vol. 7. Raven Press, New York, 1984

55. Linton SJ: Behavioral remediation of chronic pain: a status report. Pain 24:125, 1986

56. Chapman SL: A review and clinical perspective on the use of EMG and thermal biofeedback for chronic headaches. Pain 27:1, 1986

57. Sanders SH: Component analysis of a behavioral treatment program for chronic low-back pain. Behav Ther 14:697, 1983

58. Linton SJ, Götestam KG: A controlled study of the effects of applied relaxation and applied relaxation plus operant procedures in the regulation of chronic pain. Br J Clin Psychol 23:291, 1984

59. Sorbi M, Tellegen B: Differential effects of training in relaxation and stress-coping in patients with migraine. Headache 26:473, 1986

60. Attanasio V, Andrasik F, Blanchard EB: Cognitive therapy and relaxation training in muscle contraction headache: efficacy and cost-effectiveness. Headache 27:254, 1987

61. Cameron R: Behavior and cognitive therapies. p. 79. In Roy R, Tunks E (eds): Chronic Pain: Psychosocial Factors in Rehabilitation. Williams & Wilkins, Balti-more, 1982

62. Turner JA, Chapman CR: Psychological interventions for chronic pain: a critical review. I. Relaxation train-ing and biofeedback. Pain 12:1, 1982

63. Kerns RD, Turk DC, Holzman AD: Psychological treatment for chronic pain: a selective review. Clin Psychol Rev 3:15, 1983

64. O'Brien CP, Weisbrot MM: Behavioral and psycholog-ical components of pain management. In Brown RM, Pinkert TM, Ludford JP (eds): Contemporary Research in Pain and Analgesia, 1983. NIDA Research Monograph 45, Washington DC, 1983

65. Turk DC, Meichenbaum D, Genest M: Pain and Behavioral Medicine: A Cognitive-Behavioral Per-spective. Guilford, New York, 1983

66. Keefe FJ, Bradley LA: Behavioral and psychological approaches to the assessment and treatment of chronic pain. Gen Hosp Psychiatry 6:49, 1984

67. Trifiletti RJ: The psychological effectiveness of pain management procedures in the context of behavioral medicine and medical psychology. Genet Psychol Monogr 109:251, 1984

68. Turk DC, Flor H: Etiological theories and treatments for chronic back pain. II. Psychological models and interventions. Pain 19:209, 1984

69. Bell NW, Abramowitz SI, Folkins CH et al: Biofeed-back, brief psychotherapy, and tension headache. Headache 23:162, 1983

70. Lacroix JM, Clarke MA, Carson Bock J, Doxey NCS: Muscle-contraction headaches in multiple-pain patients: treatment under worsening baseline condi-tions. Arch Phys Med Rehabil 67:14, 1986

71. Flor H, Haag G, Turk DC: Long-term efficacy of EMG biofeedback for chronic rheumatic back pain. Pain 27:195, 1986

72. Holroyd KA, Penzien DB: Pharmacological versus non-pharmacological prophylaxis of recurrent migraine headache: a meta-analytic review of clinical trials. Pain 42:1, 1990

73. Flor H, Fydrich T, Turk DC: Efficacy of multidisciplinary pain treatment centers: a meta-analytic review. Pain 49:221, 1992

74. Bigos SJ, Bowyer OR, Braen GR et al: Acute low back problems in adults. Clinical Practice Guideline Number 14. US Dept of Health and Human Services, Rockville, Maryland, 1994

75. Flor H, Turk DC: Etiological theories and treatments for chronic back pain. I. Somatic models and interventions. Pain 19:105, 1984

76. Nachemson AL: Newest knowledge of low back pain: a critical look. Clin Orthop 279:8, 1992

77. Malmivaara A, Hakkinen U, Aro T et al: The treatment of acute low back pain—bed rest, exercises, or ordinary activity? N Engl J Med 332:351, 1995

78. Mitchell RI, Carmen GM: Results of a multicenter trial using an intensive active exercise program for the treatment of acute soft tissue and back injuries. Spine 15:514, 1990

79. Manniche C, Lundberg E, Christensen I et al: Intensive dynamic back exercises for chronic low back pain: a clinical trial. Pain 47:53, 1991

80. Meade TW, Dyer S, Browne W et al: Low back pain of mechanical origin: randomised comparison of chiropractic and hospital outpatient treatment. BMJ 300:1431, 1990

81. Koes BW, Bouter LM, van Mameren H et al: A randomized clinical trial of manual therapy and physiotherapy for persistent back and neck complaints: subgroup analysis and relationship between outcome measures. J Manipulative Physiol Ther 16:211, 1993

82. Anderson R, Meeker WC, Wirick BE et al: A meta-analysis of clinical trials of spinal manipulation. J Manipulative Physiol Ther 15:181, 1992

83. Gross AR, Aker PD, Goldsmith CH, Peloso P: Conservative management of mechanical neck disorders: a systematic overview and meta-analysis. Online J Curr Clin Trials, in press, 1996

84. Ward NG, Bloom GL, Friedel RO: The effectiveness of tricyclic antidepressants in the treatment of coexisting pain and depression. Pain 7:331, 1979

85. Hameroff SR, Cork RC, Scherer K et al: Doxepin effects on chronic pain, depression and plasma opioids. J Clin Psychiatry 43:22, 1982

86. Carette S, Bell MJ, Reynolds WJ et al: Comparison of amitriptyline, cyclobenzaprine, and placebo in the treatment of fibromyalgia: a randomized, double-blind clinical trial. Arthritis Rheum 37:32, 1994

87. Turkington RW: Depression masquerading as diabetic neuropathy. JAMA 21:1147, 1980

88. McQuay HJ, Carroll D, Glynn CJ: Low dose amitriptyline in the treatment of chronic pain. Anaesthesia 47:646, 1992

89. McQuay HJ, Carroll D, Glynn CJ: Dose-response for analgesic effect of amitriptyline in chronic pain. Anaesthesia 48:281, 1993

90. Max MB, Lynch SA, Muir J et al: Effects of desipramine, amitriptyline, and fluoxetine on pain in diabetic neuropathy. N Engl J Med 326:1250, 1992

91. Watson CP, Chipman M, Reed K et al: Amitriptyline versus maprotiline in post-herpetic neuralgia: a randomized, double-blind, crossover trial. Pain 48:29, 1992

92. Lascelles RG: Atypical facial pain and depression. Br J Psychiatry 112:651, 1966

93. Turkewitz LJ, Casaly JS, Dawson GA, Wirth O: Phenelzine therapy for headache patients with concomitant depression and anxiety. Headache 32:203, 1992

94. Bánk J: A comparative study of amitriptyline and fluvoxamine in migraine prophylaxis. Headache 34:476, 1994

95. Manna V, Bolino F, Di Cicco L: Chronic tension-type headache, mood depression and serotonin: therapeutic effects of fluvoxamine and mianserine. Headache 34:44, 1994

96. Onghena P, Van Houdenhove B: Antidepressant-induced analgesia in chronic non-malignant pain: a meta-analysis of 39 placebo-controlled studies. Pain 49:205, 1992

97. Zitman FG, Linssen ACG, Edelbroek PM, Stijnen T: Low dose amitriptyline in chronic pain: the gain is modest. Pain 42:35, 1990

98. Pheasant H, Bursk A, Goldfarb J et al: Amitriptyline and chronic low-back pain: a randomized double-blind crossover study. Spine 8:552, 1983

99. Quimby LG, Gratwick GM, Whitney CD, Block SR: A randomized trial of cyclobenzaprine for the treatment of fibromyalgia. J Rheumatol, suppl. 19, 16:140, 1989

100. Reynolds WJ, Moldofsky H, Saskin P, Lue FA: The effects of cyclobenzaprine on sleep physiology and symptoms in patients with fibromyalgia. J Rheumatol 18:452, 1991

101. Jaeschke R, Adachi J, Guyatt G et al: Clinical usefulness of amitriptyline in fibromyagia: the results of 23

N-of-1 randomized controlled trials. J Rheumatol 18:447, 1991

102. Lake AE III, Saper JR, Madden SF, Kreeger C: Comprehensive inpatient treatment for intractable migraine: a prospective long-term outcome study. Headache 33:55, 1993

103. Kudrow L: Paradoxical effects of frequent analgesic use. p. 335. In Critchley M, Friedman AP, Gorini S, Sicuteri F (eds): Advances in Neurology. Vol. 33. Headache: Physiopathological and Clinical Concepts. Raven Press, New York, 1982

104. Spierings EL, Miree LF: Non-compliance with follow-up and improvement after treatment at a headache center. Headache 33:205, 1993

105. Hering R, Steiner TJ: Abrupt outpatient withdrawal of medication in analgesic-abusing migraineurs. Lancet 337:1442, 1991

106. Raskin NH: Repetitive intravenous dihydroergotamine as therapy for intractable migraine. Neurology 36:995, 1986

107. Robbins L, Remmes A: Outpatient repetitive intravenous dihydroergotamine. Headache 32:455, 1992

108. Silberstein SD, Silberstein JR: Chronic daily headache: long-term prognosis following inpatient treatment with repetitive IV DHE. Headache 32:439, 1992

109. Gerber WD, Diener HC, Scholz E, Niederberger U: Responders and non-responders to metoprolol, propranolol, and nifedipine treatment in migraine prophylaxis: a dose-range study based on time-series analysis. Cephalalgia 11:37, 1991

110. Leone M, Grazzi L, La Mantia L, Bussone G: Flunarizine in migraine: a minireview. Headache 31:388, 1991

111. Gawel MJ, Kreeft J, Nielson RF et al: Comparison of the efficacy and safety of flunarizine to propranolol in the prophylaxis of migraine. Can J Neurol Sci 19:340, 1992

112. Sorensen PS, Larsen BH, Rasmussen MJ et al: Flunarizine versus metoprolol in migraine prophylaxis: a double-blind, randomized parallel group study of efficacy and tolerability. Headache 31:650, 1991

113. Mastrosimone F, Iaccarino C, de Caterina G: Efficacy and tolerance of cyclandelate versus pizotifen in the prophylaxis of migraine. J Med 23:1, 1992

114. Lamsudin R, Sadjimin T: Comparison of the efficacy between flunarizine and nifedipine in the prophylaxis of migraine. Headache 33:335, 1993

115. Ziegler DK, Hurwitz A, Preskorn S et al: Propranolol and amitriptyline in prophylaxis of migraine. Arch Neurol 50:825, 1993

116. Scharff L, Marcus DA: Interdisciplinary outpatient group treatment of intractable headache. Headache 34:73, 1984

117. Graff-Radford SB, Reeves JL, Jaeger B: Management of chronic head and neck pain: effectiveness of altering factors perpetuating myofascial pain. Headache 27:186, 1987

118. Dao TTT, Lavigne GJ, Charbonneau A et al: The efficacy of oral splints in the treatment of myofascial pain of the jaw muscles: a controlled clinical trial. Pain 56:85, 1994

119. Spinhoven P, Linssen AC, Van Dyck R, Zitman FG: Autogenic training and self-hypnosis in the control of tension headache. Gen Hosp Psychiatry 14:408, 1992

120. Llacqua GE: Migraine headaches: coping efficacy of guided imagery training. Headache 34:99, 1994

121. Magni G, Moreschi C, Rigatti-Luchini S, Merskey H: Prospective study on the relationship between depressive symptoms and chronic musculoskeletal pain. Pain 56:289, 1994

122. Atkinson JH, Slater MA, Grant I et al: Depressed mood in chronic low back pain: relationship with stressful life events. Pain 35:47, 1988

123. Brown GK: A causal analysis of chronic pain and depression. J Abnormal Psychology 99:127, 1990

124. Sullivan MJL, Reesor K, Mikail S, Fisher R: The treatment of depression in chronic low back pain: review and recommendations. Pain 50:5, 1992

125. Engel GL: Psychogenic pain and the pain-prone patient. Am J Med 26:899, 1959

126. Blumer D, Heilbronn M: Chronic pain as a variant of depressive disease: the pain-prone disorder. J Nerv Ment Dis 170:381, 1982

127. Egle UT, Kissinger D, Schwab R: Parent-child relations as a predisposition for psychogenic pain syndrome in adulthood. A controlled, retrospective study in relation to G.L. Engel's "pain-proneness." [German language]. Psychother Psychosom Med Psychol 41:247, 1991

128. Gamsa A: Is emotional disturbance a precipitator or a consequence of chronic pain? Pain 42:183, 1990

129. Haythornthwaite JA, Sieber WJ, Kerns RD: Depression and the chronic pain experience. Pain 46:177, 1991

7
Chronic Airflow Limitation

David G. Stubbing

Chronic airflow limitation (CAL) or as it is frequently called *chronic obstruction pulmonary disease* (COPD) is one of the most frequent causes of impairment, disability, and handicap, particularly in countries in which cigarette smoking has been common. The prevalence of CAL and the death rate have continued to increase in the last half of this century so that by the late 1980s, CAL was the fourth leading cause of death in both Canada[1] and the United States.[2]

Even more important are the annual health costs from nearly 900,000 hospitalizations and more than 6 million hospital days in the United States[3] or 1 million hospital days in Canada.[4] The magnitude of the problem is expected to continue, as there is little evidence that the increase in knowledge about the health effects of cigarette smoking will have any effect on long-term smoking rates.

CAL is the irreversible abnormality of lung function characteristic of the obstructive lung diseases encompassed by the term COPD. The major conditions resulting in airflow limitation include smoking-induced chronic bronchitis and emphysema, chronic asthma, and bronchiectasis. Respiratory rehabilitation programs were developed to try to reduce the disability and handicap that occur in these patients, who account for the largest percentage of patients in any respiratory rehabilitation program.

DEFINITIONS IN PULMONARY REHABILITATION

Rehabilitation was defined in 1942 by the Council of Rehabilitation as "the restoration of the individual to the fullest medical, mental, emotional, social, and vocational potential of which he/she is capable." Rehabilitation should aim to improve health by minimizing impairment, disability, and handicap.

Pulmonary Rehabilitation was defined in 1974 by the American College of Chest Physicians as "an art of medical practice wherein an individually tailored, multidisciplinary program is formulated, which through accurate diagnosis, therapy, emotional support, and education, stabilizes or reverses both physio- and psychopathology of pulmonary diseases and attempts to return the patient to the highest possible functional capacity allowed by his pulmonary handicap and overall life situation."[5]

Impairment, Disability, and Handicap

The World Health Organization (WHO) has defined impairment, disability, and handicap for use in chronic illnesses.[6]

Impairment is any loss or abnormality of function.
Disability is any restriction or lack (resulting from impairment) of ability to perform an activity in the manner or within the range considered normal for a human being.
Handicap is a disadvantage for a given individual resulting from an impairment or disability that limits or prevents the fulfillment of a role that is normal (depending on the age, sex, social, and cultural factors) for that individual.

Unfortunately, in respiratory circles, these definitions have not been widely used in practice. The best ways to assess impairment, disability, and handicap in individuals with respiratory disease are not clear; and the relationship between the measures that have been used is poor.[7–10] This difficulty in assessing subjects is twofold: in addition to the airflow limitation seen in individuals with CAL, the chronic condition also results in impaired function of many other organ systems, the measurement of which has generally been lacking.

Other impairments frequently present in individuals with COPD include the following:

1. Impaired peripheral muscle function,[11] in part due to reduction in activity
2. Impaired nutrition[12]
3. Impaired cardiac function, primarily right ventricular dysfunction due to pulmonary artery hypertension as a result of chronic hypoxemia.[13]
4. Impaired respiratory muscle function,[14,15] in part due to the altered geometry of the chest as a result of hyperinflation
5. Impaired ability to cope[16] with depression, anxiety, and panic.

There are undoubtedly other impairments (e.g., impaired peripheral nerve function[17]), but their impact on the disability and handicap is not yet known.

MEASUREMENTS

Impairment of Lung Function

The standard measures used to evaluate lung function are expiratory flow rates, lung volumes, diffusing capacity, and blood gases. The forced expired volume in 1 second (FEV_1) is the best measure of flow rates and the measure of lung function impairment which best relates to the individual's disability.[9,10]

The measurement of diffusing capacity for carbon monoxide (DCO) also correlates with the degree of disability, but even when multiple linear regression with FEV_1 and DCO are combined, they only explain approximately 50 percent of the variability in the measures of disability.[10] There is no significant relationship between other standard measures of lung function or blood gases and measures of disability.

Disability

The disability faced by individuals with significant respiratory impairment is limitation of the ability to perform activities because of breathlessness (Fig. 7-1). The best measure of disability is the *maximum exercise capacity* (Wmax) obtained from a progressive maximum exercise test. Maximum oxygen consumption and maximum power output are measured.

In respiratory rehabilitation, two other outcome measures to assess the degree of pulmonary disability and any changes that occur with treatment are in common use: the distance walked test and the shuttle walk test.

The *distance walked* (WD) in a set period of time, usually 6 or 12 minutes, has been generally accepted.[18] Some studies also have used the endurance of individuals during a submaximal cycle exercise test at a fixed proportion of the maximum exercise capacity.[19–21] In the 6- or 12-minute walk test, patients are asked to cover as much ground as possible while walking in an enclosed corridor receiving maximum encouragement.[22] The 6-minute walk distance (6'WD) correlates well with measurements of maximum exercise capacity,[23] is reproducible[24] once the individual has learned to perform it properly, and is responsive to interventions.[23]

The *shuttle walking test*,[25] during which an individual walks on a circuit at a gradually increasing pace, also can be used as a measure of disability. There is a good relationship between the results of the shuttle walk test and a 6-minute walk test in individuals with CAL.[26]

Handicap

In studies of respiratory rehabilitation, handicap has generally been assessed as quality of life using either generic instruments that provide an estimate of health-related quality of life or specific instruments developed for individuals with chronic lung disease. Most of the standard questionnaires that are used include assessment of dyspnea, activity limitation, or symptoms, not just a measure of handicap.

Sickness Impact Profile

The Sickness Impact Profile is a generic instrument that may provide a valid measure of handicap in

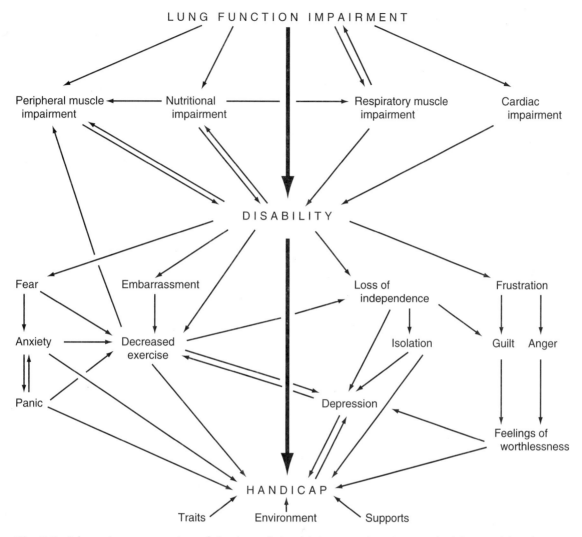

Fig. 7-1. Schematic representation of the interrelationships among impairment, disability, and handicap in individuals with severe chronic airflow limitation.

patients with CAL.[8] It does not appear to be as responsive to change as are specific instruments.

The Chronic Respiratory Disease Questionnaire

The most widely accepted specific instrument for measuring handicap in chronic airflow limitation is the Chronic Respiratory Disease Questionnaire (CRDQ). This interviewer-administered questionnaire aims to assess quality of life in four domains:

dyspnea, fatigue, emotional function, and mastery. It appears to be reproducible, valid, and responsive.

The St. George's Respiratory Questionnaire

The St. George's Respiratory Questionnaire is another disease-specific instrument. It is a self-administered 76-item questionnaire that measures quality of life in three domains: symptoms, activity, and impact on daily life. It, too, seems more valid and responsive than the generic sickness impact profile.[27]

The Psychosocial Adjustment to Illness Scale

The Psychosocial Adjustment to Illness Scale (PAIS-SR) is used in our center as a measure of handicap in individuals with airflow limitation. A 46-item self-report questionnaire that assesses psychosocial adjustment to chronic illness, it has been validated by Derogatis et al.[28] and Morrow et al.[29] In our hands, the handicap as measured by the PAIS-SR correlates well with disability[10] and is responsive to intervention.[30] Scores of PAIS-SR also correlate well with scores from the CRDQ.[31]

Other Impairments

Peripheral Muscle Function

Peripheral muscle function can be measured directly and is impaired in individuals with CAL. The severity of the impairment is related to the lung function abnormality.[11]

Nutritional Impairment

Nutrition impairment is common in CAL, in part because of decreased caloric intake and in part because of an increased metabolic rate.[32-34] Malnourishment is frequent,[12] and lung function impairment[12,15,32] and disability are more severe in the malnourished patient. Other individuals show nutritional problems such as obesity, which aggravates the disability caused by the lung impairment.

Respiratory Ventricular Dysfunction

Right ventricular dysfunction resulting from pulmonary artery hypertension is a consequence of chronic hypoxemia. Pulmonary artery pressures and right ventricular function can be measured directly, but few studies have assessed the effects of this impairment on disability and handicap in CAL.

Respiratory Muscle Function

Respiratory muscle function can be assessed by measuring maximum static inspiratory (PImax) and expiratory pressures (PEmax). The degree of impairment is related to measurements of lung function and maximum exercise capacity.[35]

Psychosocial Adjustment Problems

Psychosocial adjustment problems are common in the presence of severe impairment in lung function. Major psychiatric problems are also common in individuals with significant CAL, but the prevalence of psychiatric disorders varies among studies. Using the Beck Depression Inventory, Light et al.[36] found that 42 percent of 45 patients exhibited depression, whereas Karajgi et al.[37] found only 18 percent had significant depression, a value not significantly different from that in the general population. Anxiety and panic disorders are also common, with prevalence rates ranging from 24 to 34 percent in different studies.[37,38]

Using the PAIS-SR, we found that significant psychosocial adjustment problems occurred in approximately 60 percent of 40 consecutive patients who entered our rehabilitation program. The severity of the psychosocial adjustment correlated significantly with the degree of disability, but not with the degree of lung function impairment.[10]

PROGRAM FORMAT— ASSESSING THE LITERATURE

Assessing the effectiveness of respiratory rehabilitation and comparing different studies are also difficult because of variations among programs with regard to format, admission criteria, or specific areas covered during classes. Some programs are based on a 5-day-a-week attendance, but the length of stay may be prescribed or alternatively tailored for each individual. Patients may either stay in hospital or travel each day from home. In other programs, individuals may attend as few as 2 half-days a week for exercise and education, but may come for as long as 12 weeks. Some studies have only assessed individuals with severe impairment and disability, whereas others have included individuals whose impairment or disability may be mild to moderate. Some programs accept only those who are motivated, whereas others accept any persons disabled by breathlessness unless they are unable to learn in the language of the program or have a medical contraindication to exercise.

Although rehabilitation provides comprehensive care for individuals with CAL, is performed by a multidisciplinary and interdisciplinary team, and provides interventions that are tailored to each individual's requirements, in general the expertise of the staff determines the educational input patients receive. Activities may include exercise training regimens for peripheral and respiratory muscles and education about the use of medication and oxygen, improving nutrition, energy conservation techniques, pacing of activities, breathing retraining, breathing control, panic and anxiety control with relaxation, effective use of leisure time, and infection prevention and management.

Some research studies have evaluated the effectiveness of a multidisciplinary program; others have tried to assess the effectiveness of the various components that make up the total program.

MULTIDISCIPLINARY RESPIRATORY REHABILITATION

Many studies of respiratory rehabilitation in patients with CAL have assessed only the exercise component of a rehabilitation program. Although there is a general consensus that a multidisciplinary rehabilitation program is beneficial, most of the published data are from small or uncontrolled studies.[39] Most studies agree that although rehabilitation has little effect on measures of lung function impairment, disability is lessened as demonstrated by an increase in exercise capability. Only the recent studies have attempted to assess handicap as an outcome measure, and in general they agree that handicap, too, is reduced. Three recent randomized controlled studies merit careful assessment.

Goldstein et al.[19] randomized 89 stable patients with airflow limitation to receive either an 8-week inpatient rehabilitation program or no active intervention. The mean age was 66 years, mean FEV_1 was 34 percent predicted, and there were nearly equal numbers of men and women. Outcome measures including assessment of impairment, disability, and handicap were made at baseline, 8, 16, and 24 weeks.

Seventy-eight subjects completed the study. Seven of those who withdrew were from the treatment group and four were from the control group. The rehabilitation program had no effect on measurements of lung function impairment, but disability and handicap were reduced by the intervention.

Disability was assessed by two measures of exercise capability. The 6'WD increased after rehabilitation, and the changes persisted to 24 weeks. There was no change in the control group ($P < .01$). Another measure of disability, submaximal exercise endurance at a fixed workload of approximately 60 percent of baseline maximum power output, increased significantly in the treatment group, but did not change in the control group ($P < .001$).

Handicap was assessed using the CRDQ. At baseline, control and treatment groups were similar. Over the course of the study there was no change in the control group, but in the treatment group there was a significant improvement in the CRDQ score in the domains of dyspnea ($P < .01$), fatigue ($P = .05$), emotional function ($P < .05$), and mastery ($P < .01$), which persisted to 24 weeks, indicating a lessening of handicap (or an improvement in quality of life). When those who withdrew from the study were included in the final analysis, using the assumption that they had not changed from baseline to 24 weeks, results were not altered.

Toshima et al.[40] evaluated 350 patients with CAL and randomized 129 of these to either a comprehensive rehabilitation program or to a control group who received education only. Ten subjects withdrew before treatment. The mean age was 62 years, mean FEV_1 was 1.3 L, and approximately one-fourth of each group was female. The rehabilitation group attended 12 sessions in 8 weeks. At each session, they undertook regular exercise in a supervised setting and received education classes and individualized teaching about the disease, instruction in physical and respiratory therapy, and psychosocial support. The control group received classroom instruction about living, coping with, and improving health in the presence of lung disease. There were four sessions in the 8-week study. The major differences between the regimen for the two groups were more intensive and individualized educational input for the treatment group plus the exercise program.

The authors did not report the effects of the treatment programs on lung function impairment or on handicap. However significant improvement in disability occurred as shown by an increase in treadmill endurance time in the treatment group but not in the control group.

Wijkstra et al.[41] also recently reported the results of a randomized trial of rehabilitation. Forty-five patients with moderately severe airflow limitation (FEV_1, 1.3) were randomly allocated to an intervention (n = 30) or to a control group (n = 15). The intervention group undertook a home-based rehabilitation program after an initial 2-day hospitalization for evaluation. The rehabilitation program involved exercises for 30 minutes, twice a day for 12 weeks, according to an individualized protocol. They learned and practiced relaxation techniques, breathing retraining, upper and lower limb exercise training, and inspiratory muscle training. They visited the physiotherapist for instruction twice a week, and both a nurse and general practitioner visited their homes once a month for education about living with lung disease. The control group had no intervention.

Follow-up at 12 weeks included assessment of measures of lung function impairment, disability, and handicap. Impairment as assessed by FEV_1 did not change in the treatment group, but fell slightly in the control group. Disability as measured by maximum power output on a cycle ergometer showed a 10 percent increase in the treatment group ($P < .05$) and a 9 percent decline in the control group. Handicap measured by the CRDQ showed a highly significant improvement in all domains of dyspnea, fatigue, emotion, and mastery ($P < .001$), with no change in the control group. The change of the score in the domains of dyspnea, emotion, and mastery differed significantly between the two groups ($P < .01$). Long-term assessment of the benefits of this 12-week program was not performed.

In summary, results of these randomized controlled trials (RCTs) confirm the impression of many earlier studies that a multidisciplinary rehabilitation program lessens the disability even though there is no change in measures of lung function impairment. Measures of other impairments, such as peripheral muscle function or respiratory muscle function, have not been assessed.

The study of Goldstein et al.[19] indicates that the benefits persist for at least 16 weeks after the rehabilitation program has been completed. Guyatt et al.,[23] however, recently reported the results of a follow-up study of rehabilitation and suggested that improvements in disability and handicap revert toward baseline levels within 6 months. We have prospectively studied 122 individuals with CAL (FEV_1 = 1.0 ± 0.41) following a multidisciplinary rehabilitation program.[42] Fifty-nine individuals have been followed for 12 months. The rehabilitation program was an individually tailored, university, hospital-based program. Patients attended 5 days a week for an average of 4.6 weeks. At discharge from the program, patients were encouraged to maintain their own exercise regimen. They were seen by the physiotherapist and respirologist at 2, 6, and 12 months after discharge from the program when outcome measures were recorded.

Although the rehabilitation program had no effect on lung function impairment, there was a significant improvement in disability as measured by the 6'WD and a significant improvement in handicap as measured by the PAIS-SR and the CRDQ. At 12 months, improvement in disability persisted ($P < .001$), as did the improvement in handicap ($P < .05$), but over the course of follow-up there was a trend back toward baseline handicap scores.

INDIVIDUAL COMPONENTS OF RESPIRATORY REHABILITATION

Comprehensive care of the individual with CAL involves a multidisciplinary rehabilitation program involving many disciplines and interventions. Because of the wide range of activities to which an individual is exposed and because exercise alone can result in an improvement in both disability and handicap, it is difficult to determine the effects of the individual components of a rehabilitation program. In part, this problem arises because some of the interventions have general rather than specific objectives; therefore, simple measures of outcome are difficult to develop. Nevertheless, attempts have been made to assess the individual value of some of the components of rehabilitation including the following:

1. Pharmacologic therapy including oxygen
2. Exercise training of peripheral and ventilatory muscles

3. Ventilatory muscle rest
4. Nutrition
5. General education about lung disease
6. Breathing retraining and control
7. Energy conservation during activity
8. Psychosocial interventions

Pharmacologic Therapy Including Oxygen

Most rehabilitation programs admit individuals who are in a stable condition and who have already received maximum medical therapy. Nevertheless, there is still a role for assessment of drug use and education about medications. Even though CAL is irreversible, bronchodilating agents including β_2-agonists and anticholinergics usually result in a modest improvement in lung function. By reducing impairment in this way disability also may be lessened.

In addition to prescribing the appropriate inhaled medications, the patient must be taught the best technique for delivering the drug from a metered-dose inhaler. Several studies have shown that this technique is difficult for many, even after they have been adequately trained.[43–45] Spacer devices have been developed to simplify the technique so that the actuation of the canister and the act of inspiration do not have to occur simultaneously. Spacer devices not only optimize drug delivery to the lung, but also minimize oropharyngeal deposition, which may reduce the potential for side effects, particularly with the high dose inhaled corticosteroids.[46] Dry powder inhalers also remove the requirement of coordinating actuation of the device with breathing. Oropharyngeal drug deposition, however, cannot be minimized, and careful attention must be paid to rinsing the mouth after using inhaled corticosteroids with this delivery system.

Bronchodilators

Anticholinergics and sympathomimetics are equally effective at improving lung function in CAL. Anticholinergics should be used regularly, but it is unclear whether β_2-agonists should be taken on a fixed regimen or used only when needed. In light of the evidence suggesting that regular β_2-agonists may result in worsening lung function in asthma,[47] studies are in progress to assess whether this regimen is appropriate for COPD.

Even in the absence of a measurable effect of bronchodilators on expiratory flow rates, improvement in other measures of impairment or disability may occur to merit the regular prescription of bronchodilating agents. O'Donnell and Webb[48] showed that functional residual capacity fell after the use of an anticholinergic bronchodilating agent, even if FEV_1 did not increase. There was an associated improvement in disability, as shown by a 6'WD, with this change in impairment.

Methylxanthines have been used as bronchodilators in CAL for many years, but with the introduction of potent inhaled bronchodilators their use has fallen into disfavor in many countries, in part because of the adverse effects that frequently occur.

Eaton et al.[49] performed a randomized, blinded, cross-over trial of theophylline versus placebo in 14 subjects with severe irreversible airflow obstruction. Theophylline levels in the therapeutic range were achieved, and although there was significant improvement in measures of lung function impairment, there was no change in 12'WD or in the oxygen cost diagram, which was used to assess breathlessness. Mahler et al.[50] performed a similar trial in 12 individuals who had somewhat less severe airflow limitation. Therapeutic levels of theophylline were also achieved, but there was no improvement in measures of lung function impairment or disability, although scores for dyspnea on two questionnaires, the Baseline Dyspnea Index and the Transitional Dyspnea Index, improved in the theophylline group. In a randomized, double-blind trial, Guyatt et al.[51] compared the effects of placebo, theophylline, salbutamol, or combined theophylline and salbutamol therapy in 19 patients with severe airflow limitation. In all three bronchodilator groups lung function improved, as did measures of disability and handicap. There was no further improvement in measures of lung function, disability (6'WD) or handicap (CRDQ) with a combination of both salbutamol and theophylline.

These studies suggest that the use of theophylline, either alone or in combination with other bronchodilating agents, has little advantage over the use of bronchodilating agents alone. In view of the potential for adverse effects, there is little role for the use of theophylline in chronic stable CAL.

Steroids

Inhaled or oral corticosteroids are frequently used in individuals with CAL. In the presence of acute exacerbation, the aim is to shorten the duration of the episode and to return lung function to its usual level. Oral or parenteral corticosteroids are usually used in this situation. Long-term use of inhaled corticosteroids may play a role in slowing the decline in lung function that occurs with time. Two large trials are currently investigating this possibility. No studies have carefully assessed any potential effect of inhaled corticosteroids on disability or handicap.

Other Drugs

Other drugs including antibiotics, mucolytics and expectorants, inotropic agents, and respiratory stimulants are all used at times in individuals with CAL. They are not used specifically, however, in a rehabilitation setting to attempt to change impairment, disability, or handicap.

Narcotic agents and benzodiazepines have been used to treat the discomfort of dyspnea, but usually they are reserved for individuals with such severe impairment or disability that they can no longer benefit from rehabilitation. The evidence is weak that they might provide benefit even in end-stage lung disease.

Oxygen

Supplemental oxygen is the only treatment for CAL that has been shown to prolong life. The Nocturnal Oxygen Therapy Trial[52] performed by the National Institutes of Health and the Medical Research Council Trial[53] both showed that long-term oxygen therapy used continuously for at least 15 hours each day (overnight) improved survival in individuals with cor pulmonale who were hypoxemic during the day. Oxygen should be offered to this group of patients.

Because it is widely believed that nocturnal hypoxemia that results in an increase in pulmonary artery pressure eventually leads to cor pulmonale, oxygen has been suggested for individuals who are hypoxemic at night but who do not yet have cor pulmonale, even if they are not hypoxemic during the day. Fletcher et al.[54] performed a double-blind, 3-year trial of supplemental oxygen at 3 L/min versus a sham treatment with compressed air at 3 L/min in 38 individuals who had nocturnal oxyhemoglobin desaturation. Although there was no significant difference in mortality rate between the treatment and control groups there was a significant downward trend in pulmonary artery pressure in the treated group. Mean pulmonary artery pressure fell in the oxygen treatment group from 26.7 to 23 mmHg, whereas in the control group values went from 22.5 to 26.4 mmHg ($P < .02$). Similar trends occurred with mean systolic and diastolic pulmonary artery pressures. A larger, longer-term study is needed to determine whether there is potential for preventing the development of cor pulmonale or improving survival in patients with CAL who are hypoxemic only during sleep.

Oxygen and Exercise

Many studies have assessed the effect of oxygen on disability, but results are conflicting. Although most suggested that oxygen is beneficial either by decreasing breathlessness at equivalent work or increasing endurance time, some studies do not show any benefit and others suggest that oxygen is helpful only if significant oxyhemoglobin desaturation occurs.

Lilker et al.[55] performed a double-blind, crossover trial of oxygen in patients with cor pulmonale, and reported no change in dyspnea with the use of supplemental oxygen. Patients felt better whether they used oxygen or compressed air. Longo et al.[56] studied 27 patients with COPD who were mildly hypoxemic and found no improvement in exercise tolerance with the use of supplemental oxygen at 2 or 4 L/min.

Light et al.[57] assessed Wmax with and without 30 percent oxygen in 17 subjects with severe airflow limitation. Although the group showed a small but statistically significant difference, with Wmax increasing from 69.1 to 76.7 W, eight of the subjects showed no change at all. Those who improved exhibited a fall in oxyhemoglobin saturation during exercise when breathing room air. On the other hand, Bradley et al.[58] showed no change in Wmax, with 26 patients breathing oxygen at 5 L/min compared to compressed air at 5 L/min, although they showed an increase in endurance time. In a study by Davidson et al.[59] involving 17 patients with a mean FEV_1 0.79 ± .03, supplemental oxygen appeared to have increased endurance, even in those individuals who did not become hypoxemic with exercise.

The consensus is that although compressed air may have a placebo effect, oxygen improves endurance and reduces dyspnea at equivalent work, perhaps by decreasing minute ventilation and/or delaying the onset of respiratory muscle fatigue.[60] It is not yet clear whether it is necessary to eliminate oxyhemoglobin desaturation with exercise to achieve the maximum benefit on endurance. There is no benefit in providing supplemental oxygen before exercise[61] or to speed recovery from breathlessness after exercise.

Oxygen has been shown effective in reducing the cardiac impairment present in cor pulmonale and the resultant disability. There is no evidence, however, that handicap is minimized or that oxygen has significant psychological effects. Lahdensuo et al.[62] studied 26 hypoxemic patients before and 1, 3, and 6 months after starting supplemental oxygen. They found no improvement in depression scores on the Beck Depression Inventory and no significant improvement in coping skills during activities of daily living. In many cases, supplemental oxygen may aggravate the handicap because of the stigma patients perceive if they leave the home wearing nasal cannulae and pulling a stroller with oxygen.

Exercise

Numerous, mostly uncontrolled, studies have tried to assess the effects of exercise regimens alone in individuals with CAL (see reference 40 for review). Unfortunately most have only used measures of exercise capabilities (disability) as outcome and have ignored the potential effects of exercise on pulmonary impairment or on handicap. Some of the studies have assessed general exercise regimens, but more recently attempts have been made to assess the effects of specific endurance training of individual muscle groups, strength training, and respiratory muscle training either alone or in combination with a general exercise program.

General Exercise Training

Numerous reports of uncontrolled studies using general exercise regimens suggest there is a lessening of disability but no improvement in impairment with an exercise regimen, but truly good controlled studies are rare.

Cockcroft et al.[63] randomized 39 patients with airflow limitation, many of whom had evidence of coal workers pneumoconiosis, to either an exercise program at a rehabilitation center or to a control group. The last 19 were randomized by a method known as minimization in an attempt to achieve similar smoking habits, age range, and baseline 12'WD in the two groups. Men over the age of 70 were excluded. Results in 34 subjects were analyzed. There was a significant lessening of disability (an increase in 12'WD) in the treatment group, with no change in the control group ($P < .05$).

In a more recent study, Weiner et al.[64] randomized 36 subjects to either a control group, a general exercise training program plus sham inspiratory muscle training or a group that received both general exercise training and inspiratory muscle training. The exercise groups were supervised three times a week, but there was no contact with the control group. There were 12 patients in each group.

The control group did not show any change in impairment or disability. The group that received general exercise training alone showed a decrease in disability as measured by an improvement in the 12'WD and an increase in endurance at steady state on a cycle ergometer, although there was no evidence of change in impairment. Measures of handicap were not made.

Specific Peripheral Muscle Training

Almost all of the studies of general exercise regimens have assessed the effect of walking and cycling exercises on those tasks. More recently, interest has focused on specific exercise training aimed at improving the function of individual muscle groups. This interest has focused primarily on exercises using upper extremities, because many patients complain that activities using the arms, especially if these activities are performed overhead, result in an inordinate degree of breathlessness compared with leg activity. Studies have indicated that just elevating the unsupported arms causes a marked increase in oxygen consumption ($\dot{V}CO_2$) and carbon dioxide output ($\dot{V}CO_2$), with an increase in tidal volume, breathing frequency, and minute ventilation.[65] If the elevated arms are supported, however, these metabolic and accompanying respiratory changes do not occur.[66]

When the arms are used, the muscles not only undertake exercise but have to work against gravity. Celli et al.[67] suggested that arm activity placed an added burden on the respiratory system because some of the muscles that may have stabilized the respiratory system cannot function this way when they are supporting the arms. During unsupported arm exercise, the ventilatory load, usually supported by inspiratory rib cage muscles and accessory muscles, shifted to the diaphragm. Few studies have assessed the effects of upper extremity training on disability and handicap in CAL.

The work of Belman and Kendregan[68] suggested that specific muscle training is necessary to improve the performance of individual muscle groups. They studied 15 subjects with CAL, eight of whom undertook upper limb training and seven of whom undertook lower limb training. Training sessions were performed twice for 20 minutes, four times each week for 6 weeks. Not all subjects showed a change in endurance. In those who improved, arm training only resulted in a significant change in arm endurance, but not leg endurance, and leg training resulted in an improvement in leg endurance, but not arm endurance. Lake et al.[69] performed a randomized controlled study to assess the specificity of muscle training in patients with airflow limitation. Twenty-eight patients were randomly assigned to a control group or one of three actively treated groups. One group undertook upper limb training alone, a second group lower limb training alone, and the third group undertook both upper and lower limb training. There were three 1-hour supervised exercise sessions each week for 8 weeks. The outcome measures were performed at entry and at the end of the 8-week period.

There was a significant improvement in arm endurance in both the arm-trained group and the combined-training group. There was a significant improvement in 6′WD in both the lower-limb trained and combined exercise groups. Specific arm training did not result in any improvement in 6′WD, and specific leg training did not result in any improvement in arm endurance.

Ries et al.[21] randomized 45 patients in a multidisciplinary rehabilitation program to one of three groups. A control group received the rehabilitation program alone. The intervention groups received either high- or low-intensity upper limb training in addition to the rehabilitation program. The specific training included low-resistance, high-repetition weight lifting exercises with increasing weight over the course of the study period.

The control group did not show a significant improvement in upper limb performance, although endurance time for isokinetic arm ergometry increased from 290 ± 45 seconds to 700 ± 405 seconds. The low-intensity training also had little effect, but the group receiving high-intensity training showed a significant improvement in upper limb performance. Endurance time increased from 270 ± 98 seconds to 1,725 ± 139 seconds ($P < .05$) and Wmax also increased ($P < .05$).

Couser et al.[70] and Martinez et al.[71] both showed that specific arm training results in increased arm endurance and a reduction in the metabolic cost of arm activity. In the latter study, improvements in the metabolic cost of unsupported arm exercise decreased only in a group who undertook unsupported arm exercises. Those who underwent supported arm exercise training did not show an improvement in unsupported exercise.

Strength Training

Almost all of the aforementioned studies have looked at endurance exercise training, and the outcome measures for exercise capability also have been measures of endurance. Simpson et al.,[20] however, assessed the effect of weight training using outcome measures of strength, lung function impairment, disability, and handicap.

Thirty-four subjects with CAL were stratified on the basis of lung function impairment and oxygenation with exercise and then randomized. The treatment group undertook three training sessions a week for 8 weeks. Weight-lifting exercises consisted of 10 repetitions of single arm curl, single leg extension, and single leg press. Each of these exercises were repeated three times. The resistance was progressively increased during the 8-week study period. The control group did not have any active intervention. Three subjects withdrew from each group before completion of the study.

Significant improvement in strength was observed of all three muscle groups in the treatment group, but not in the control group. Weight training had no effect on measurements of lung function impairment or respiratory muscle strength.

Disability was assessed by three measures. Wmax did not change significantly in either group, although there was a positive trend toward a treatment effect. Similarly, the 6'WD was unchanged but with a positive trend toward a treatment effect. The 6'WD in the treatment group increased from 391 ± 22.5 m to 427 ± 27.2 m, whereas in the control group the respective distances were 369 ± 32 and 376 ± 32.1 m. The lack of a measurable treatment effect may represent a type-2 error. The submaximal exercise test measured at 80 percent of the initial Wmax, showed a significant increase in endurance time in the treatment group but not in the control group ($P < .01$).

Handicap was measured using the CRDQ. Significant improvement was seen only in the treatment group in the domains of dyspnea ($P < .01$), fatigue ($P < .05$), and mastery ($P < .01$).

This study indicates that specific strength training of individual muscle groups can improve the disability and handicap without any change in measures of lung function impairment.

Ventilatory Muscle Training

Impairment of ventilatory muscles, as measured by the ability to generate a static inspiratory or expiratory pressure, is commonly found in patients with airflow limitation. In some, it is probably due largely to the altered geometry of the rib cage as a result of hyperinflation. In others, it is aggravated by malnourishment, and some would suggest that respiratory muscles occasionally suffer from chronic fatigue. Methods for training of ventilatory muscles, therefore, have been developed, and results have been reported in numerous studies.

In many of the early publications, a resistive load was used for ventilatory muscle training with vari-able results, probably because in many subjects the objectives of training were not achieved. With resistive loads, subjects were able to adopt a pattern of long, slow breaths, which minimized the work performed against the load. Once this problem was recognized, methods for training were altered. While training, individuals were asked to reproduce a pattern of breathing that resulted in a training effect, and in other studies a threshold load was used to force the individual to develop high inspiratory pressures during training periods.

Results of these studies demonstrated that impairment of respiratory muscle function can be improved by training, but an effect on disability or handicap is not universally accepted. Harver et al.[72] studied the effect of targeted inspiratory muscle training in 19 individuals with airflow limitation. There was a significant improvement in impairment as shown by an increase in respiratory muscle strength in the intervention group. Belman and Shadmehr[73] also studied patients with targeted breathing through an inspiratory resistive load. Subjects were randomized into a high-intensity training group or a low-intensity training group, which served as controls. After 6 weeks, impairment improved significantly, as demonstrated by an increase in respiratory muscle strength and increased endurance for loaded breathing only in the high-intensity training group.

Neither of these studies assessed measurements of lung function impairment, disability, or handicap with respiratory muscle training, although earlier, Belman and Mittman[74] had shown in an uncontrolled study that ventilatory muscle training in 10 subjects with airflow limitation resulted in an improvement in arm and leg endurance.

Ventilatory muscle training using a threshold loading device also results in an improvement in respiratory muscle strength and endurance without any change in the disability experienced by these individuals. In a double-blind randomized study in 22 individuals, Larson et al.[75] assessed the effects of ventilatory muscle training at 15 or 30 percent of PImax. Daily 15-minute training sessions were undertaken for 8 weeks. Neither group demonstrated any change in lung function impairment. In the high-intensity training group (30 percent PImax) there was a significant increase in PImax ($P < .01$)

and in respiratory muscle endurance at 66 percent of initial PImax ($P < .05$). An 8 percent increase in 12'WD was statistically significant, but was not different from the nonsignificant increase that occurred in the low-intensity training group. Measurements of handicap using the profile of mood states and sickness impact profile showed no changes.

Flynn et al.[76] and Goldstein et al.[77] assessed the value of twice-a-day inspiratory muscle training on measurements of impairment and disability. Both studies showed a significant improvement in PImax, with no change in a control group. Measurements of lung function impairment and disability, including 6- or 12-minute walking distance, Wmax, and exercise cycle endurance, did not change in either the treatment or the control groups.

In summary, these studies indicate that even if inspiratory muscle training improves inspiratory muscle function, there is no change in measures of lung function impairment or disability. Any effects on handicap probably have not been adequately assessed. In these studies, however, many of the individuals in both treatment and control groups had PImax at a level not considered to indicate severe impairment. It may be that only those with severe impairment would achieve improvements in disability and/or handicap from respiratory muscle training. Further studies are necessary and enrollment should be confined to those who have both severe airflow limitation and severe impairment of respiratory muscle function.

Combined Rehabilitation and Ventilatory Muscle Training

Two studies assessed the effect of combining a rehabilitation program with inspiratory muscle training. Dekhuijzen et al.[78] studied 40 subjects with moderate airflow limitation who were entered into a rehabilitation program. They were randomized to receive rehabilitation alone or rehabilitation plus targeted flow inspiratory resistive training. Subjects attended the program for 2 hours each day, 5 days a week for 10 weeks. In addition to the usual rehabilitation interventions, the inspiratory training group undertook two 15-minute sessions each day, breathing through an incentive flow meter with an added resistance. The flow rates and resistance were adjusted to achieve 70 percent of PImax. Outcome measures of lung function and respiratory muscle impairment, disability, and handicap were made at baseline and at the end of 12 weeks.

There was no change in lung function between the two groups. Respiratory muscle impairment was reduced in both groups, but it was significantly more reduced in the inspiratory training group. Disability also improved in both groups. Both the Wmax ($P < .01$) and the 12'WD increased ($P < .01$), but the change in 12'WD was greater in the training group than in the rehabilitation alone group ($P < .05$). Results of two questionnaires, the Activities in Daily Life List and the Symptoms Check List (SCL-90) to assess components of handicap showed similar improvements in both study groups.

In a randomized controlled study, Weiner et al.[64] compared the effect of combined inspiratory muscle training involving a threshold inspiratory muscle load plus a general exercise program to general exercises alone. Both exercise groups were supervised three times a week for 6 months. The inspiratory muscle training began at a threshold load equal to 15 percent of the PImax, and this load was then incrementally increased until 60 percent of PImax was reached. The general exercise group undertook sham inspiratory muscle training with no threshold load applied.

In this study the control group showed no changes in impairment or disability. In both intervention groups, there also was no change in measures of lung function impairment, but respiratory muscle strength and respiratory muscle endurance improved in the group that received inspiratory muscle training. PImax increased from 44.2 to 57.8 cm H_2O ($P < .0005$). Disability decreased in both treatment groups. Both the 12'WD and endurance time at 66 percent of Wmax increased ($P < .001$), but the changes were significantly greater in the group that received the combined training ($P < .05$).

Ventilatory Muscle Rest

In the early 1980s Macklem[79] suggested that the permanent increase in load to the respiratory muscles from the presence of severe airflow limitation could result in the development of chronic fatigue of the ventilatory muscles, which could lead to respiratory failure. Although it is not universally accepted that chronic fatigue is present, the use of intermittent ventilatory support to rest the respiratory muscles is being assessed. The development of techniques for noninvasive ventilation has allowed this research to progress. In a controlled study, O'Donnell et al.[80] showed that the application of continuous positive airway pressure (CPAP) resulted in a statistically significant increase in exercise endurance time ($P < .01$) and a reduction in exertional dyspnea. These findings may have applications for exercise training, but CPAP cannot yet be applied in a way that could be used while individuals undertake normal daily activities.

Several studies have assessed the effect of noninvasive ventilation, either negative pressure or positive pressure applied via a nasal mask, in patients with airflow limitation and respiratory failure. A National Institutes of Health sponsored trial[81] randomized 184 patients to receive either negative pressure ventilation or sham ventilation for 12 weeks. There were no improvements in outcome measures of impairment, disability, or handicap in the ventilated group. Unfortunately, approximately two-thirds of the ventilated patients did not achieve the study objective of a significant decrease in diaphragmatic electromyographic (EMG) signal.

It has been argued that the patients most likely to respond to ventilatory muscle rest are those with the most severe impairment and the highest arterial PCO$_2$. Nevertheless, Mezzanotte et al.[82] studied a group of 13 individuals with CAL divided into two groups. Eight subjects used nocturnal nasal ventilatory support with CPAP for 1 to 3 weeks. Significant improvements in 12'WD and respiratory muscle strength were found in the treatment group, but not in the controls.

It is likely that ventilatory support to rest the respiratory muscles, probably during sleep, would be beneficial in selected individuals with airflow limitation, but the evidence suggests that the routine use of ventilatory support, even in severe CAL, is unwarranted.

Nutrition

Optimization of nutritional status is an important consideration in patients with CAL. Many individuals are obese, which adds a significant load to the respiratory system, and during activity, also adds a load to the peripheral muscles. Nutritional advice regarding weight loss is important and should be combined with an exercise program, psychosocial support, and once weight has been lost, education about preventing weight gain. No studies have evaluated the effect of weight loss alone on impairment, disability, or handicap in chronic airflow limitation; but one would expect some improvement in at least disability.

Malnutrition is also common and has received much more attention than obesity. Malnutrition aggravates impairment and disability.[12,15,32] Even some individuals whose body weight is within the ideal range may be malnourished, as shown by a reduced lean body mass. Schols et al.[12] studied 255 nonobese patients with CAL who were being assessed for rehabilitation. Although the majority were well nourished, approximately 25 percent showed a decrease in ideal body weight to less than 90 percent of that predicted and a decrease in fat-free mass. More important, 10 percent of the population who were of normal body weight were malnourished, as shown by a decreased fat-free mass. The malnourished individuals had more impairment and more disability than well-nourished individuals. The group of patients with normal body weight but decreased fat-free mass were even more disabled than underweight, malnourished individuals.

Several other studies have supported these findings, reporting impairment in respiratory muscle function and lower walking distance in malnourished individuals.[32,83] Other studies reported conflicting results, with respiratory muscle strength and endurance the same in both malnourished and well-nourished individuals with airflow limitation.[84–86]

In the malnourished patient, correction of the nutritional depletion seems warranted. Rogers et al.[87] performed a randomized controlled study of nutritional supplementation in 17 individuals with severe airflow limitation and ideal body weight less than 90 percent of that predicted. The mean body weight in each group was approximately 78 percent of ideal body weight. The treatment group received a nutritionally balanced meal plan with a calorie intake of 1.7 times the resting energy expenditure and approximately 1.5 g/k protein. A variety of nutritional supplements were incorporated into their meal plan. The control group did not receive any dietary interventions. Baseline measurements were made and repeated at 4 weeks and 4 months. The nutritional repletion resulted in statistically significant increases in body weight and 12'WD, with no change in the control group. Peripheral muscle function, as shown by hand grip force, increased significantly. PImax also increased from 36.1 cm H_2O to 48.6 cm H_2O, but this increase did not reach statistical significance. With only 15 individuals in the treatment group and 12 in the control group, this finding probably represents a type 2 error. There were no changes in the control group.

Efthimiou et al.[88] confirmed some of these findings; but once the trial period of their study was over, benefits did not persist. They assessed 14 poorly nourished patients randomized to either a treatment group or a control group and compared them with age- and FEV_1-matched individuals who were well nourished. All groups were asked to eat normally during the first 3 months and last 3 months of the trial. In the middle 3 months, the treatment group was taught to increase calorie and protein intake to values between 25 and 50 percent greater than that recommended for moderately active individuals. The control groups continued with their usual diet. At baseline PImax, PEmax, and hand grip strength were similar in both groups of malnourished patients, but less than the values in the well-nourished patients. The intervention group showed a reduction in impairment during the treatment period, with a significant improvement in respiratory muscle and hand grip strength and a reduction in disability and dyspnea. 6'WD increased significantly, whereas the controls showed no change. During the 3 months after supplementation, the outcome measures tended to revert toward baseline.

Several other studies show that if increases of more than 30 percent occur in energy intake, body weight, respiratory muscle function, and/or exercise performance improve.

General Education

Education is an integral part of respiratory rehabilitation programs. Patients are taught about their disease, how drugs should be used, how to recognize infections and treat them early to prevent worsening of lung function, and ways to cope with the disability and handicap caused by the impairment. Few studies assess the effect of the educational program alone, but instruments are available to assess knowledge,[89] and some studies have shown that patients in an education program improved their knowledge about their disease.[90] There is no evidence, however, that this improvement in knowledge alone affects impairment, disability, or handicap.

One controlled study compared individuals with COPD in two communities. One community acted as the control and the other provided a health education program consisting of three to six 2-hour sessions on living with lung disease. The education group did not show any significant change in disability or handicap.[91]

Breathing Retraining and Control

During exercise, many patients with CAL exhibit rapid, shallow breathing, which results in an increase in dead space ventilation. This pattern of breathing occurs even at low levels of exercise, resulting at least in part from dynamic hyperinflation and produces an increase in the inspiratory work of breathing. Patients are generally taught techniques aimed at changing the ventilatory pattern during exercise to one of slower frequency and larger tidal volume. Pursed-lip breathing is then added to help slow breathing frequency further and decrease dynamic airway compression.

These techniques, particularly pursed-lip breathing, have resulted in slower deeper breathing, with an improvement in oxygenation and a decrease in arterial PCO_2,[92,93] but only one study investigated the effects of breathing retraining on disability.

Casciari et al.[94] reported the effects of teaching breathing control during exercise on the pattern of breathing and the ability to undertake exercise in a group of patients with CAL. Twenty-two subjects were studied, 12 in a control group and 10 in an active treatment group. Both the control and treatment groups undertook exercise training for 3 weeks. During this time, they achieved similar improvements in exercise capacity. During the second 3 weeks, the treatment group was instructed in breathing control techniques in addition to continuing the progressive exercise regimen, whereas the control group continued exercise without other instructions.

During the breathing retraining, the treatment group exhibited a statistically significant increase in exercise capacity compared with the control group ($P < .05$). During active exercise, they were able to use larger tidal volumes and to breathe slower. This study demonstrated the positive effect on disability of breathing retraining in which subjects with CAL are taught to adopt a pattern of longer, slower breaths.

Energy Conservation

One of the roles of the occupational therapist is to teach techniques for conserving energy during activities of daily living. The aim is to teach methods of performing tasks with the lowest metabolic cost, thereby reducing the ventilatory requirement and the dyspnea that accompany that task. For example, sitting down for tasks requiring arm activities should make the breathlessness less troublesome if sitting reduces the oxygen consumption of the lower extremities and trunk muscles.

No controlled studies have assessed breathlessness during activities of daily living before and after education about energy conservation techniques, perhaps because of the difficulty in finding a valid reproducible, responsive, and reliable method of assessing these activities.

Two studies have assessed the effect of an energy conservation technique during walking using a wheeled walker. Honeyman et al.[95] performed an RCT in 11 patients with CAL. Six-minute walking distance, breathlessness, and oxyhemoglobin saturation were assessed when individuals walked with or without a wheeled walker. The use of the walker resulted in an increase in 6'WD (a decrease in disability) and at the same time a reduction in both breathlessness and hypoxemia. Wesmiller et al.[96] also studied patients with CAL, with and without the use of a wheeled walker. They also showed, that at least in the severely disabled (i.e., those whose 12'WD was less than 1,000 feet), a significant improvement in walking distance occurred.

When walking on a treadmill, arm support reduces the oxygen cost of the workload.[97,98] By supporting the arms and allowing the subject to adopt a tripod position that stabilizes the rib cage muscles,[99] the walker probably reduced oxygen consumption during ambulation.

Psychosocial Interventions

Because of the high prevalence of depression, anxiety, and panic in patients with CAL, psychosocial support and interventions play an important role in respiratory rehabilitation programs. Drug treatment has been tried for depression and anxiety, and patients are generally taught coping skills and relaxation techniques.

Agle et al.[16] assessed depression, anxiety, and body preoccupation in 24 patients entering a rehabilitation program. Those who improved exercise capability had fewer psychological symptoms at entry to the program than poor responders; they also showed more improvement in psychological symptoms. Toshima et al.[100] showed that although rehabilitation resulted in an improvement in disability and self-efficacy, there was no effect on depression.

Light et al.[101] studied 12 patients with severe airflow limitation who had significant depression based on their score on the Beck Depression Inventory. Patients randomly received two 6-week treatment periods, one with placebo and the other with a tricyclic antidepressant (doxepin hydrochloride). Three patients were unable to tolerate the antidepressant phase of the study. Although depression scores varied for each individual during the study, the tricyclic antidepressive had no effect on depression score or on measures of impairment or disability. However, a significant relationship between change in depression score over time and change in 12'WD was noted. If depression score improved 12'WD increased; if depression score deteriorated, the disability worsened.

Active relaxation techniques have been studied to see whether improvement occurred in disability or handicap. Renfroe,[102] studied progressive muscle relaxation in 12 patients and compared the results to a control group who were told to try relaxing but were not taught how. The treatment group, but not the control group, showed improvement in breathlessness and anxiety at the end of each relaxation session. However, there did not appear to be any long-term effect, suggesting that relaxation has to be practiced when it is needed. Yoga also has been studied in a randomized trial in 24 patients with CAL.[103] The control group was given standard physiotherapy instruction. The intervention group using yoga showed a significant improvement in Wmax, but the control group did not. The intervention group also increased their ability to cope with their breathing disorder.

More work is needed to determine whether active relaxation and yoga, or other coping strategies such as biofeedback and autosuggestion have any long-term role in improving disability or handicap in patients with CAL.

PATIENT SELECTION

Motivation and Goal Setting

Although the accepted practice is to admit into a rehabilitation program only patients who are motivated to take part and who recognize the existence of their disability and handicap, I do not know of any studies that have evaluated the effects of motivation on outcome. Moreover, motivation can change and the benefits that will occur during participation in a rehabilitation program may provide the motivation to encourage the patient to work to maintain these benefits.

Similarly, goal setting is routinely mentioned as part of the preparation for rehabilitation. In general, respiratory patients seem to have generic goals rather than specific goals. These goals include improving breathing, becoming less dyspneic, being able to walk more, or being less anxious. These goals often are implied rather than detailed. The effect of the setting of specific goals in respiratory rehabilitation has not been studied. If specific goals are set and achieved, the patient may receive psychological benefits as well as physical ones. On the other hand, when goals are set but not achieved, the effect may be detrimental.

Severity of Impairment, Disability, and Handicap

Several studies have tried to define physiologic factors that indicate a likely benefit from rehabilitation or factors suggesting that individuals will not improve because they are too ill. Niederman et al.[104] assessed 33 patients before and after rehabilitation and showed that the degree of lung function impairment at entry did not correlate with improvements in disability after the rehabilitation program. ZuWallack et al.[105] showed similar results and also suggested that the severity of the disability at entry did not affect outcome measures of disability after rehabilitation. Neither study assessed changes in handicap.

We have followed 131 consecutive patients with airflow limitation admitted to our rehabilitation program[42] (Fig. 7-2). They were stratified according to severity of lung function impairment, disability, and handicap. Although the lung function impairment did not change during the study, 6'WD and PAIS-SR improved, whether impairment was severe or mild and whether initial disability was severe or mild. Whether the PAIS-SR showed severe or mild handicap, improvement occurred in both 6'WD and PAIS-SR score (Fig. 7-3).

These studies show that the initial severity of impairment, disability, or handicap does not preclude improvement in disability and handicap with rehabilitation.

Foster et al.[106] showed that even in the presence of respiratory failure with an elevated arterial PCO_2, there was still a significant improvement in disability as measured by a 6'WD. We confirmed these findings in our follow-up study group, which included 30 individuals with elevated arterial PCO_2.[107] Six-minute walking distance improved from 281.5 ± 93 m to 350.8 ± 96 m ($P < .001$). Handicap, which was measured using the PAIS-SR, also improved significantly ($P < .05$).

OTHER BENEFITS OF RESPIRATORY REHABILITATION

It has been suggested that general benefits from comprehensive rehabilitation programs may include a reduction in the number of hospitalizations, reduced cost, and improvement in survival. Several studies have suggested that the number of hospital days spent in the year after rehabilitation is less than in the year before rehabilitation. However, it may be that an acute event resulting in hospitalization led to the referral for rehabilitation in the first place.

Sneider et al.[108] retrospectively analyzed the hospitalizations of 150 randomly selected patients from each of three groups. One group was interviewed, but not entered into a rehabilitation program. Another received education but no exercise, and the third group completed a multidisciplinary rehabilitation program. The rehabilitation group showed a decrease of 1.8 hospital days/year, whereas the other two groups showed an increase in hospital days per year. Many other studies suggest that rehabilitation may have dramatic effects on the number of hospital days and hospital costs for these individuals and that despite the high cost of a rehabilitation program, net savings accrue (see reference 40 for review).

The other potential improvement that has been assessed is increased survival, but no prospective randomized controlled studies have evaluated whether pulmonary rehabilitation has any impact on survival. Several long-term follow-up studies, however, have suggested that patients who undertake a comprehensive rehabilitation program have an improved survival, even at 10-year follow-up.[108–110]

SUMMARY

In the stable patient with CAL, multidisciplinary respiratory rehabilitation reduces disability and handicap, even when there is no change in lung function impairment. Some of the benefits may accrue because of reduction of peripheral muscle function impairment, nutritional impairment, or other unmeasured or unmeasurable impairments. Other purported benefits of respiratory rehabilitation

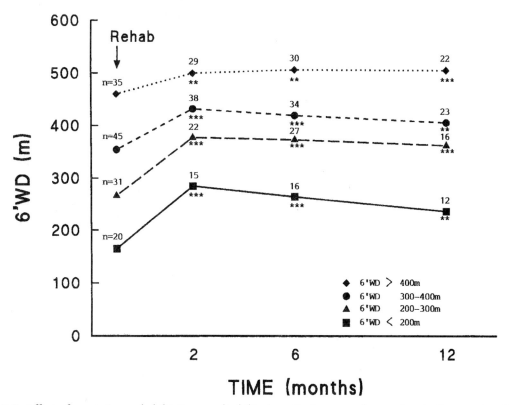

Fig. 7-2. Effect of respiratory rehabilitation on disability in patients grouped according to the severity of disability before rehabilitation. 6'WD, 6-minute walking distance in meters. **, $P < .01$; ***, $P < .001$.

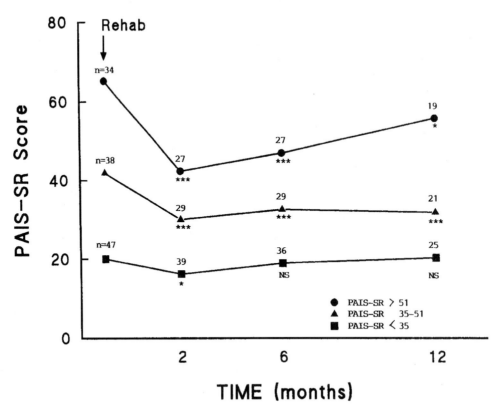

Fig. 7-3. Effect of respiratory rehabilitation on handicap in patients grouped according to the severity of handicap before rehabilitation. PAIS-SR, Psychosocial Adjustment to Illness Scale—Self-Report; NS, not significant; *, $P < .05$; ***, $P < .001$.

include an improvement in survival and a reduction in hospitalization and hospital costs.

Although each component of a respiratory rehabilitation program may confer some benefit, a multidisciplinary program is probably more effective than single interventions. More effort is needed to develop effective ways of assessing impairment, disability, and handicap so that unanswered questions can be tested.

REFERENCES

1. Health Reports: Mortality Summary 1989, p. 16. Statistics Canada, Ottawa. Vol. 3:S12, 1991

2. Bureau of the Census: Statistical Abstract of the United States, p. 95. United States Department of Commerce. Washington, DC, 1994

3. Vital and Health Statistics: Detailed Diagnosis and Procedure, National Hospital Discharge Survey, 1992. p. 17. United States Department of Health and Human Services. Hyattsville, MD, 1994

4. Health Reports: Hospital Morbidity 1989–90. p. 32. Statistics Canada. Ottawa. Vol. 4:S1, 1992

5. American Thoracic Society: Pulmonary rehabilitation. Am Rev Respir Dis 124:663, 1981

6. World Health Organization: International Classification of Impairments, Disabilities and Handicaps: A Manual of Classification Relating to the Consequences of Disease. World Health Organization, Geneva, 1980

7. Guyatt GH, Berman LB, Townsend M et al: A measure of quality of life for clinical trials in chronic lung disease. Thorax 42:773, 1987

8. Williams SJ, Bury MR: Impairment, disability and handicap in chronic respiratory illness. Soc Sci Med 29:609, 1989

9. Jones PW, Baveystock CM, Littlejohns P: Relationships between general health measured with the Sickness Impact Profile and respiratory symptoms, physiological measures and mood in patients with chronic airflow limitation. Am Rev Respir Dis 140:1538, 1989

10. Stubbing DG, Haalboom PA: Relationship between impairment, disability and handicap in chronic lung disease. Am Rev Respir Dis 147:A475, 1993

11. Allard C, Jones NL, Killian KJ: Static peripheral skeletal muscle strength and exercise capacity in patients with chronic airflow limitation. Am Rev Respir Dis 138:A90, 1989

12. Schols AMWJ, Soeters PB, Dingemans AMC et al: Prevalence and characteristics of nutritional depletion in patients with stable COPD eligible for pulmonary rehabilitation. Am Rev Respir Dis 147:1151, 1993

13. Bishop JM, Cross KW: Use of other physiological variables to predict pulmonary arterial pressure in patients with chronic obstructive pulmonary disease: multi-centre study. Eur Heart J 2:519, 1981

14. Sharp JT, Van Lith P, Nuchprayoon CV et al: The thorax in chronic obstructive lung disease. Am J Med 44:30, 1968

15. Rochester DF, Braun NMT: Determinants of maximal inspiratory pressure in chronic obstructive pulmonary disease. Am Rev Respir Dis 132:42, 1985

16. Agle DP, Baum GL, Chester EH et al: Multidiscipline treatment of chronic pulmonary insufficiency. 1. Psychologic aspects of rehabilitation. Psychosom Med 35:41, 1973

17. Jarratt JA, Morgan CN, Twomey JA et al: Neuropathy in chronic obstructive pulmonary disease: a multicentre electrophysiological and clinical study. Eur Respir J 5:517, 1992

18. Butland JA, Pang J, Gross BR et al: Two-, six-, and twelve-minute walking tests in respiratory disease. BMJ 284:1607, 1982

19. Goldstein RS, Gort EH, Stubbing D et al: Randomized control trial of respiratory rehabilitation. Lancet 344:1394, 1994

20. Simpson K, Killian K, McCartney N et al: Randomized control trial of weightlifting exercise in patients with chronic airflow limitation. Thorax 47:70, 1992

21. Ries AL, Ellis B, Hawkins RW: Upper extremity exercise training in chronic obstructive pulmonary disease. Chest 93:688, 1988

22. Guyatt GH, Pugsley SO, Sullivan MJ et al: Effect of encouragement on walking test performance. Thorax 39:818, 1984

23. Guyatt GH, Thompson PJ, Berman LB et al: How should we measure function in patients with chronic heart and lung disease? J Chronic Dis 38:517, 1985

24. Knox AJ, Morrison JFJ, Muers MF: Reproducibility of walking test results in chronic obstructive airways disease. Thorax 43:388, 1988

25. Singh SJ, Morgan MDL, Scott S et al: Development of a shuttle walking test of disability in patients with chronic airways obstruction. Thorax 47:1019, 1992

26. Singh SJ, Morgan MDL, Hardman AE et al: Comparison of oxygen uptake during a conventional treadmill test and the shuttle walking test in chronic airflow limitation. Eur Respir J 7:2016, 1994

27. Jones PW, Quirk FH, Baveystock CM, Littlejohns P: A self-complete measure of health status for chronic airflow limitation. Am Rev Respir Dis 145:1321, 1992

28. Derogatis LR, Lopez MC: Pais and Pais-SR scoring manual I. Johns Hopkins University School of Medicine, Baltimore, 1983

29. Morrow GP, Chiarello RJ, Derogatis LR: A new scale of assessing patients' psychosocial adjustment to medical illness. Psychol Med 9:605, 1978

30. Stubbing DG, Barr P, Haalboom P: Long-term follow-up of the effects of respiratory rehabilitation on disability and handicap in patients with chronic airflow limitation. Am J Respir Crit Care Med 149:A268, 1994

31. Stubbing DG, Barr P, Haalboom P: Comparison of the Chronic Respiratory Disease Questionnaire (CRDQ) and the Psychosocial Adjustment to Illness Scale—Self-Report (PAIS-SR) as measures of handicap in patients with chronic airflow limitation. Am J Respir Crit Care Med 149:A268, 1994

32. Donahoe M, Rogers RM, Wilson DO, Pennock BE: Oxygen consumption of the respiratory muscles in normal and malnourished patients with chronic obstructive pulmonary disease. Am Rev Respir Dis 140:385, 1989

33. Goldstein S, Askanazi J, Weissman C et al: Energy expenditure in patients with chronic obstructive pulmonary disease. Chest 91:222, 1987

34. Fitting JW, Frascarolo PH, Jéquier E, Leuenberger PH: Energy expenditure and ribcage-abdominal motion in chronic obstructive pulmonary disease. Eur Respir J 2:840, 1989

35. Killian KJ: Limitation of exercise by dyspnea. Can J Sport Sci 12:S1,53S, 1987

36. Light RW, Merrill EJ, Despars JA et al: Prevalence of depression and anxiety in patients with COPD: relationship to functional capacity. Chest 87:35, 1985

37. Karajgi B, Rifkin A, Doddi S, Kolli R: The prevalence of anxiety disorders in patients with chronic obstructive pulmonary disease. Am J Psychiatry 147:200, 1990

38. Yellowees PM, Persjh L, Bowden JJ et al: Psychiatric morbidity in subjects with chronic airflow obstruction. Med J Aust 146:305, 1987

39. Ries AL: Position paper of the American Association of Cardiovascular and Pulmonary Rehabilitation. Scientific basis of pulmonary rehabilitation. J Cardiopulmonary Rehabil 10:418, 1990

40. Toshima MT, Kaplan RM, Ries AL: Experimental evaluation of rehabilitation in chronic obstructive pulmonary disease: short-term effects on exercise endurance and health status. Health Psychol 9:237, 1990

41. Wijkstra PJ, Van Altena R, Kraan J et al: Quality of life in patients with chronic obstructive pulmonary disease improves after rehabilitation at home. Eur Respir J 7:269, 1994

42. Stubbing DG, Barr P, Haalboom P, Vaughan R: Is the effect of respiratory rehabilitation in COPD independent of the degree of impairment, disability or handicap? Am Rev Respir Dis 151:A688, 1995

43. Orehek J, Gayrard P, Grimaud CH, Sharpin J: Patient error in use of bronchodilator metered aerosols. BMJ 1:76, 1976

44. Epstein SW, Manning CPR, Ashley MJ, Corey PN: Survey of the clinical use of pressurized aerosol inhalers. Can Med Assoc J 128:813, 1979

45. Shim C, Williams MH: The adequacy of inhalation of aerosol from canister nebulizers. Am J Med 69:891, 1980

46. Corr D, Dolovich M, McCormack D et al: Design and characteristics of a portable breath actuated particle size selective medical aerosol inhaler. J Aerosol Sci 13:1, 1982

47. Sears MR, Taylor DR, Print CG et al: Regular inhaled beta-agonist treatment in bronchial asthma. Lancet 336:1391, 1990

48. O'Donnell DE, Webb KA: The efficacy of adjunct high dose anticholinergic therapy in relieving breathlessness in patients with severe chronic airflow limitation. Am Rev Respir Dis 149:A286, 1994

49. Eaton ML, McDonald FM, Church TR et al: Effects of theophylline on breathlessness and exercise tolerance in patients with chronic airflow obstruction. Chest 82:538, 1982

50. Mahler D, Matthay RA, Synder PE et al: Sustained release theophylline reduces dyspnea in non-reversible obstructive airways disease. Am Rev Respir Dis 131:22, 1985

51. Guyatt GH, Townsend M, Pugsley SO et al: Bronchodilators in chronic airflow limitation: effects on airway function, exercise capacity and quality of life. Am Rev Respir Dis 135:1069, 1987

52. Nocturnal Oxygen Therapy Trial Group: Continuous or nocturnal oxygen therapy in hypoxemic chronic obstructive lung disease. Ann Intern Med 93:391, 1980

53. Medical Research Council Working Party: Long-term domiciliary oxygen therapy in chronic hypoxic cor pulmonale complicating chronic bronchitis and emphysema. Lancet 1:681, 1981

54. Fletcher EC, Luckett RA, Goodnight-White S et al: A double-blind trial of nocturnal supplemental oxygen for sleep desaturation in patients with chronic obstructive pulmonary disease and a daytime PaO_2 above 60 mmHg. Am Rev Respir Dis 145:1070, 1992

55. Lilker ES, Karnick A, Learner L: Portable oxygen in chronic obstructive lung disease with hypoxemia and cor pulmonale. A controlled double-blind cross-over study. Chest 68:236, 1975

56. Longo AM, Moser KM, Luchsinger PC: The role of oxygen therapy in the rehabilitation of patients with chronic obstructive pulmonary disease. Am Rev Respir Dis 103:690, 1971

57. Light RW, Mahutte CK, Stansbury DW et al: Relationship between improvement in exercise performance with supplemental oxygen and hypoxic ventilatory drive in patients with chronic airflow obstruction. Chest 95:751, 1989

58. Bradley BL, Garner AE, Billiu D et al: Oxygen assisted exercise in chronic obstructive lung disease. Am Rev Respir Dis 118:239, 1978

59. Davidson AC, Leach R, George RJD, Geddes DM: Supplemental oxygen and exercise ability in chronic obstructive airways disease. Thorax 43:965, 1988

60. Bye PTP, Esau SA, Levy RD et al: Ventilatory muscle function during exercise in air and oxygen in patients with chronic airflow limitation. Am Rev Respir Dis 132:236, 1985

61. McKeon JL, Murree-Allen K, Saunders NA: Effects of breathing supplemental oxygen before progressive exercise in patients with chronic obstructive lung disease. Thorax 43:53, 1988

62. Lahdensuo A, Ojanen M, Ahonen A et al: Psychosocial effect of continuous oxygen therapy in hypoxaemic chronic obstructive pulmonary disease patients. Eur Respir J 2:977, 1989

63. Cockcroft AE, Saunders MJ, Berry G: Randomized control trial of rehabilitation in chronic respiratory disability. Thorax 36:200, 1981

64. Weiner P, Azgad Y, Gamam R: Inspiratory muscle training combined with general exercise reconditioning in patients with COPD. Chest 102:1352, 1992

65. Martinez F, Couser J, Celli B: Respiratory response to arm elevation in patients with chronic airflow limitation. Am Rev Respir Dis 143:476, 1991

66. Dolmage TE, Maestro L, Avendano MA, Goldstein RS: The ventilatory response to arm elevation of patients with chronic obstructive pulmonary disease. Chest 104:1097, 1993

67. Celli BR, Rassulo J, Make BJ: Dyssynchronous breathing during arm but not leg exercise in patients with chronic airflow obstruction. N Engl J Med 314:1485, 1986

68. Belman MJ, Kendregan BA: Exercise training fails to increase skeletal muscle enzymes in patients with chronic obstructive pulmonary disease. Am Rev Respir Dis 123:256, 1981

69. Lake FR, Henderson K, Briffa T et al: Upper-limb and lower-limb exercise training in patients with chronic airflow obstruction. Chest 97:1077, 1990

70. Couser JI, Martinez FJ, Celli BR: Pulmonary rehabilitation that includes arm exercise reduces metabolic and ventilatory requirements for simple arm elevation. Chest 103:37, 1993

71. Martinez FJ, Vogel PD, Dupont DN et al: Supported arm exercise vs unsupported arm exercise in the rehabilitation of patients with severe chronic airflow obstruction. Chest 103:1397, 1993

72. Harver A, Mahler DA, Daubenspeck JA: Targeted inspiratory muscle training improves respiratory muscle function and reduces dyspnea in patients with chronic obstructive disease. Ann Intern Med 111:117, 1989

73. Belman MJ, Shadmehr R: Targeted resistive muscle training in chronic obstructive pulmonary disease. J Appl Physiol 65:2726, 1988

74. Belman MJ, Mittman C: Ventilatory muscle training improves exercise capacity in chronic obstructive pulmonary disease patients. Am Rev Respir Dis 121:273, 1980

75. Larson JL, Kim MJ, Sharp JT et al: Inspiratory muscle training with a pressure threshold breathing device in patients with chronic obstructive pulmonary disease. Am Rev Respir Dis 138:689, 1988

76. Flynn MG, Barter CE, Nosworthy JC et al: Threshold pressure training, breathing pattern and exercise performance in chronic airflow obstruction. Chest 95:535, 1989

77. Goldstein RS, De Rosie J, Long S et al: Applicability of a threshold loading device for inspiratory muscle training in patients with COPD. Chest 96:564, 1989

78. Dekhuijzen PNR, Folgering HTM, van Herwaarden CLA: Target-flow inspiratory muscle training during pulmonary rehabilitation in patients with COPD. Chest 99:128, 1991

79. Macklem PT: The clinical relevance of respiratory muscle research. J. Burns Amberson Lecture. Am Rev Respir Dis 134:812, 1986

80. O'Donnell DE, Sanii R, Younes M: Improvement in exercise endurance in patients with chronic airflow limitation using continuous positive airway pressure. Am Rev Respir Dis 138:1510, 1988

81. Shapiro SH, Ernst P, Gray-Donald K et al: Effect of negative pressure ventilation in severe pulmonary disease. Lancet 340:1425, 1992

82. Mezzanotte WS, Tangel DJ, Fox AM et al: Nocturnal nasal continuous positive airway pressure in patients with chronic obstructive pulmonary disease. Chest 106:1100, 1994

83. Rochester DF, Braun NMT: Determinants of maximal inspiratory pressure in chronic obstructive pulmonary disease. Am Rev Respir Dis 132:42, 1985

84. Lewis MI, Belman MJ, Dorr-Uyemura L: Nutritional supplementation in ambulatory patients with chronic obstructive pulmonary disease. Am Rev Respir Dis 135:1062, 1987

85. Knowles JB, Fairbarn MS, Wiggs BJ et al: Dietary supplementation and respiratory muscle performance in patients with COPD. Chest 93:977, 1988

86. Gray-Donald K, Gibbons L, Shapiro SH, Martin JG: Effect of nutritional status on exercise performance in patients with chronic obstructive pulmonary disease. Am Rev Respir Dis 140:1544, 1989

87. Rogers RM, Donahoe M, Costantino J: Physiologic effects of oral supplemental feeding in malnourished patients with chronic obstructive pulmonary disease. Am Rev Respir Dis 146:1511, 1992

88. Efthimiou J, Fleming J, Gomes C, Spiro SG: The effect of supplementary oral nutrition in poorly nourished patients with chronic obstructive pulmonary disease. Am Rev Respir Dis 137:1075, 1988

89. Hopp JW, Lee JW, Phils R: Development and validation of a pulmonary rehabilitation knowledge test. J Cardiopulmonary Rehabil 9:273, 1989

90. Neish CM, Hopp JW: The role of education in pulmonary rehabilitation. J Cardiopulmonary Rehabil 8:439, 1988

91. Howland J, Nelson EC, Barlow PB et al: Chronic obstructive airway disease: impact of health education. Chest 90:233, 1986

92. Thoman RL, Stoker GL, Ross JC: The efficacy of pursed-lips breathing in patients with chronic

obstructive pulmonary disease. Am Rev Respir Dis 93:100, 1966

93. Mueller RE, Petty TL, Filley GF: Ventilation and arterial blood gas changes induced by pursed lips breathing. J Appl Physiol 28:784, 1970

94. Casciari RJ, Fairshter RD, Harrison A et al: Effects of breathing retraining in patients with chronic obstructive pulmonary disease. Chest 79:393, 1981

95. Honeyman P, Barr P, Stubbing DG: Effect of a walking aid on disability, oxygenation and breathlessness in patients with chronic airflow limitation. J Cardiopulmonary Rehabil 16:63, 1996

96. Wesmiller SW, Hoffman LA: Evaluation of an assistive device for ambulation in oxygen dependent patients with COPD. J Cardiopulmonary Rehabil 14:122, 1994

97. Von Duvillard ST, Pivirotto JM: The effect of front handrail and non-handrail support on treadmill exercise in healthy women. J Cardiopulmonary Rehabil 11:164, 1991

98. Parillo D, Wygand J, Otto RM et al: The cardiovascular and metabolic response to supported vs non-supported treadmill walking. J Cardiopulmonary Rehabil 11:301, 1991

99. Sharp JT, Drutz WS, Moisan T et al: Postural relief of dyspnea and severe chronic obstructive pulmonary disease. Am Rev Respir Dis 122:201, 1980

100. Toshima TM, Blumberg E, Ries AL, Kaplan RM: Does rehabilitation reduce depression in patients with chronic obstructive pulmonary disease? J Cardiopulmonary Rehabil 12:261, 1992

101. Light RW, Merrill EJ, Despars J et al: Doxepin treatment of depressed patients with chronic obstructive pulmonary disease. Arch Intern Med 146:1377, 1986

102. Renfroe KL: Effect of progressive relaxation on dyspnea and state anxiety in patients with chronic obstructive pulmonary disease. Heart Lung 17:408, 1988

103. Tandon MK: Adjunct treatment with yoga in chronic severe airways obstruction. Thorax 33:514, 1978

104. Niederman MS, Clemente PH, Fein AM et al: Benefits of a multidisciplinary pulmonary rehabilitation program. Chest 99:798, 1991

105. ZuWallack RL, Patel K, Reardon JZ et al: Predictors of improvement in the twelve-minute walking distance following a six-week outpatient pulmonary rehabilitation program. Chest 99:805, 1991

106. Foster S, Lopez D, Thomas HM: Pulmonary rehabilitation in COPD patients with elevated PCO_2. Am Rev Respir Dis 138:1519, 1988

107. Stubbing DG, Barr P, Haalboom P, Vaughan R: Effect of respiratory rehabilitation in patients with severely impaired lung function or respiratory failure. Am Rev Respir Dis 151:A684, 1995

108. Sneider R, O'Malley JA, Cahn M: Trends in pulmonary rehabilitation at Eisenhower Medical Centre: an eleven-years' experience 1976–1987. J Cardiopulmonary Rehabil 8:453, 1988

109. Haas A, Cardon H: Rehabilitation in chronic obstructive pulmonary disease: a five year study of 252 male patients. Med Clin North Am 53:593, 1969

110. Sahn SA, Nett LM, Petty TL: Ten year follow-up of a comprehensive rehabilitation program for severe COPD. Chest 77:311, 1980

8

Cardiac Rehabilitation

Robert S. McKelvie

Cardiac rehabilitation is defined by the World Health Organization as "the sum of activity required to ensure cardiac patients the best possible physical, mental, and social conditions so that they may by their own efforts regain as normal as possible a place in the community and lead an active life."[1] Rehabilitation of cardiac patients consists of two components, exercise training and counseling.[2] The training component consists of a prescribed exercise program designed to improve the patient's functional work capacity and confidence. Counseling is made up of several components including psychological, nutritional, and vocational. It is clear from this description that a multidisciplinary team including individuals from physical or occupational therapy, kinesiology, psychology, nutrition, and medicine is necessary for an effective cardiac rehabilitation program. This chapter provides information about the physiologic, psychological, and cardiovascular risk reduction benefits associated with cardiac rehabilitation. Practical aspects of rehabilitation are also discussed.

RATIONALE FOR CARDIAC REHABILITATION

Effects of Physical Training

Physical inactivity causes a reduction in functional capacity in 1 to 3 weeks as a result of changes in both systemic and peripheral variables. On the other hand, it takes several months to improve the fitness level.[3,4] Patients who have undergone angioplasty or coronary artery bypass surgery or who have experienced myocardial infarction all have some physical deconditioning. This deconditioning can exacerbate symptoms of fatigue, shortness of breath, and even angina, independent of any deterioration in the cardiac status. Therefore, the clinical course of cardiac patients undergoing cardiac surgery is a strong rationale for participation in a cardiac exercise rehabilitation program to improve their functional capacity.

When considering the effects of physical training, it is important to consider the two different types of workload being performed during an activity: the external workload and the internal workload. The external workload is represented by the power output of a required activity, which determines the oxygen demand for the activity.[5] For example, during cycle ergometry a power output of 400 kilopond-meter/min requires an oxygen uptake (VO_2) of approximately 800 ml/min.[6] Therefore, an identical external workload produces similar VO_2 demands in different individuals.[7] Internal workload is the product of heart rate and systolic blood pressure, known as the rate pressure product (RPP), which determines the myocardial VO_2.[8,9] The internal workload is not directly determined by the external workload.[5]

The exercise heart rate and blood pressure responses are linearly related to the VO_2 during exercise for an individual at a given level of fitness (Fig. 8-1).[5] Maximum heart rate is not greatly affected by training, but the relationship between the heart rate and VO_2 is altered.[10] After training, at any given submaximal external work rate, the heart rate is lower resulting in a decreased RPP and myocardial VO_2. Therefore, after training the lower myocardial VO_2 at a given submaximal workload results in a reduced coronary artery blood flow requirement.[9,11]

Exercise training increases maximum oxygen uptake (VO_2max) in healthy individuals and patients with heart disease.[5,12–14] This increase is realized through a combination of central and peripheral adaptations.[5,15] For patients with heart disease, earlier studies suggested that the increase in VO_2max was mediated by peripheral changes in skeletal muscle resulting in a decreased myocardial VO_2 secondary to a reduction in adrenergic efferent stimuli.[16,17] In support of this theory are the facts that for a given submaximal workload after training, reductions occur in heart rate,[16,18–21] systemic arterial pressure,[16,18–20] and cardiac output,[16,22] and increased arteriovenous oxygen difference.[22]

Although the peripheral adaptations after exercise training of patients with heart disease are well established, the central adaptations have not been as clearly defined. Furthermore, central adaptations are not necessarily required to achieve the reduction in anginal symptoms observed in patients with heart disease after training. In fact, the reduction in RPP and increase in diastolic period (due to a lower heart rate) explains the reduction in anginal symptoms at a given submaximal workload after training.[18,21,23–27]

Some investigators do support the theory that central adaptations also take place after training in patients with heart disease. Thompson et al.[28] had patients train with one limb and then determined the exercise response while they performed with the untrained limb. They found improvements in exercise performance for both the trained and untrained muscle groups following exercise training, suggesting that some central adaptation is associated with exercise training.

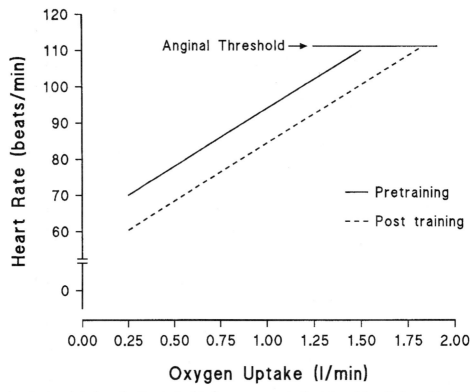

Fig. 8-1. The heart rate, plotted on the Y-axis, in this figure represents the internal (cardiac) workload and the oxygen uptake, plotted on the X-axis, represents the external (total body) workload. As can be seen after training, a greater external workload can be achieved before the internal workload is reached, which precipitates angina. Therefore, exercise training does not necessarily change the original threshold, but it changes the relationship between heart rate (internal workload) and oxygen uptake (external workload).

Studies have demonstrated an improvement in left ventricular function following exercise training.[12,29–34] The improvement is observed when individuals have trained for a minimum of 6 months[33] but not with shorter periods of exercise training.[21,35] Therefore, the peripheral adaptations occur early during the training period, whereas central adaptations may only occur with more prolonged training.

After training, an increase in stroke volume and ejection fraction at a constant afterload occurs, suggesting an increase in myocardial contractility.[12,29,31–33] Other studies have found that after training, there is a mean velocity of circumferential shortening and systolic time interval indices of left ventricular performance improve during an isometric handgrip at a constant blood pressure.[30,34] The results of these studies suggest an improvement of left ventricular function after exercise, suggesting an improvement in myocardial perfusion, although this improvement has been difficult to demonstrate.

Indirect evidence to support the theory of improvement in myocardial perfusion after exercise training has existed for many years.[18] Several studies have demonstrated less ST segment depression at the same RPP after training.[32,36,37] Exercise thallium testing has been used to assess patients and has demonstrated an improvement in myocardial perfusion after training.[12,38–40] Ferguson et al.[40] measured coronary sinus blood flow and left ventricular myocardial oxygen uptake after training. They found an increase in maximal coronary sinus flow and left ventricular myocardial oxygen uptake, indicating an improvement in myocardial blood flow after training.

Despite these studies angiographic studies failed to demonstrate collateral vessel development in patients with coronary artery disease (CAD).[41–45] Interestingly, Sim and Neill[43] observed an increase in the RPP at the onset of angina, but no change when angina was produced by ventricular pacing. These investigators suggested exercise training may reduce coronary vasoconstriction during exercise. This theory is supported by laboratory studies demonstrating a decrease in coronary vasomotor reactivity after exercise training in dogs.[46] More recently, angiographic evidence has suggested that combining exercise training with a low-fat diet may improve myocardial perfusion by regression of coronary atherosclerosis.[47,48] It is now widely recognized that a sedentary life-style is an independent risk factor for the development of CAD.[49,50] Although exercise training has a beneficial independent effect, it also appears to have an impact on other known risk factors for CAD.[51,52]

Effects of Exercise Training on Serum Lipids

Generally, exercise training has a favorable effect on serum lipid profile.[53–55] The beneficial effect of exercise training on serum lipids appears dependent on the net energy expenditure rather than the intensity of exercise.[54,56] Exercise training produces an increase in high-density lipoprotein (HDL) cholesterol, which tends to level off after 6 to 12 months of training.[57] Even with unsupervised exercise training, a 10 percent increase in HDL cholesterol and HDL cholesterol/total cholesterol ratio has been found.[54] This increase is similar to the degree of change observed with drug therapy and translates into a 30 percent reduction in CAD risk.[58] Although several long-term studies of exercise training in healthy sedentary men suggest a benefit on lipid profiles,[56,57,59,60] however, other studies have not shown similar benefit.[61,62] The disparity in findings among these studies may result from several factors including the short periods of observation, the uncontrolled nature of some of the studies, the inclusion of subjects with predominantly low HDL cholesterol, and the use of only a few subjects and even fewer women.[63] A meta-analysis performed by Tran and Weltman[55] demonstrated that exercise training had a beneficial effect on plasma lipid profile. Even when body weight did not change, cholesterol and low-density lipoprotein (LDL) cholesterol declined significantly. The greatest decrease in serum lipid level was observed when exercise training was combined with weight loss. Serum cholesterol levels increased slightly when weight gain occurred during exercise training. Therefore, a combination of exercise training and weight loss has a more beneficial effect on serum lipid levels than exercise training alone.

Effects of Exercise Training on Hypertension

Studies of the effects of exercise training on established hypertension reported an average reduction of 11 mmHg for systolic pressure and 8 mmHg for diastolic pressure.[64] These studies had certain limitations including small sample size,[65–67] lack of a control group,[68,69] and doubtful adequacy of the exercise program.[67,70] Nonetheless, meta-analyses demonstrated a significant reduction in systolic and diastolic blood pressure.[71] The effects of exercise may be most beneficial in obese hypertensive patients.[72,73] Exercise training must be habitual to maintain the beneficial effects on blood pressure.[67,74]

Effects of Exercise Training on Glucose Intolerance

Regular physical activity has a beneficial effect in patients with non-insulin-dependent diabetes mellitus.[75–78] Studies have demonstrated significant decreases in glycosylated hemoglobin levels indicating effective control of the diabetes after as little as 6 weeks of training.[75,76] Insulin levels considered to be atherogenic are also decreased after exercise training.[79,80] Therefore, exercise training has significant effects on both plasma glucose and insulin levels in patients with diabetes.

Effects of Exercise Training Independent of Other Risk Factors

Although some of the beneficial effects of exercise training are related to changes in risk factors, there is also an independent effect of exercise to reduce the effects of CAD. Evidence suggests that exercise training increases the activity of the fibrinolytic system[81] and may reduce hypercoagulable states,[82,83] thus reducing the probability of inappropriate coagulation. Furthermore, regular physical activity may inhibit platelet aggregation.[84]

Studies have demonstrated a beneficial effect on the autonomic nervous system after exercise training.[85,86] Plasma catecholamine levels are reduced[87,88] and an increase in heart rate variability suggesting an increase in vagal tone[86,88,89] is observed in patients who participate in regular exercise training. This change in autonomic balance in favor of the parasympathetic nervous system may reduce patient risk for developing a serious ventricular arrhythmia.[90]

Psychological Effects of Exercise Training

CAD not only may cause physical limitations but also may produce a significant degree of psychological debility. The goal of a well-designed cardiac rehabilitation program is to reduce the physical and psychological limitations associated with CAD.

Several studies have examined the effects of exercise training on anxiety levels.[91–100] Controversy exists regarding the effects of exercise training on anxiety, but generally controlled trials have found a significant decrease in anxiety levels in the group involved in regular physical activity.[95–99] Reasons for not showing a beneficial effect with exercise training have been small sample sizes, inadequate exercise intensity, and lack of a control group. King et al.[100] reported that exercise did not change anxiety levels in 120 sedentary men and women; however, the subjects were not anxious before the training. This fault highlights the need to include only anxious subjects at baseline, especially when the sample size is small.

Some studies have compared the effects of exercise training with psychotherapy or relaxation techniques on depression.[101–104] Furthermore, North et al.[105] reported the results of a meta-analysis study, which included 80 trials that examined the effects of exercise on depression. They found that regular habitual exercise decreased the level of depression. Both aerobic and anaerobic exercises reduced depression as effectively as psychotherapy. The best strategy for depressed patients is a combination of exercise and psychotherapy, which was better than exercise alone in reducing depression.

Friedman and Rosenman[106] identified behavior characteristics associated with an increased risk of CAD and labeled as type A personality disorder. Several criteria are used to define type A behavior, but the two main diagnostic components are impatience and free-floating hostility (i.e., easily aroused irritation or anger). Also, it would appear that insecurity or low self-esteem precede and sustain the presence of type A behavior.[107] Little research has been published on the effects of exercise training on type A behavior, and results are inconsistent. Although some investigations demonstrated that exercise has a beneficial effect on type A behavior,[108–110] others have not.[111,112] This inconsistency may be related to methodology; for example, type A behavior has specific diagnostic criteria and cannot be properly assessed by questionnaires administered by inexperienced nonmedical personnel. Also the key component to diagnosing type A behavior is the videotaped structured interview. Studies often do not use this approach, and their questionnaires omit questions concerning the presence of free-floating hostility.[107] A combined approach of exercise and counseling is the best way to decrease the amount of type A behavior.

Potential Improvements with Exercise Rehabilitation

Regular exercise training increases peak exercise performance by approximately 25 to 30 percent.[12,18,22,29,41] The increase in performance for an individual patient depends on factors such as the pretraining level of fitness, the intensity of training, and duration of the exercise program. More recently, a combination of aerobic and resistance (weight lifting) training has been advocated for patients with CAD.[113] The effects of combined resistance and aerobic training was compared to the effects of aerobic training alone in a group of CAD patients who had already participated for 3 months in an aerobic training program.[114] After training, patients in the combined group had a 15 percent increase in peak incremental exercise test performance, a 30 percent increase in muscle strength, and a 109 percent increase in endurance exercise capacity. The group training aerobically showed no significant change for any of these end points. These results clearly suggest that a combined program of aerobic and resistance training may be most beneficial for CAD patients with well-maintained left ventricular function.

Summary

As outlined in previous sections, exercise rehabilitation can be expected to produce beneficial effects on risk factors for CAD such as hypertension, glucose intolerance, and hyperlipidemia. Furthermore, regular physical activity may decrease levels of anxiety and depression in patients manifesting these symptoms.

SECONDARY PREVENTION

Although it is important that cardiac rehabilitation improves functional capacity, it would be even more important if evidence demonstrated a reduction in morbidity and mortality. Such a reduction would encourage clinicians to refer patients to a cardiac exercise rehabilitation program. Furthermore, the overall benefits of cardiac rehabilitation would certainly justify the cost and the patient effort involved in maintaining these programs.

Over the last 20 years, more than 4,700 patients have been randomized to trials of cardiac rehabilitation.[12,115–131] These studies typically involved supervised exercise training programs with two to four sessions a week lasting 20 to 60 minutes each. The extent of the nonexercise interventions varied significantly, but in most studies the patients in the exercise group received some degree of risk factor modification. Length of exercise training varied considerably from months to years. Although these studies have shown a trend toward lower mortality among survivors of myocardial infarction involved in the exercise rehabilitation, they have been unable to rigorously test the hypothesis that rehabilitation reduces overall mortality because of their small sample size.

Meta-Analysis

Another approach to investigate the impact of cardiac rehabilitation on significant clinical outcomes such as morbidity and mortality is to pool data from smaller trials of similar design in which sufficient methodologic detail has been provided to ensure comparability. This methodologic approach of meta-analyses represents a way to increase statistical power for primary end points and subgroups, resolve uncertainty when studies disagree, improve estimates of effect size, and answer questions not posed at the start of individual studies.[132] The strength of this form of analyses is based on the quality of the component studies and data available and not the number of accumulated patient years. Trials included in a meta-analysis must be similar in general design, entry criteria, and intervention. Furthermore, trials selected for analyses must represent an unbiased sample from the literature.

Early studies that pooled data to examine the effect of cardiac rehabilitation on morbidity and mortality found on average a 25 percent reduction in mortality for patients involved in the rehabilitation group.[133–135] These studies, however, were limited because all available trials were not included in the analyses and direct comparisons were made between patients in different trials. More recent meta-analyses studies have used data from all available randomized trials meeting specific inclusion criteria.[136,137]

Oldridge et al.[136] used five criteria to include trials in a meta-analysis: (1) documented myocardial infarction, (2) randomization of patients, (3) rehabilitation (defined as some combination of exercise and risk factor modification), (4) follow-up study (≥ 24 months after randomization), and (5) documentation of outcome to include at least two of all causes of death, cardiovascular mortality, and nonfatal recurrent myocardial infarction. Thirteen trials were included in the meta-analysis. In one of these trials, however, patients were allocated in groups according to their time of enrollment. Another trial did not meet the 24-month follow-up criterion. In still another trial, patients were randomized into control or treatment based on their hospital of origin. After these trials were excluded 10 trials including 4,347 patients were available for meta-analysis. The pooled odds ratios (OR) of 0.76 (95 percent confidence intervals [CI], 0.63 to 0.92) for all-cause death and of 0.75 (95 percent CI, 0.62 to 0.93) for cardiovascular death were significantly lower in the rehabilitation group than in the control group. There was no significant difference for nonfatal recurrent myocardial infarction between the two groups.

Using a similar form of meta-analysis and inclusion criteria as those of Oldridge et al.[136] O'Connor and colleagues performed another meta-analysis.[137] The end points in their study were total mortality, cardiovascular mortality, sudden death, and fatal and nonfatal myocardial infarction. For each end point, an OR and 95 percent CI were calculated for the combined trials. Twenty-two studies including 4,554 patients were available for the meta-analysis. Significant reductions in total mortality (OR = 0.80; 95 percent CI = 0.66 to 0.96), cardiovascular mortality (OR = 0.78; 95 percent CI = 0.63 to 0.96), and fatal

reinfarction (OR = 0.75; 95 percent CI = 0.59 to 0.95) were observed for the rehabilitation group but not the comparison group at an average follow-up of 3 years. At 1 year there was a significant reduction in sudden death for the rehabilitation group compared to the comparison group (OR = 0.63; 95 percent CI = 0.41 to 0.97). There was no significant reduction between the groups for nonfatal reinfarction.

These meta-analyses demonstrate consistent results that suggest an exercise-based rehabilitation program reduces mortality but not nonfatal recurrent infarction. These studies have also led to the recommendation that middle-aged men should be involved in exercise-based rehabilitation programs after a myocardial infarction.[138]

Persisting Problems

Many more issues relating to cardiac rehabilitation must be explored. Whether some patients would benefit more than others from rehabilitation remains unclear. The optimal timing for rehabilitation, the most efficacious dose (intensity, frequency, and duration), and the type of training (low intensity versus high intensity; aerobic training versus combined aerobic and resistance training) all must be determined. The effects of cardiac rehabilitation should be studied in patients after angioplasty, coronary artery bypass surgery, and thrombolytic therapy, as well as in patients with silent ischemia and congestive heart failure. Studies so far have randomized few women (approximately 3 percent); the effects of cardiac rehabilitation in women, therefore, requires further investigation. In addition, most patients were less than 70 years old; therefore, data on the effects of exercise rehabilitation in elderly persons are lacking. Finally, many studies were performed before the widespread use of beta-blockers and calcium-channel blockers. How exercise rehabilitation interacts with these drugs and other forms of therapy also needs investigation.

Although these meta-analyses demonstrated a reduction in mortality, they did not elucidate the physiologic mechanisms responsible for the effect. Potential mechanisms include an increase in myocardial blood flow, decrease in myocardial work, increase in myocardial function, and increase in electrical stability of the myocardium (Table 8-1). Further studies are required to determine which of

Table 8-1. Biologic Mechanisms by Which Exercise May Contribute to the Primary or Secondary Prevention of Coronary Heart Disease[a]

Maintain or increase myocardial oxygen supply
 Delay progression of coronary atherosclerosis (possible)
  Improve lipoprotein profile (increase HDL-C/LDL-C ratio) (probable)
  Improve carbohydrate metabolism (increase insulin sensitivity) (probable)
  Decrease platelet aggregation and increase fibrinolysis (probable)
  Decrease adiposity (usually)
 Increase coronary collateral vascularization (unlikely)
 Increase epicardial artery diameter (possible)
 Increase coronary blood flow (myocardial perfusion) or distribution (possible)
Decrease myocardial work and oxygen demand
 Decrease heart rate at rest and submaximal exercise (usually)
 Decrease systolic and mean systemic arterial pressure during submaximal exercise (usually) and at rest (possible)
 Decrease cardiac output during submaximal exercise (probable)
 Decrease circulating plasma catecholamine levels (decrease sympathetic tone) at rest (probable) and at submaximal exercise (usually)
Increase myocardial function
 Increase stroke volume at rest and in submaximal and maximal exercise (likely)
 Increase ejection fraction at rest and during exercise (likely)
 Increase intrinsic myocardial contractility (possible)
 Increase myocardial function resulting from decreased "afterload" (probable)
 Increase myocardial hypertrophy (probable); but this may not reduce CHD risk
Increase electrical stability of myocardium
 Decrease regional ischemia at submaximal exercise (possible)
 Decrease catecholamines in myocardium at rest (possible) and at submaximal exercise (probable)
 Increase ventricular fibrillation threshold due to reduction of cyclic AMP (possible)

Abbreviations: HDL-C, high-density lipoprotein cholesterol; LDL-C, low-density lipoprotein cholesterol; CHD, coronary heart disease; AMP, adenosine monophosphate.

[a]Expression of likelihood that effect will occur for an individual participating in endurance type training program for 16 weeks or longer at 65% to 80% of functional capacity for 25 minutes or longer per session (300 kcal) for three or more sessions per week ranges from unlikely, possible, likely, probable, to usually. (From Haskell et al,[141] with permission)

these mechanism(s) is most responsible for the reduction in mortality after exercise rehabilitation.

CONCLUSIONS

Cardiac rehabilitation is comprised of two components: exercise training and risk factor modification. Exercise training of patients with cardiac disease significantly improves functional capacity. Regular training also results in improvements in other risk factors for CAD such as hypertension and hypercholesterolemia. Meta-analyses have demonstrated that cardiac rehabilitation significantly reduces total mortality, cardiovascular mortality, and fatal reinfarction in patients involved in rehabilitation. Nonfatal reinfarction rates are not significantly reduced. The reduction in mortality associated with exercise training is independent of alterations in other risk factors.

It is unlikely that further prospective randomized controlled trials (RCTs) of cardiac exercise rehabilitation will be performed for several reasons. First, it is difficult to recruit enough patients who would be willing to be randomized to an exercise or control group. Second, event rates are relatively low among the randomized population; thus a long follow-up period and large sample size would be required. Finally, analysis would be complex because of confounding effects of contemporary alterations in lifestyle and other risk factors for cardiovascular disease.[139] It has been estimated that at least 4,000 patients would need to be randomized into a prospective RCT to reliably distinguish between no effect and the most plausible alternative of a 20 percent reduction in cardiovascular-related mortality.[137]

Many more studies are required to better define the role of cardiac rehabilitation for the treatment of cardiac disease. Future studies need to include more women and individuals over the age of 70 years. Studies need to be designed to assess which types of exercise training are most beneficial, as well as the effects on quality of life. Further work is required to better define the mechanism(s) responsible for the reduction in mortality associated with cardiac rehabilitation. With the advent of technology such as positron emission tomography scanning, studies will be designed to better evaluate myocardial perfusion after cardiac rehabilitation.

Although much more work is needed in the area of cardiac rehabilitation, data strongly suggest that middle-aged men should participate in cardiac rehabilitation programs after an acute myocardial infarction. Even though future studies are required in other groups of patients with CAD (e.g., postangioplasty, postoperative coronary artery bypass surgery, stable angina, or congestive heart failure) the relative safety of training in supervised exercise programs[140] and the well-known general physiologic responses to training outlined in this chapter support the use of regular training in a broad range of patients with cardiac disease.

REFERENCES

1. Report of the World Health Organization Expert Committee on Disability Prevention and Rehabilitation: Rehabilitation of patients with cardiovascular disease: report of a WHO Expert Committee. WHO Tech Rep Series No 270, 1964
2. Greenland P, Chu JS: Efficacy of cardiac rehabilitation services with emphasis on patients after myocardial infarction. Ann Intern Med 109:650, 1988
3. Saltin B, Blomqvist G, Mitchell JH et al: Response to submaximal and maximal exercise after bed rest and training. Circulation suppl. VII, 38:VII, 1968
4. Saltin B, Rowell LB: Functional adaptations to physical activity and inactivity. Fed Proc 39:1506, 1980
5. Clausen JP: Circulatory adjustments to dynamic exercise and effects of physical training in normal subjects and in-patients with coronary artery disease. p. 39. In Sonnenblick EH, Lesch M (eds): Exercise and Heart Disease. Grune & Stratton, Orlando, 1977
6. McKelvie RS, Jones NL: Cardiopulmonary exercise testing. Clin Chest Med 10:277, 1989
7. Rowell LB: Human Circulation: Regulation During Physical Stress. p. 213. Oxford University Press, New York, 1986
8. Amsterdam EA, Hughes III JL, DeMaria AN et al: Indirect assessment of myocardial oxygen consumption in the evaluation of mechanisms and therapy of angina pectoris. Am J Cardiol 33:737, 1974
9. Gobel FL, Nordstrom LA, Nelson RR et al: The rate pressure product as an index of myocardial oxygen consumption during exercise in patients with angina pectoris. Circulation 57:549, 1978
10. Åstrand P-O, Rodahl K: Physical training. Textbook of Work Physiology. p. 412. Physiological Bases of Exercise. 3rd Ed. McGraw-Hill, Toronto, 1986
11. Klocke FJ: Coronary blood flow in man. Prog Cardiovasc Dis 19:117, 1976
12. Froelicher V, Jensen D, Genter F et al: A randomized trial of exercise training in patients with coronary artery disease. JAMA 252:1291, 1984
13. Myers J, Ahnve S, Froelicher V et al: A randomized trial of the effects of 1 year of exercise training on computer-measured ST segment displacement in patients with coronary artery disease. J Am Coll Cardiol 4:1094, 1984
14. Froelicher V, Jensen D, Sullivan M: A randomized trial of the effects of exercise training after coronary artery bypass surgery. Arch Intern Med 145:689, 1985
15. Mitchell JH, Blomqvist G: Maximal oxygen uptake. N Engl J Med 284:1018, 1971
16. Clausen JP, Trap-Jensen J: Effects of training on the distribution of cardiac output in patients with coronary artery disease. Circulation 42:611, 1970
17. Clausen JP, Trap-Jensen J, Lassen NA: Evidence that the relative exercise-bradycardia induced by training can be caused by extracardiac factors. In Larsen OA, Malmborg RO (eds): Coronary Heart Disease and Physical Fitness. p. 27. University Park Press, Baltimore, 1971
18. Redwood DR, Rosing DR, Epstein SE: Circulatory and symptomatic effects of physical training in patients with coronary artery disease and angina pectoris. N Engl J Med 286:959, 1972
19. Clausen JP, Larsen OA, Trap-Jensen J: Physical training in the management of coronary artery disease. Circulation 40:143, 1969
20. Ehsani AA, Heath GW, Hagberg JM et al: Effects of 12 months of intense exercise training on ischemic ST-segment depression in patients with coronary artery disease. Circulation 64:1116, 1981
21. Detry JM, Bruce RA: Effects of physical training on exertional ST segment depression in coronary heart disease. Circulation 44:390, 1971
22. Detry J-MR, Rousseau M, Vandenbroucke G et al: Increased arteriovenous oxygen difference after

physical training in coronary heart disease. Circulation 44:109, 1971

23. Frick MH, Katila M: Haemodynamic consequences of physical training after myocardial infarction. Circulation 37:192, 1968

24. Kavanagh T, Shephard RJ: Conditioning of postcoronary patients: comparison of continuous and interval training. Arch Phys Med Rehabil 56:72, 1975

25. Clausen JP: Circulatory adjustments to dynamic exercise and effect of physical training in normal subjects and patients with coronary artery disease. Prog Cardiovasc Dis 18:459, 1976

26. Detry JMR, Rousseau MT, Brasseur LA: Early hemodynamic adaptations to physical training in patients with healed myocardial infarction. Eur J Cardiol 2:307, 1975

27. Ferguson RJ, Côté P, Gauthier P, Bourassa MG: Changes in exercise coronary sinus blood flow with training in patients with angina pectoris. Circulation 58:41, 1978

28. Thompson PD, Cullinane E, Lazarus B, Carleton RA: Effect of exercise training on the untrained limb exercise performance of men with angina pectoris. Am J Cardiol 48:844, 1981

29. Paterson DH, Shephard RJ, Cunningham D et al: Effects of physical training on cardiovascular function following myocardial infarction. J Appl Physiol 47:482, 1979

30. Ehsani AA, Martin WH, Heath GW, Coyle EF: Cardiac effects of prolonged and intense exercise training in patients with coronary artery disease. Am J Cardiol 50:246, 1982

31. Hagberg JM, Ehsani AA, Holloszy JO: Effect of 12 months of intense exercise training on stroke volume in patients with coronary artery disease. Circulation 67:1194, 1983

32. Ehsani AA, Biello DR, Schultz J et al: Improvement of left ventricular contractile function by exercise training in patients with coronary artery disease. Circulation 74:350, 1986

33. Jensen D, Atwood JE, Froelicher V et al: Improvement in ventricular function during exercise studied with radionuclide ventriculography after cardiac rehabilitation. Am J Cardiol 46:770, 1980

34. Martin WH, Heath G, Coyle EF et al: Effect of prolonged intense endurance training on systolic time intervals in patients with coronary artery disease. Am Heart J 107:75, 1984

35. Verani S, Hartung GH, Hoepfel-Harris J et al: Effects of exercise training on left ventricular performance and myocardial perfusion in patients with coronary artery disease. Am J Cardiol 47:797, 1981

36. Laslett LJ, Paumer L, Amsterdam EA: Increase in myocardial oxygen consumption indexes by exercise training at onset of ischemia in patients with coronary artery disease. Circulation 71:958, 1985

37. Ehsani AA, Heath GW, Hagberg JM et al: Effects of 12 months of intense exercise training on ischemic ST-segment depression in patients with coronary artery disease. Circulation 64:1116, 1981

38. Sebrechts CP, Klein JL, Ahnve S et al: Myocardial perfusion changes following 1 year of exercise training assessed by thallium-201 circumferential count profiles. Am Heart J 112:1217, 1986

39. Schuler G, Schlierf G, Wirth A et al: Low-fat diet and regular supervised physical exercise in patients with symptomatic coronary artery disease: reduction of stress induced myocardial ischemia. Circulation 77:172, 1988

40. Ferguson RJ, Taylor AW, Côté P et al: Skeletal muscle and cardiac changes with training in patients with angina pectoris. Am J Physiol 243:H830, 1982

41. Ferguson RJ, Petitclerc R, Choquette G et al: Effect of physical training on treadmill exercise capacity, collateral circulation and progression of coronary disease. Am J Cardiol 34:764, 1974

42. Conner JF, LaCamera F, Swanick EJ et al: Effects of exercise on coronary collateralization—angiographic studies of six patients in a supervised exercise program. Med Sci Sports Exerc 8:145, 1976

43. Sim DN, Neill WA: Investigation of the physiological basis for increased exercise threshold for angina pectoris after physical conditioning. J Clin Invest 54:763, 1974

44. Nolewajka AJ, Kostuk WJ, Rechnitzer PA, Cunningham DA: Exercise and human collateralization: an angiographic and scintigraphic assessment. Circulation 60:114, 1979

45. Kennedy CC, Spiekerman RE, Lindsay MI et al: One year graduated exercise program for men with angina pectoris. Mayo Clin Proc 51:231, 1976

46. Bove AA, Dewey JD: Proximal coronary vasomotor reactivity after exercise training in dogs. Circulation 71:620, 1985

47. Ornish D, Brown SE, Scherwitz LW et al: Can lifestyle changes reverse coronary heart disease? The Lifestyle Heart Trial. Lancet 336:129, 1990

48. Schuler G, Hambrecht R, Schlierf G et al: Myocardial perfusion and regression of coronary heart disease in patients on a regimen of intensive physical exercise and low fat diet. J Am Coll Cardiol 19:34, 1992

49. Powell KE, Thompson PD, Caspersen CJ, Kendrick JS: Physical activity and the incidence of coronary heart disease. Annu Rev Public Health 8:253, 1987

50. AHA Medical/Scientific Statement: Statement on Exercise: benefits and recommendations for physical activity programs for all Americans. A Statement for Health Professionals by the Committee on Exercise and Cardiac Rehabilitation of the Council on Clinical Cardiology. Circulation 86:340, 1992

51. Oberman A: Rehabilitation of patients with coronary heart disease. In Braunwald E (ed): Heart Disease: A Textbook of Cardiovascular Medicine. p. 1395. WB Saunders, Philadelphia, 1988

52. Vermeulen A, Lie KI, Durrer D: Effects of cardiac rehabilitation after myocardial infarction: changes in coronary risk factors and long-term prognosis. Am Heart J 105:798, 1983

53. Williams PT, Krauss RM, Vranizan KM et al: The effects of long distance running and weight loss on plasma low-density lipoprotein subfraction concentrations in men. Arteriosclerosis 9:623, 1989

54. Marti B, Suter E, Riesen WF et al: Effects of long-term, self-monitored exercise on the serum lipoprotein and apolipoprotein profile in middle-aged men. Atherosclerosis 81:19, 1990

55. Tran ZV, Weltman A: Differential effects of exercise on serum lipid and lipoprotein levels seen with changes in body weight. JAMA 254:919, 1985

56. Williams PT, Krauss RM, Vranizan KM, Wood PD: Changes in lipoprotein subfraction during diet-induced and exercise-induced weight loss in moderately overweight men. Circulation 81:1293, 1990

57. Thompson PD, Cullinane EM, Sady SP et al: Modest change in high-density lipoprotein concentration and metabolism with prolonged exercise training. Circulation 78:25, 1988

58. Manninen V, Elo MO, Frick H et al: Lipid alterations and decline in the incidence of coronary heart disease in the Helsinki Heart Study. JAMA 260:641, 1988

59. Baker TT, Allen D, Lei LY, Willcox K: Alterations in lipid and protein profiles of plasma lipoproteins in middle-aged men consequent to an aerobic exercise program. Metabolism 35:1037, 1986

60. Wood PD, Stefanick ML, Dreon DM et al: Changes in plasma lipids and lipoproteins in overweight men during weight loss through dieting as compared with exercise. N Engl J Med 319:1173, 1988

61. Raz I, Rosenblit H, Kark JD: Effects of moderate exercise on serum lipids in young men with low HDL-cholesterol. Arteriosclerosis 8:245, 1988

62. Wood PD, Haskell WL, Blair SN et al: Increased exercise level and plasma lipoprotein concentrations: a one-year randomized, controlled study in sedentary middle-aged men. Metabolism 31:31, 1983

63. Chandrashekhar Y, Anand IS: Exercise as a coronary protective factor. Am Heart J 122:1723, 1991

64. Hagberg JM, Seals DR: Exercise training and hypertension. Acta Med Scand Suppl 711:131, 1986

65. Mann GV, Garrett HL, Fabri A et al: Exercise to prevent coronary heart disease: an experimental study of the effects of training on risk factors for coronary disease in men. Am J Med 46:12, 1969

66. Kukkonen K, Rauramaa R, Vontilainer E, Lansimies E: Physical training of middle aged men with borderline hypertension. Ann Clin Res 34:139, 1982

67. Roman O, Camuzzi AL, Villalon E, Klenner C: Physical training program in arterial hypertension: a long-term prospective follow-up. Cardiology 67:230, 1981

68. Boger JL, Kasch FW: Exercise therapy in hypertensive men. JAMA 211:1668, 1970

69. Choquette G, Ferguson RJ: Blood pressure reduction in "borderline" hypertensives following physical training. Can Med Assoc J 108:699, 1973

70. Johnson WP, Grover JA: Hemodynamic and metabolic effects of physical training in four patients with essential hypertension. Can Med Assoc J 96:842, 1967

71. Hagberg JM: Exercise fitness and hypertension. In Bouchard C et al (eds): Exercise, Fitness and Health: A Consensus of Current Knowledge. Human Kinetics Books, Champaign, IL, 1990

72. Franklin B, Buskirk E, Hodgson J et al: Effects of physical conditioning on cardiorespiratory function, body composition and serum lipids in relatively normal-weight and obese middle-aged women. Int J Obesity 3:97, 1979

73. Krotkiewski M, Mandrovkas K, Sjostrom L et al: Effects of long-term physical training on body fat, metabolism and blood pressure and obesity. Metabolism 28:650, 1979

74. Kiyonaga A, Arakawa K, Tanaka H et al: Blood pressure and hormonal responses to aerobic exercise. Hypertension 7:125, 1985

75. Trovati M, Carta Q, Cavalot F et al: Influence of physical training on blood glucose control, glucose tolerance, insulin secretion, and insulin action in non-insulin-dependent diabetic patients. Diabetes Care 7:416, 1984

76. Schneider SH, Amorosa LF, Khachadurian AK et al: Studies on the mechanisms of improved glucose control during regular exercise in type II (non-insulin-dependent) diabetes. Diabetologia 26:355, 1984

77. Rauramaa R: Relationship of physical activity, glucose tolerance, and weight management. Prev Med 13:37, 1984

78. Heath GW, Gavin JR, Hinderliter JM et al: Effects of exercise and lack of exercise on glucose toler-

ance and insulin sensitivity. J Appl Physiol 55:512, 1983

79. Stout RW: Blood glucose and atherosclerosis. Arteriosclerosis 1:227, 1981

80. Oberman A: Exercise and the primary prevention of cardiovascular disease. Am J Cardiol 55:10D, 1985

81. Ferguson EW, Bernier LL, Banta GR et al: Effects of exercise and conditioning on clotting and fibrinolytic activity in men. J Appl Physiol 62:1416, 1987

82. Lee G, Amsterdam EA, DeMaria AM et al: Effect of exercise on hemostatic mechanisms. In Amsterdam EA, Wilmore JH, DeMaria AM (eds): Exercise in Cardiovascular Health and Disease. Yorke Medical Books, New York, 1977

83. Donahue RP, Abbott RD, Reed DM, Yano K: Physical activity and coronary heart disease in middle-aged and elderly men: the Honolulu heart program. Am J Public Health 78:683, 1988

84. Watts EJ, Weir P: Reduced platelet aggregation in long distance runners. Lancet 1:1013, 1098, 1989

85. Cooksey JD, Reilly P, Brown S et al: Exercise training and plasma catecholamines in patients with ischemic heart disease. Am J Cardiol 42:372, 1978

86. Pagani M, Somers V, Furlan R et al: Changes in autonomic regulation induced by physical training in mild hypertension. Hypertension 12:600, 1988

87. Ehsani AA, Health GW, Martin WH et al: Effects of intense exercise training on plasma catecholamines in coronary patients. J Appl Physiol 57:154, 1984

88. Coats AJS, Adamopoulos S, Radaelli A et al: Controlled trial of physical training in chronic heart failure: exercise performance, hemodynamics, ventilation, and autonomic function. Circulation 85:2119, 1992

89. Seals DR, Chase P: Influence of physical training on heart rate variability and baroreflex circulatory control. J Appl Physiol 66:1886, 1989

90. Billman GE, Schwartz PJ, Stone HL: The effects of daily exercise on susceptibility to sudden cardiac death. Circulation 69:1181, 1984

91. Wood D: The relationship between state anxiety and acute physical activity. Am Correct Thers J 31:67, 1977

92. Kowal D, Patton J, Vogel J: Psychological states and aerobic fitness of male and female recruits before and after basic training. Aviat Space Environ Med 49:603, 1978

93. Morgan W: Anxiety reduction following acute physical activity. Psychiatr Ann 9:141, 1979

94. Molloy DW, Beerschoten DA, Barrie MJ et al: Acute effects of exercise on neuropsychological function in elderly subjects. J Am Geriatr Soc 36:29, 1988

95. Lichtman S, Poser E: The effects of exercise on mood and cognitive functioning. J Psychosom Res 27:43, 1983

96. Blumenthal JA, Williams RS, Needels TL et al: Psychological changes accompany aerobic exercise in healthy middle-aged adults. Psychosom Med 44:529, 1982

97. Simons C, Birkimer J: An exploration of factors predicting effects of aerobic conditioning on mood state. J Psychosom Res 32:63, 1988

98. Fasting K, Gronningsaeter H: Unemployment, trait anxiety, and physical exercise. Scand J Sport Sci 8:99, 1986

99. Moses J, Steptoe A, Mathews A et al: The effects of exercise training on mental well-being in the normal population: a controlled trial. J Psychosom Res 33:47, 1989

100. King AC, Taylor CB, Haskell WL et al: The influence of regular aerobic exercise on psychological health: a randomized, controlled trial of healthy middle-aged adults. Health Psychol 8:305, 1989

101. Griest JH, Klein MH, Eischens RR et al: Running as treatment for depression. Compr Psychiatry 20:41, 1979

102. Klein MH: A comparative outcome study of group psychotherapy vs exercise treatments for depression. Int J Mental Health 13:148, 1985

103. McCann I, Holmes D: The influence of aerobic exercise on depression. J Pers Soc Psychol 46:1142, 1984

104. McNeil JK, LeBlanc EM, Joyner M: The effect of exercise on depressive symptoms in moderately depressed elderly. Psychol Aging 6:487, 1991

105. North TC, McCullagh P, Tran ZV: Effect of exercise on depression. Exerc Sport Sci Rev 18:379, 1990

106. Friedman M, Rosenman RH: Association of specific overt behavior pattern with blood and cardiovascular findings. JAMA 169:1286, 1959

107. Friedman M: Type A behavior: its diagnosis, cardiovascular relation and the effect of its modification on recurrence of coronary artery disease. Am J Cardiol 64:12C, 1989

108. Blumenthal JA, William RS, William RB et al: Effects of exercise on the type A (coronary prone) behavior pattern. Psychosom Med 42:289, 1980

109. Blumenthal JA, Emery CF, Walsh MA et al: Exercise training in healthy type A middle-aged men: effects on behavioral and cardiovascular responses. Psychosom Med 50:418, 1988

110. Lobitz WC, Brammell HL, Stoll S et al: Physical exercise and anxiety management training for cardiac stress management in a non-patient population. J Cardiovasc Rehabil 3:683, 1983

111. Jasnoski M, Holmes DS: Influence of initial aerobic fitness, aerobic training and changes in aerobic fitness on personality functioning. J Psychosom Res 25:553, 1981

112. Roskies E, Seraganian P, Oslasohn R et al: The Montreal Type A Intervention Project: major findings. Health Psychol 5:45, 1986

113. McKelvie RS, McCartney N: Weightlifting training in cardiac patients: considerations. Sports Med 10:355, 1990

114. McCartney N, McKelvie RS, Haslam DRS, Jones NL: Usefulness of weightlifting training in improving strength and maximal power output in coronary artery disease. Am J Cardiol 67:939, 1991

115. Kenetala E: Physical fitness and feasibility of physical rehabilitation after myocardial infarction in men of working age. Ann Clin Res, supp. 9, 4:1, 1972

116. Sanne H: Exercise tolerance and physical training of non-selected patients after myocardial infarction. Acta Med Scand, suppl. 551:1, 1973

117. Wilhelmsen L, Sanne H, Elmfeldt D et al: A controlled trial of physical training after myocardial infarction: effects on risk factors, nonfatal reinfarction, and death. Prev Med 4:491, 1975

118. Kallio V: Results of rehabilitation in coronary patients. Adv Cardiol 24:153, 1978

119. Kallio V, Hamalainen H, Hakkila J, Luurila OJ: Reduction in sudden deaths by a multifactorial intervention program after acute myocardial infarction. Lancet 2:1091, 1979

120. Carson P, Phillips R, Lloyd M et al: Exercise after myocardial infarction: a controlled trial. J R Coll Phys Lond 16:147, 1982

121. Vermeulen A, Lie KI, Durrer D: Effects of cardiac rehabilitation after myocardial infarction: changes in coronary risk factors and long-term prognosis. Am Heart J 105:798, 1983

122. Shaw LW: Effects of a prescribed supervised exercise program on mortality and cardiovascular morbidity in patients after a myocardial infarction. The National Exercise and Heart Disease Project. Am J Cardiol 48:39, 1981

123. Rechnitzer P, Cunningham DA, Andrew GM et al: Relation of exercise to the recurrence rate of myocardial infarction in men. Ontario Exercise-Heart Collaborative Study. Am J Cardiol 51:65, 1983

124. Lamm G, Denolin H, Dorssiev D, Pisa Z: Rehabilitation and secondary prevention of patients after acute myocardial infarction: WHO Collaborative Study. Adv Cardiol 31:107, 1982

125. Mara S, Paolillo V, Spadaccini F, Angelino PF: Long-term follow-up after a controlled randomized post-myocardial infarction rehabilitation program: effects on morbidity and mortality. Eur Heart J 6:656, 1985

126. Hare DL, Worcester M, Goble AJ: The effects of early exercise training on outcome one year after myocardial infarction, abstracted. The Cardiac Society of Australia and New Zealand, August:412, 1983

127. Bethell HJN: Rehabilitation of coronary patients. Practitioner 226:477, 1982

128. Miller NH, Haskell WL, Berra K, DeBusk RF: Home versus group exercise training for increasing functional capacity after myocardial infarction. Circulation 70:645, 1984

129. Palatsi I: Feasibility of physical training after myocardial infarction and its effect on return to work, morbidity and mortality. Acta Med Scand, suppl. 599:4, 1976

130. Hakkila J: Morbidity and mortality after myocardial infarction. p. 159. In Kellerman JJ, Denolin H (eds): Critical Evaluation of Cardiac Rehabilitation. S Karger, Basel, 1977

131. Blumenthal JA, Rejeski WJ, Walsh-Riddle M et al: Comparison of high- and low-intensity exercise training early after acute myocardial infarction. Am J Cardiol 61:26, 1988

132. Sacks HS, Berrier J, Reitman D et al: Meta-analyses of randomized controlled trials. N Engl J Med 316:450, 1987

133. May GS, Eberlein KA, Furberg CD et al: Secondary prevention after myocardial infarction: a review of long-term trials. Prog Cardiovasc Dis 24:331, 1982

134. Shephard RJ: The value of exercise in ischemic heart disease: a cummulative analysis. J Cardiac Rehabil 3:294, 1983

135. Naughton JP: Contributions of exercise clinical trials to cardiac rehabilitation. Clin Sports Med 3:545, 1984

136. Oldridge NB, Guyatt GH, Fischer ME, Rimm AA: Cardiac rehabilitation after myocardial infarction: combined experience of randomized clinical trials. JAMA 260:945, 1988

137. O'Connor GT, Buring JE, Yusuf S et al: An overview of randomized trials of rehabilitation with exercise after myocardial infarction. Circulation 80:234, 1989

138. Oberman A: Does cardiac rehabilitation increase long-term survival after myocardial infarction? Circulation 80:416, 1989

139. Bittner V, Oberman A: Efficacy studies in coronary rehabilitation. Cardiol Clin 11:333, 1993

140. Van Camp SP, Peterson RA: Cardiovascular complications of outpatient cardiac rehabilitation programs. JAMA 256:1160, 1986

141. Haskell WL, Leon AS, Caspersen CJ et al: Cardiovascular benefits and assessment of physical activity and physical fitness in adults. Med Sci Sports Exerc 24:S206, 1992

9

Lower Extremity Amputations

Sikhar N. Banerjee

Amputations of extremities have been performed since the dawn of civilization. Hippocrates was the first to describe amputation surgery for saving lives. Before the introduction of anesthesia by Morton in 1847, amputation of extremities was a gruesome procedure, and the majority of patients died as a result of the trauma of surgery and sepsis.

After World War II, all countries were confronted with a large number of young people with amputations of extremities resulting from war injuries. This tragedy provided impetus for research and development in amputation surgery and prosthetics. In the United States, the Veterans Administration spearheaded this effort, which resulted in the development of quadrilateral and patellar tendon-bearing sockets at the University of California Biomechanics Laboratory and hip disarticulation and Syme's prosthesis at the Ontario Crippled Children's Center. Amputation surgery and postoperative care have undergone major changes in the last 30 years, and many new prosthetic components have been introduced to improve function of lower extremity amputees.

Faced with many alternative management methods, a clinician must make decisions regarding treatment options that will enhance the patient's function and state of well-being. Ideally, a treatment option should be supported by a Level I evidence regarding its efficacy. Unfortunately, many treatment methods lack Level I evidence and management decisions are based on weaker evidence, but irrespective of the strength of the evidence, the treatment method must have a strong biologic basis.

RIGID PLASTER CAST OR SOFT DRESSING AND WEIGHT-BEARING

In 1969 Berlmont et al.[1] reported the benefits of a rigid plaster cast application in the operating room and early weight-bearing on the plaster pylon. Weiss[2] in 1969 emphasized the use of myoplasty to maintain neuromuscular pattern in the residual limb. Burgess et al.[3] applied these principles in elderly dysvascular patients and delayed weight-bearing when necessary, depending on the medical status of the patient and degree of vascular insufficiency of the residual limb. Burgess et al.[4] reported results of 193 amputations in 177 patients. Primary healing was achieved in 156 or 81 percent of the amputations, and 150 or 78 percent healed at the below-knee level. Sarmiento et al.[5] reported a retrospective chart review of 625 cases of major lower extremity amputations, 85 percent of which were for peripheral vascular disease. The authors compared the outcome in 328 patients (experimental group) during a 4-year period (1964 to 1968) with 297 patients (control group) who underwent amputations in the previous 4 years (1960 to 1963).

During the 1964 to 1968 level-selection method, the surgical technique was changed and 172 of 328 patients underwent immediate postsurgical fitting. The experimental group required revision from a below-knee to an above-knee level in 7.5 percent compared to 47.6 percent in the control group ($P < .01$). In addition, 64 percent of the experimental group was ambulatory with a prosthesis, and only

19 percent was ambulatory in the control group. The authors did not find any significant difference in the healing rate within the experimental group when patients fitted with immediate prosthesis were compared with those who did not undergo immediate fitting. It is not clear whether these two groups were comparable or how decisions were made regarding immediate prosthetic fitting. One cannot draw any conclusion from this study regarding efficacy of rigid dressing or immediate postoperative prosthetic fitting.

In a study of 182 patients with diabetes who underwent below-knee amputation, Mooney et al.[6] assigned patients in a sequential manner every 2 months to one of three treatment methods: soft dressing, plaster shell, and plaster pylon with delayed weight-bearing. All surgeries were performed by second-year residents. Flaps were made of equal lengths and myoplasty was performed in most patients. The healing rate was 74 percent for patients treated with plaster pylon and 65 and 59 percent, respectively, for plaster shell and soft dressing healing rates. However, healing time was shortest for the plaster shell group and longest for the plaster pylon group. The authors concluded that rigid dressing and ambulation do not deter healing, but early ambulation is a deterrent to healing. The study provides a weak Level III evidence regarding efficacy of rigid dressing, as the patients were not randomly assigned to treatment groups, and statistical analysis regarding the significance of the observed differences was not reported.

Moore et al.[7] compared the healing, revision, and complication rates of two groups of patients undergoing below-knee amputations for peripheral vascular disease. A retrospective chart review was performed for 55 patients undergoing below-knee amputation using standard technique between 1961 and 1966 and 53 below-knee amputations with immediate application of plaster pylon and ambulation. The standard surgical technique consisted of circular incision and application of a posterior plaster splint. The surgical technique was modified for the immediate postoperative prosthetic (IPOP) fitting group by using a long posterior flap, myodesis in the majority of patients, and the use of Hemovac drains in some patients. A plaster pylon was applied in the operating room.

The primary healing rate was 85 percent in the IPOP group and 53 percent in the standard technique group; 11 percent of patients in the IPOP group required revision to a higher level compared to 24 percent in the standard technique group. All patients in the IPOP group were ambulatory with a prosthesis compared to 81 percent in the standard group. The authors concluded that long posterior flap, rigid dressing, and immediate postoperative prosthesis accounted for improved results. This study provides a Level IV evidence regarding efficacy of rigid dressing as the study used a historical control. The authors did not provide statistical analysis. Use of equal flaps may account for the high failure of healing rate in the standard technique group.

In the early 1970s, Warren et al.[8] formed the Boston Interhospital Amputation Study to evaluate the feasibility of IPOP in community hospitals. A total of 53 surgeons and 18 hospitals participated in the 2.5 year study, which included 75 lower extremity amputations. Following skin closure, an immediate postoperative plaster prosthesis was applied and weight-bearing was delayed until the first cast change 1 week after surgery. The overall healing rate was 90 percent, of which 58 percent was primary and 32 percent was secondary healing. At the end of the follow-up period, 56 of 75 enrolled patients were ambulatory with a prosthesis. The authors concluded that the immediate postoperative plaster technique can make a real contribution to the rehabilitation of lower extremity amputations if a smoothly functioning team can be organized with the surgeon as an active member of the team.

Cohen et al.[9] in a retrospective chart review reported a 97.3 percent healing rate in 38 patients undergoing below-knee amputations with conventional technique and soft dressing. In nine patients where IPOP technique was applied, only two patients achieved primary healing. The authors concluded that IPOP does not increase the percentage of patients rehabilitated or decrease the failure rate of below-knee amputation. It is difficult to draw any definitive conclusion from this retrospective chart review because of the small number of patients undergoing IPOP procedures and the level of experience and competence of the prosthetist and physical therapist.

Mooney et al.[10] reported the results of 190 consecutive below-knee amputations for peripheral vascular disease using long posterior flaps and application of rigid plaster dressing in the operating room and delayed weight-bearing with plaster pylon. Of 190 patients, 174 (91 percent) achieved primary healing and another eight patients had delayed healing, resulting in an overall healing rate of 96 percent. Eighty-eight percent of patients were successfully fitted with a prosthesis and became ambulatory. The authors attributed the use of long posterior flaps and delayed weight-bearing as important factors in achieving a high success rate.

In a nonrandomized trial, Nicholas et al.[11] compared the healing rate, length of hospital stay, and successful use of a prosthesis in a group of 27 patients undergoing below-knee amputation for peripheral vascular disease. Thirteen patients had a rigid dressing applied in the operating room, and 14 patients were treated with a soft dressing. There was no significant difference in length of hospital stay, healing rate, or successful use of a prosthesis; but the sample size for this trial was too small to detect a significant difference between groups. As the patients were not randomized, comparability of the groups cannot be guaranteed.

Baker et al.[12] reported the results of a randomized trial involving 51 patients undergoing below-knee amputation for peripheral vascular disease. The patients were randomly assigned to rigid plaster or soft dressing groups. A long posterior flap, myoplasty, and meticulous hemostasis were carried out in all patients. A plaster pylon was added 2 to 6 weeks after surgery and gait training was initiated. In the rigid dressing group, 66.6 percent of the patients achieved primary healing, 21.6 percent achieved secondary healing, and 14.8 percent required above-knee amputation. In the soft dressing group, corresponding rates were 58.3, 25.0, and 16.7 percent, respectively. Even though there was a trend toward a better healing rate for the rigid dressing, these differences were not statistically significant. A small sample size is most likely the reason for the lack of statistically significant difference.

Malone et al.[13] carried out a retrospective chart review of 133 patients who underwent below-knee amputation at the San Francisco and Tucson VA Hospitals between 1966 and 1978. A trial of 142 below-knee amputations were done, predominantly for peripheral vascular disease, using xenon skin blood flow for level selection, long posterior flaps, and immediate postoperative prosthetic fitting technique. The authors reported 0 percent postoperative mortality, an 89 percent healing rate, and 100 percent prosthetic rehabilitation in unilateral below-knee amputees and a 93 percent rehabilitation of all bilateral below-knee amputees. The authors surveyed costs for the amputation surgery and rehabilitation in all 172 VA hospitals in the United States and concluded that if all hospitals use the immediate postoperative prosthetic fitting program projected savings would be $80 million over 5 years.

Kane et al.[14] reviewed 52 consecutive below-knee amputations for peripheral vascular disease. Thirty-four patients received a rigid plaster cast with IPOP and 18 were treated with a soft dressing. Even though there was a trend toward less stump necrosis (21 versus 17 percent) and infection (21 versus 33 percent) in the IPOP group, the difference was not statistically significant because of the small sample size. The authors concluded that the IPOP method had little if any effect on the early rehabilitation of vascular amputees.

Conclusion

The surgical technique and postoperative care for lower extremity amputations have undergone major changes since World War II with the introduction of the long posterior flap for below-knee amputation and rigid plaster dressing with delayed weight-bearing for dysvascular amputees (Table 9-1). Most published reports have claimed efficacy for rigid plaster dressing when compared to soft dressing, but since 1970 only one randomized controlled trial, that of Baker et al.,[12] has been reported comparing rigid dressing with soft dressing. Even though there was a trend toward better healing with the rigid dressing, the differences were not statistically significant because of the small sample size (type II error). Despite this lack of evidence, the use of long posterior flaps and application of rigid dressing following below-knee amputation have become a standard method of treatment in many centers, primarily

Table 9-1. Summary of Studies Comparing Rigid with Soft Dressing

Author	Sample Size	Design	Statistical Analysis	Conclusion	Level of Evidence Recommend Grade	Strength/ Weakness
Sarmiento et al.[5] (1970)	625	Retrospective chart review with historical control	Yes	Better healing and ambulation rate in rigid dressing group	Level IV Grade C	Nonrandomized Surgical technique different for each group
Burgess et al.[4] (1971)	177	Case series No control group	No	Better healing with rigid dressing	Level V Grade C	Lack of control group
Mooney et al.[6] (1971)	182	Cohort control	No	Healing rate and time better with plaster dressing	Level III Grade C	Nonrandomized Nonstatistical analysis
Moore et al.[7] (1972)	108	Retrospective chart review Historical control	No	Better healing and ambulation rate with rigid dressing	Level IV Grade C	Nonrandomized Historical control No statistical analysis
Warren et al.[8] (1973)	75	Case series	No	Excellent healing rate	Level V Grade C	No control group
Cohen et al.[9] (1974)	47	Retrospective chart review	No	Poor healing with rigid dressing	Level IV Grade C	Nonrandomized small number of patients in rigid dressing group
Mooney et al.[10] (1976)	190	Case series	No	Excellent healing (96%)	Level V Grade C	No control group
Nicholas et al.[11] (1976)	27	Cohort control	No	No difference between groups	Level III Grade C	Nonrandomized small sample
Baker et al.[12] (1977)	51	Randomized control	Yes	No difference between groups	Level II Grade B	Small sample
Malone et al.[13] (1979)	133	Case series Retrospective chart review	No	Better healing Reduced cost	Level V Grade C	No control group
Kane et al.[14] (1980)	52	Cohort control	Yes	No difference between groups	Level III Grade C	Small sample

because it is based on sound biologic principles. The use of a long posterior flap improves healing because of better blood flow in the posterior flap, and the rigid dressing reduces edema, thereby maintaining the integrity of the small vessels and reducing the intensity of postoperative pain.

IMMEDIATE OR DELAYED WEIGHT-BEARING

Several investigators have recommended the application of a rigid dressing and immediate weight-bearing. Whether immediate weight-bearing reduces the time between surgery and prosthetic fitting when compared with delayed weight-bearing remains controversial. The latter is a common practice specifically for dysvascular amputees. Thorpe et al.[15] reported a randomized trial involving 24 patients undergoing above-knee amputation for osteosarcoma. The patients were randomly assigned by a two-by-two factorial method to receive a rigid plaster dressing with quadrilateral brim by either a physical therapist or prosthetist. The patients were then randomly assigned to receive either immediate weight-bearing (within 24 hours) or delayed weight-bearing after suture removal. Both groups attended physical therapy twice a day according to established protocol. The patients fitted with a plaster cast by the physical therapists and those treated with delayed ambulation required significantly less analgesics. However, there was no difference in time among all groups from the day of surgery to fitting of a trial prosthesis. The authors concluded that delayed ambulation is preferable because of reduced analgesic intake and because rigid dressings can be applied by the physical therapists.

OTHER METHODS OF RESIDUAL LIMB CARE

Controlled Environment Treatment

Redhead and Snowdon[16] at the Biomechanical Research and Development unit at Rochampton developed a unique approach to wound healing called controlled environment treatment (CET). The bare residual limb, after surgery, is placed in a transparent plastic sleeve, which is connected through a flexible hose to a console with an air compressor controlling air pressure, temperature, humidity, and sterility. The treatment is continued 24 hours a day until healing of the residual limb is achieved.

After the initial presentation of CET in 1974 at the First World Congress of International Society of Prosthetics and Orthotics, several reports regarding its efficacy have been published. Burgess[17] reported results of 20 patients treated by CET; 17 achieved primary healing and two required revision to the above-knee level. Troup[18] reported results of CET treatment of 100 patients with various clinical problems including 47 patients undergoing lower extremity amputations; 30 (64 percent) achieved primary healing, leading the author to conclude that CET was effective in promoting wound healing by reducing edema and maintaining a sterile environment. Ruckley et al.[19] compared the healing rate following below-knee amputation in 60 patients randomized to rigid plaster dressing or CET. Primary healing was achieved in 21 (70 percent) of the patients treated with plaster dressing and 18 (60 percent) treated by CET. Four (13 percent) in each group required revision to the above-knee level. The authors concluded that CET treatment offers no advantage over rigid plaster dressing for either healing or rehabilitation.

Pneumatic Sleeve

Little[20] introduced the use of a pneumatic weight-bearing prosthesis, which consisted of an inflatable plastic bag mounted in an aluminum frame pylon connected to a solid ankle cushion heel (SACH) foot. The plastic bag is inflated to 25 mmHg and the dressing is changed 48 hours after surgery. Patients were allowed partial weight-bearing within the parallel bars, and all eight patients achieved primary healing of the residual limb. Subsequently, pneumatic prosthesis has been used for edema reduction and prosthetic gait training. All authors (Table 9-2) have claimed success in achieving primary healing and later ambulation with a prosthesis. However, controlled clinical trial comparing pneumatic prosthesis with rigid plaster or soft dressing has not been performed.

RESIDUAL LIMB HEALING AND ANTIBIOTICS

Wound infection is a common complication after lower extremity amputation for peripheral vascular disease, and many require amputation at a higher level. Robbs et al.[25] reported the results of a controlled trial comparing a combination of Amoxycillin and flucloxacillin given before surgery and continued for 48 hours with a control group who received antibiotics only if a wound infection became apparent during the postoperative period. The patients

Table 9-2. Summary of Studies on Pneumatic Prosthesis

Author	Design	IPOP/Late	Outcome
Little[20] (1971)	Case series n = 9	IPOP	7 primary healing
Barraclough et al.[21] (1972)	Case series n = 10	IPOP	6 primary healing 1 revision 3 deaths
Kerstein[22] (1974)	Case series n = 11	IPOP	All primary healing
Redhead et al.[23] (1972)	Case series n = 11	IPOP and Late	80 ambulatory
Monga et al.[24] (1984)	Case series n = 24	IPOP and Late	14 primary healing 7 secondary healing 3 already healed

were not randomized. Twenty-four patients received an antibiotic combination and 22 patients served as controls. The incidence of sepsis in the experimental and control groups were 33.3 and 72.7 percent, respectively, and the difference was significant ($P < .025$). Since then, several good controlled trials have been reported, firmly establishing efficacy of perioperative antibiotics in preventing wound infection following lower extremity amputation (Table 9-3).

Conclusion

There is strong evidence based on four randomized trials that perioperative antibiotics significantly reduce wound infection after lower extremity amputations for peripheral vascular disease.

NUTRITIONAL STATUS AND HEALING OF RESIDUAL LIMB

The majority of patients undergoing lower extremity amputations are dysvascular and elderly and more prone to malnutrition. Poor nutritional status always has been assumed to be associated with increased postoperative mortality, morbidity, and rehabilitation time.

Dickhaut et al.[31] studied the specific effects of malnutrition in 23 patients with diabetes undergoing Syme's amputations. A patient was diagnosed to be malnourished when serum albumin was less than 3.5 g/100 ml and/or total lymphocyte count was less than 1500/cm³. All patients met Wagner's criteria for Syme's amputation. The healing rate among well-nourished patients was 86 percent compared to 25 percent for the malnourished group. There was a highly significant relationship between nutritional status and healing in both groups ($P \leq .0035$ and $\leq .0096$). Kay et al.[32] and Pedersen et al.[33] reported similar complications and poor wound healing among malnourished patients as indicated by low serum albumin and lymphocyte count. However, from these studies it is not clear whether malnutrition causes increased complications or that they occur concurrently. Therefore, a study is needed to establish whether correction of malnutrition will reduce postoperative mortality and morbidity in patients undergoing lower extremity amputation.

RESIDUAL LIMB PAIN

All patients experience varying degrees of pain in the residual limb during the first 2 to 3 weeks after surgery. Persistent pain in the residual limb warrants further investigation to rule out infection, neuroma formation, bony spur, persistent ischemia, or heterotrophic ossification. Correction of the underlying cause will reduce or eliminate pain in most patients. However, some patients will continue to experience persistent pain in the residual limb, and many treatment methods have been advocated with varying

Table 9-3. Summary of Studies of Perioperative Antibiotics in Lower Extremity Amputation

Author	Sample	Design	Antibiotic	Result	Level of Evidence Recommend Grade
Robbs et al.[25] (1981)	46	Cohort control	Amoxycillin Flucloxacillin (A-CA)	Significant reduction of sepsis	Level III Grade C
Huizinga et al.[26] (1983)	44	Cohort control	Amoxycillin & Flucloxacillin (A-CA) or Penicillin	Significant reduction of sepsis with A-CA	Level III Grade C
Moller et al.[27] (1985)	50	Randomized control	Meticillin	Significant reduction of sepsis	Level I Grade A
Sonne Holm et al.[28] (1985)	152	Randomized control	Cefoxitin	Significant reduction of sepsis	Level I Grade A
Friss[29] (1987)	457	Randomized control	Cefuroxime or Penicillin G	Both equally effective	Level I Grade A
Norlin et al.[30] (1990)	35	Randomized control	Cefotaxime	Significant reduction of sepsis	Level I Grade A

degrees of success. If the residual limb is sensitive to touch or pressure, a program of desensitization with massage, vibration, and transcutaneous nerve stimulation may reduce sensitivity and discomfort. No controlled studies have been reported.

Capsaicin

Capsaicin, an alkaloid from hot pepper, has been known to have analgesic property by depleting substance P in small-diameter pain fibers. Rayner et al.[34] reported complete relief of pain with local application of 0.025 percent capsaicin cream in a 47-year-old diabetic with bilateral below-knee amputations. The patient suffered from persistent burning pain in both residual limbs for 2 years. The pain had been refractory to analgesics, amitriptyline, and temazepam. The capsaicin cream was applied to both residual limbs four times a day; after 7 days there was complete pain relief. The pain returned after use of the capsaicin cream was discontinued. The capsaicin was compared with a placebo cream by applying capsaicin cream to one residual limb and placebo cream to the other. Capsaicin completely relieved the pain, but the placebo cream had no effect.

Weintraub et al.[35] reported a single case study involving a below-knee amputee with residual limb pain. The study design was a double-blind crossover trial with 0.075 percent capsaicin cream and placebo. The patient experienced significantly more pain (i.e., severe burning) with capsaicin cream than with the placebo associated. The strength of capsaicin was three times greater than that used in the earlier case report.

PHANTOM LIMB PAIN

All patients undergoing amputations of extremities will experience phantom sensations, and some will experience disabling pain in the phantom limb. The reported incidence of phantom limb pain varies from 59 to 90 percent.[36–38] Sherman[39] reviewed published treatments of phantom pain and concluded that none of the treatments are efficacious and treatment effects are no more than placebo effect. Davis[40] reported that some of the medical treatment of phantom pain was effective in controlling pain.

Epidural Block

Bach et al.[41] pretreated 11 patients who were to undergo below-knee amputation with epidural block with morphine hydrochloride and/or bupivacaine, 0.25 percent, 72 hours before amputation. Fourteen patients undergoing amputation served as controls and did not receive preoperative epidural block. During postoperative periods, all patients received analgesics. At the end of a week, three (27 percent) of the experimental group, and nine (64 percent) of the control group experienced phantom pain, but the difference was not significant ($P < .10$). However, at the end of 6 months, none of the patients in the experimental group had phantom pain compared to five (38 percent) of the control group ($P < .05$).

During 1-year follow-up, all patients in the experimental group were pain free and two (27 percent) in the control group were still having pain ($P < .20$). Preoperative continuous epidural block may be effective in reducing the incidence of phantom pain, but because of the small sample size and nonrandomized nature of the trial, no definite conclusion can be drawn.

Calcitonin

Jaeger et al.[42] studied 161 consecutive patients with limb amputations during a 2-year period. Twenty-one patients developed phantom limb pain and were treated with 200 IU Salmon calcitonin intravenously in a placebo-controlled, double-blind, crossover trial. After 1 week, 19 (90 percent) experienced at least 50 percent pain relief of whom 16 (76 percent) were pain free. Saline (placebo) infusion did not reduce pain. At 2-year follow-up, 15 (71 percent) reported that they had never experienced phantom pain since their initial treatment with calcitonin.

Mexiletine

Mexiletine, an antiarrhythmic drug, is effective in the treatment of neurogenic and central pain syndromes (e.g., diabetic neuropathy and thalamic pain). Davis[43] reported an open label trial involving 31 lower extremity amputees with phantom pain. All were treated with mexiletine with a maximum dose of 900 mg/day in divided doses. For patients who did not experience significant pain relief with mexiletine alone, a clonidine TTS1 patch was added. All patients were followed up to 1 year.

Twelve patients (39 percent) experienced excellent pain relief with reduction of 6 points on a visual analog scale (VAS), and six patients (19 percent) had good pain relief with a 4-point drop in VAS score. The remaining 13 patients had minimal pain relief with mexiletine alone and a clonidine patch was added; 11 of these 13 experienced excellent pain relief. All patients at 1-year follow-up were maintaining low VAS score (1.13). The most common side effects of mexiletine were nausea and upper gastrointestinal symptoms, which were resolved by adjusting the dosage and taking the drug with food.

β-Adrenergic Blockade

The analgesic effect of the β-adrenergic blocking drug propranolol was discovered serendipitously by Oille.[44] In a letter to the editor, he reported that while treating a 74-year-old man for angina and tachycardia with propranolol, 120 mg/day, over 2 months, the patient was completely freed of the distressing phantom pain he had suffered for 62 years. Ahmad[45] reported a similar experience with two patients who experienced complete relief of phantom pain while being treated with propranolol for angina. Marsland et al.[46] reported excellent pain relief with β-adrenergic blocking drugs in three traumatic lower extremity amputees without cardiovascular disease; two were treated with propranolol, 80 mg/day, and one patient with metoprolol, 100 mg, three times a day. All experienced pain relief 48 hours after initiation of therapy and remained pain free at 6-month follow-up. No controlled trial has been reported regarding efficacy of β-adrenergic blocking drugs in the treatment of phantom limb pain.

Carbamazepine

Carbamazepine is an anticonvulsant but has been used for pain relief in several central pain syndromes (e.g., trigemina neuralgia, thalamic syndrome). In a letter to the editor, Elliott et al.[47] reported that five patients with phantom limb pain were treated with carbamazepine, 400 to 600 mg/day, for 6 weeks. It was found to be effective in alleviating lancinating type of phantom pain in all patients. All were able to reduce or discontinue the medication after 8 weeks without recurrence of pain. Patterson[48] reported treatment of phantom pain with carbamazepine in a patient with above-elbow amputation who suffered from severe lancinating phantom pain for 25 years and had been treated unsuccessfully with antidepressants and neuroleptics. The patient was treated with increasing dosage of carbamazepine until a serum level of 8 to 12 mg/ml was reached. At 10 mg/ml the pain relief was complete. The patient discontinued the drug after 3 weeks and the phantom pain promptly returned. Carbamazepine therapy was resumed and the patient experienced complete pain relief. The author did not provide follow-up data.

Antidepressants

Antidepressants have been used widely for treatment of chronic pain including phantom limb pain. Panerai et al.[49] studied analgesic effects of tricyclic antidepressants chlorimipramine and nortriptyline in a group of 39 patients suffering from central pain states, 28 of whom were suffering from phantom limb pain. The study was a double-blind within patient 3 × 3 Latin square trial. After 1 week of placebo washout patients were randomly assigned for 2 weeks in each sequence:

1. Clorimipramine (CIM)—nortriptyline (NOR)—placebo
2. NOR—placebo—CIM
3. Placebo—CIM—NOR

The dosage of each drug was 25 mg one to four times a day. Pain intensity was evaluated by the patient on a visual analog scale.

Twenty-four patients completed the study. At the end of the second and third weeks, both antidepressants were superior to the placebo ($P < .0001$), and chlorimipramine was more effective than nortriptyline ($P < .0001$). The side effects were moderately severe and commonly seen with antidepressant treatment. Although both antidepressants were effective in reducing pain, the tricyclic antidepressant active through the serotoninergic system (CIM) was superior to that active through the noradrenergic system (NOR).

The antinociceptive effects of antidepressants were not related to their effects on depression score. It appears from this trial that tricyclic antidepressants are effective in reducing discomforts in patients with central pain such as phantom limb pain. The authors did not provide subgroup analysis of patients with phantom limb pain, and it is not clear how many of the 28 patients with phantom limb pain completed the study.

Peripheral Stimulation

Peripheral stimulation with massage, vibration, and electrical stimulation has been known to reduce pain in many pain states.

Winnem[50] treated 11 lower limb amputees with transcutaneous electrical nerve stimulation (TENS) for phantom pain. Each patient received a TENS treatment for 15 minutes twice a day for 5 days. Treatment started initially with high-frequency (100 Hz) TENS and then, if the patient did not experience pain relief, with low-frequency (2 Hz) TENS. When pain relief was not achieved with either high- or low-frequency TENS applied to the residual limb, electrodes were placed on the contralateral lower limb around the corresponding spinal dermatome segment. Two of the 11 patients experienced complete pain relief, and five others experienced definite improvement, resulting in reduction of analgesic by 50 percent. All patients were followed for 3 to 12 months.

Lundeberg[51] studied 24 patients with chronic phantom limb pain who were unresponsive to TENS. All were treated with vibratory and placebo stimulation. Vibratory stimulation was applied to the residual limb through an electromechanical vibrator for 25 minutes twice a day at a frequency of 100 Hz. Seventy-five percent of patients experienced significant pain relief, with vibratory stimulation compared to 44 percent with placebo stimulation. Of 21 patients who started treatment with vibratory stimulation, only seven were still using the treatment at the end of 2 years. Most patients discontinued treatment because of minimal pain reduction or development of tolerance. Lundeberg[51] concluded that vibratory stimulation may alleviate phantom limb pain, but the study presents several fatal flaws. Patients were not randomly assigned to treatment, and the author did not provide statistical analysis. In addition, at the end of 2 years, only 30 percent of the patients were experiencing pain relief with vibratory stimulation compared to 44 percent of patients who experienced pain relief with placebo stimulation.

Finsen et al.[52] studied the effects of TENS on residual limb healing and phantom limb pain in 51 patients randomly assigned to three treatment groups following lower limb amputation: Group A, sham TENS and chlorpromazine; Group B, sham TENS only; Group C, active TENS. TENS stimulation was given 30 minutes twice a day for 2 weeks during the postoperative period using a low frequency (7 pulses/2 sec). All patients were followed for at least 1 year.

The healing rate among below-knee amputees was significantly higher ($P < .05$) in Group C (active TENS). Analgesic intake also was lower in this group, but the differences were not statistically significant during the first 4 weeks.

Phantom pain was not different in the three groups. At 6 weeks, none of the patients in Group C (active TENS) complained of phantom pain, although 36 and 58 percent of patients in Groups A and B, respectively, complained of phantom pain. At the end of 1 year, there was no significant difference in incidence of phantom pain among the groups. The intensity of phantom pain was mild in all groups, and Group C patients did not use any analgesics for phantom pain.

The authors concluded that healing rates following amputation are significantly improved with TENS, and the prevalence of phantom pain was significantly lowered by TENS after 4 months but not after 1 year. Overall intensity and incidence of phantom pain in this group of patients were considerably lower than in other published reports.

Dorsal Column Stimulation

In 1967, Shealy[52a] introduced dorsal column stimulation for treatment of chronic pain. Since then conflicting reports regarding its efficacy have been reported. In early stages of development, the electrodes were implanted through open laminectomy, but in recent years percutaneous technique has been developed.

Nelson et al.[53] reported excellent pain relief in four of five patients treated with dorsal column stimulation and followed for 7 to 25 months. Wester[54] reported results of dorsal column stimulation in 35 patients with chronic pain of various etiologies, five of whom suffered from phantom limb pain. Follow-up was accomplished through questionnaire and the follow-up period was 4 to 60 months. Four patients with phantom limb pain experienced only minimal reduction of pain. In a review of 96 patients with chronic pain of various causes treated by dorsal column stimulation during a 10-year period, Kumar et al.[55] reported no pain relief in two patients with phantom limb pain. Permanent implantation was not carried out in these patients.

Dorsal Root Entry Zone Lesions and Postamputation Pain

Saris et al.[56] reviewed records of 28 patients who underwent the dorsal root entry zone (DREZ) procedure for postamputation pain and were followed 6 months to 5 years, with an average of 2.0 years. A good outcome was defined by reduction of 3 units on a visual analog scale of 0 to 10. The patient reported feeling better and would have had the operation if the results were known ahead of time. Of the 22 patients in the study, only eight (36 percent) reported good results. However, in a subgroup analysis of nine patients who had phantom limb pain alone, six (67 percent) reported good results. The authors concluded that the DREZ procedure is indicated if a patient experiences phantom pain alone or pain associated with root avulsion.

Relaxation Training

Phantom pain is often associated with anxiety and muscle tension that usually exacerbates pain. Sherman et al.[57] reported the results of treatment of 16 lower extremity amputees with phantom pain. Ten patients suffered from chronic phantom pain, with a mean duration of 12 years, and two underwent amputation 1 and 5 weeks before the start of treatment. All patients attended weekly sessions consisting of training in progressive muscle relaxation, electromyographic feedback of residual limb and forehead muscles, and reassurance regarding normal phantom sensation and relation between anxiety and pain. The two recent amputees experienced complete elimination of pain after three sessions and

remained pain free after 1 year. Eight patients with chronic phantom pain became pain free after attending six treatment sessions and remained free of pain at 1- and 3-year follow-up. Four other patients experienced a significant reduction of discomfort and did not desire further treatment. Two patients did not experience any pain relief. The authors concluded that muscle relaxation training is an effective method of treatment for phantom limb pain.

Summary

Table 9-4 presents the current status and recommendations for treatments. Figure 9-1 presents a useful algorithm for clinical decision making.

RESIDUAL LIMB VOLUME REDUCTION

After lower extremity amputation, swelling of the residual limb interferes with early prosthetic fitting. Bandaging with elastic crepe bandage is the most frequently used method for reduction of stump volume. However, proper bandaging requires a skilled therapist, and improper bandaging can cause skin breakdown in the residual limb.

Manella[58] compared the effectiveness of elastic shrinker socks and elastic crepe bandage in reducing stump volume. Twelve amputees were randomly assigned to a shrinker sock or elastic bandage group, and subjects were instructed on a standard bandaging technique. The residual limb volume was calculated from sequential circumferential measurements and length using anthropometric technique. At the end of 4 weeks, the elastic shrinker group achieved significantly higher volume reduction when compared with the elastic bandage group ($P < .03$). The elastic bandage group experienced an increase in residual limb volume, raising the possibility of improper bandaging by excessive proximal compression.

In a study of 15 below-knee amputees, Mueller[59] compared the effectiveness of a removable rigid dressing and elastic bandage. Patients were randomly assigned to treatment groups and studied for 3 weeks. Residual limb and sequential circumference and lengths were measured three times a week, and volume calculation was made using

Table 9-4. Summary of Studies of Treatment for Phantom Limb Pain

Author	Sample Size	Design	Statistical Intervention	Analysis	Level of Evidence Recommend Grade
Bach et al.[41] (1988)	25	Cohort control	Epidural Morphine and/or Bupivacaine (0.25%)	Yes	Level III Grade C
Jaeger et al.[42] (1992)	21	Randomized crossover	Salmon Calcitonin 200 IU/g.v.	No	Level II Grade B
Davis[43] (1993)	31	Case series	Mexiletine 900 mg/day	Yes	Level V Grade C
Oille[44] (1970)	1	Single case study	Propranolol 120 mg/day	No	Level V Grade C
Ahmad[45] (1979)	2	Case study	Propranolol 40 mg/day	No	Level V Grade C
Marsland et al.[46] (1982)	3	Case study	Propranolol 80 mg/day	No	Level V Grade C
Elliott et al.[47] (1976)	5	Case study	Carbamazepine 400–600 mg/day	No	Level V Grade C
Patterson[48] (1988)	1	Single case study	Carbamazepine 200 mg QID	No	Level V Grade C
Panerai et al.[49] (1990)	28	Double-blind randomized crossover	Chlorimipramine 25 mg QID Nortriptylene 25 mg QID	Yes	Level I Grade A
Winnem[50] (1982)	11	Case series	TENS	No	Level V Grace C
Lundeberg[51] (1985)	24	Nonrandomized placebo control	Vibration	No	Level III Grade C
Finsen et al.[52] (1988)	51	Randomized control	TENS	Yes	Level I Grade A
Nelson et al.[53] (1975)	5	Case series	Dorsal column stimulation	No	Level V Grade C
Wester[54] (1987)	5	Case series	Dorsal column stimulation	No	Level V Grade C
Kumar et al.[55] (1991)	2	Case series	Dorsal column stimulation	No	Level V Grade C
Saris et al.[56] (1985)	28	Case series	DREZ	No	Level V Grade C
Sherman et al.[57] (1979)	16	Case series	Relaxation Biofeedback	No	Level V Grade C

anthropomorphic technique. The removable rigid dressing group achieved significantly more volume reduction than the elastic bandage group ($P < .05$). The author concluded that removable rigid dressing is more effective than elastic bandage in reducing residual limb volume in below-knee amputees.

EXERCISE IN LOWER EXTREMITY AMPUTEES

Both strengthening and conditioning exercise programs are integral parts of preprosthetic and prosthetic training programs for lower extremity amputees. The majority of lower extremity amputees are elderly and dysvascular, with generalized muscle weakness and limited exercise tolerance. Kavanagh[60] reported that 50 percent of 62 dysvascular amputees had resting electrocardiographic (ECG) abnormalities and 18 of 27 patients developed ST-segment depression on exercise testing. Cruts et al.[61] and Roth et al.[62] reported similar resting and exercise testing ECG abnormalities. Miller et al.[63] reported the results of a conditioning exercise program in 10 dysvascular amputees with significant heart disease as indicated by exercise testing. The exercise program consisted of 10 minutes of exercise twice a day using a bicycle and arm ergometer monitored with continuous ECG. Seven patients achieved average reduction of resting heart rate of 10.7 beats/min after

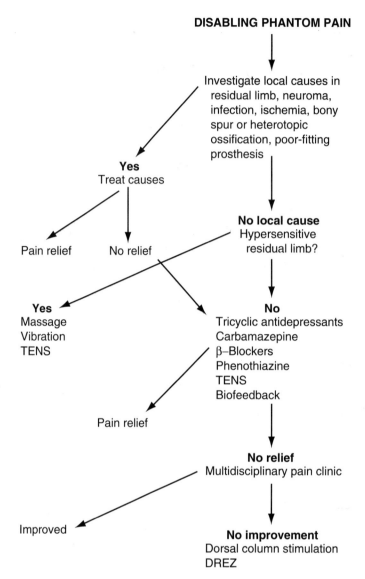

Fig. 9-1. Suggested algorithm for treatment of phantom pain.

a hospital stay of 32 days. All patients were able to walk 90 feet without excessive rise of heart rate or cardiac symptoms.

Pitetti et al.[64] studied the effects of 15 weeks of aerobic exercise training in 10 traumatic amputees. Before the start of the program, each patient underwent exercise testing in an Air-Dyne ergometer for maximum exercise capacity and walking test on a treadmill, keeping the heart rate around 60 to 80 percent of estimated maximum heart rate. Similar testing was carried out after completion of a 15-week home program according to a standard protocol with increasing intensity and duration of exercise each week. Ten patients (seven unilateral and three bilateral) completed the program, and seven patients served as controls who underwent exercise testing but did not participate in the prescribed home exercise program.

After completion of the program, there was a significant decrease in heart rate ($P \le .001$, $\le .005$,

≤ .007) at all three levels of submaximal exercise and a significant increase in work capacity accompanied by increase in oxygen consumption ($P \leq .001$). On the treadmill testing the heart rate and oxygen consumption reduced significantly in all grades of inclines. In the control group there was no significant change in either resting heart rate or heart rate and oxygen consumption while walking on the treadmill.

Klingenstierna et al.[65] studied the effects of isometric training of knee flexors and extensors in eight below-knee (traumatic and dysvascular) amputees for 8 to 12 weeks. The subjects exercised at three preset angular velocities. Isometric and isokinetic muscle strengths were measured before and after training. Needle muscle biopsies were taken from vastus lateralis, and computed tomography (CT) scan of the thigh at the level of biopsy was performed before and after training. Functional ability was measured by objective measurement of range of motion, circumference of thighs, and walking on flat surface and stairs. At the end of training program, in the amputated leg there was a significant increase in knee extension torque at all velocities and knee flexion torque at 180 degrees/s and in the nonamputated leg in extension at 180 degrees/s and 240 degrees/s and isometric strength at 60-degree knee angle. There was an increase in type II fibers in the residual limb only. Patients' walking ability increased significantly with or without gait aid ($P \leq .01$), and the walking distance doubled in most patients.

Conclusion

A graduated exercise program of progressively increasing intensity both for improvement of strength and aerobic capacity can improve amputee patients' functional capabilities and cardiovascular function. Controlled trials involving larger groups of patients are necessary to establish the efficacy of different types of exercises.

ABOVE-KNEE PROSTHESIS: OPEN OR LOCKED KNEE

Many dysvascular amputees experience difficulties in controlling a prosthetic knee, and some suffer falls because of buckling of the prosthetic knee. Isakov et al.[66] in a crossover trial involving 17

above-knee amputees measured walking speed, heart rate, and oxygen consumption when walking with an open and locked prosthetic knee. The dysvascular amputees achieved a higher walking speed, reduced heart rate, and oxygen consumption while walking with a locked knee when compared with walking with an open knee.

QUADRILATERAL OR CAT-CAM SOCKET

The ischial weight-bearing quadrilateral socket has been the accepted socket design for above-knee amputees for many years. Because of the narrow anteroposterior and wide mediolateral diameter of the socket, however, many patients experience discomfort in the groin area and mediolateral stability is less than optimal, resulting in significant Trendelenburg gait. Ivan Long[66a] introduced a normal shape/normal alignment socket (NSNA), and later Sabolich[66b] designed a contoured adducted trochanteric controlled alignment method (CAT-CAM). Both sockets have narrow mediolateral and wide anteroposterior diameter to provide better mediolateral stability and improve comfort. Both sockets have enjoyed popularity, but few clinical trials have been carried out to support the claims of superiority.

Flandry et al.[67] studied five mature unilateral traumatic above-knee amputees who had used quadrilateral sockets from 3 months to 9 years. All 5 patients were fitted with CAT-CAM socket, and the knee and ankle units were the same as those used with the quadrilateral sockets. The evaluation of each socket included the following:

1. Functional level of ambulation graded I to VI through questionnaire; grade I is nonambulatory and grade VI is able to walk 5 blocks and negotiate stairs, ramps, curbs, etc.
2. Amputees' subjective assessment by a questionnaire regarding comfort, balance, and stability—maximum score 12 points.
3. Observational gait analysis by a physician and physical therapist.
4. Femoral shaft adduction angle measured in weight-bearing position with anteroposterior roentgenograph.

5. Instrumented gait analysis for velocity, stride, length, and coronal body torque.
6. Energy cost of walking.

After fitting with a CAT-CAM socket, the patients needed a readjustment period of 2 weeks to 1 month, after which all measurements were made. Three patients were grade VI functional ambulators and there was no change in their level of ambulation. The other two patients advanced one grade in the functional level of ambulation. Four patients preferred the CAT-CAM socket based on improved comfort, balance, and stability. Most observed gait deviations with the quadrilateral socket were eliminated by conversion to the CAT-CAM socket. Adduction angle of residual limb improved with the CAT-CAM conversion and in four patients ranged from 4 to 12 degrees, with a mean improvement of 6.5 degrees. Mean walking velocity increased by 4.1 m/min with the CAT-CAM socket. All patients achieved a reduction in oxygen cost of ambulation with the CAT-CAM socket and a mean reduction of 21 percent when compared to oxygen consumption with the quadrilateral socket.

Gailey et al.[68] studied 20 unilateral mature nondysvascular above-knee amputees. They were wearing either a CAT-CAM (n = 10) or quadrilateral socket (n = 10). Ten nonamputee control subjects participated in the study. All subjects were asked to walk on an indoor track at one of two designated speeds (33.5 and 67 m/min) for 8 minutes. Heart rate and oxygen uptake were measured in all subjects during the last 3 minutes of each trial.

At a slower speed, both quadrilateral and CAT-CAM groups showed significantly higher heart rates ($P \leq .01$) and VO_2 ($P \leq .05$) when compared with control subjects. However, there was no significant difference between quadrilateral and CAT-CAM groups in heart rate and oxygen consumption. At higher speeds, VO_2 was significantly lower for CAT-CAM socket users than those using the quadrilateral socket ($P \leq .01$). There was no significant difference in heart rate between the two groups.

Both studies indicate that the CAT-CAM socket may be superior to the quadrilateral socket in terms of comfort, speed of walking, and energy cost. Controlled trials with a larger diverse patient population are necessary to be able to generalize these study results.

PROSTHETIC ANKLE AND FOOT

Since the introduction of the SACH foot almost 40 years ago, many new ankle-foot systems have been developed to improve comfort and minimize gait deviation of amputees. Many ankle-foot systems have claimed energy storing and releasing properties that make running and sports activities easier for the amputee.

Ehara et al.[69] reported a detailed biomechanical study of 14 different ankle-foot systems while a traumatic unilateral below-knee amputee walked on an instrumented walkway using 14 different ankle-foot systems. The subject walked on the walkway with two walking speeds, (100 and 130 steps/min) six times at each speed. The ankle joint power (P) was calculated from the ankle joint moment and angular velocity. A negative value of P indicated energy stored in the ankle joint, and positive value of P is the power released from the system. Energy is stored during midstance between neutral ankle angle and maximum dorsiflexion to toe off. Energy efficiency of each ankle-foot system was calculated from energy stored and released during walking. The flex walk ankle-foot system had the highest energy efficiency of 67.25 percent. The SACH foot had an efficiency of 18.85 percent.

Menard et al.[70] studied eight unilateral traumatic below-knee amputees and nine control subjects. All amputees were provided with two identical prostheses, one with a Seattle and the other with the Flex Foot. Clinical gait analysis and force plate analysis of ground reaction force (GRF) with each prosthesis were carried out while the patient walked on a level surface at the natural cadence. The patients were also asked to express their preference regarding the prosthetic foot.

GRF analysis showed that the amputated limb had a weaker propulsion and the nonamputated limb had a stronger propulsion when compared with the control subjects. This difference was similar with both prostheses. During walking with the Flex Foot, there was a larger vertical force component during the last 10 percent of stance phase.

Three months after the studies, four patients continued to use the Flex Foot and two used the Seattle Foot. The remaining two patients used both the Flex and Seattle Foot. The authors concluded that the Flex Foot would be useful for sports activities that require jumping, but the Seattle Foot, or comparable energy storing foot, would be ideal for routine activities.

Lehman et al.[71] studied nine unilateral below-knee amputees and compared biomechanical properties, metabolic demand, and shock absorption of the Flex and Seattle Foot versus the SACH foot. Each patient was fitted with a patellar tendon-bearing socket with a rubber sleeve suspension. The prosthetic foot was changed for each biomechanical and metabolic study.

The Flex Foot had the greatest forefoot compliance, with the largest midstance phase and the greatest ankle range. Both the Seattle and Flex foot produced better push off. However, no metabolic energy saving was detected with the Seattle or Flex Foot during walking or running when compared with the SACH foot. Even though there was better propulsion with the Seattle and Flex Foot, no energy saving occurred, most likely because the stored energy was not released at the appropriate time.

Conclusion

Many new ankle-foot systems have been introduced in recent years, and claims of energy storing capability are not always justified. Even the ankle-foot systems that are highly efficient in releasing stored energy may not provide lowered metabolic cost to the amputee. It appears that, for certain sports activities, flexible, highly compliant ankle-foot systems may be ideal; but for routine activities, less flexible systems may be adequate.

COMPUTER AIDED DESIGN AND MANUFACTURE OF CAD-CAM PROSTHETIC SOCKET

In the 1970s, James Foort of the Medical Research Unit of the University of British Colombia proposed the concept of computer-aided design (CAD) and manufacture of prosthetic sockets. Since then, several CAD-CAM systems have been developed and the systems are still undergoing modification.

Holden et al.[72] reported a pilot study comparing CAD-CAM with conventional sockets. Ten unilateral mature below-knee amputees were randomly assigned to three groups of prosthetics, with two prosthetists of comparable experience in each

group. One prosthetist fitted a patient with a CAD-CAM socket and the other with a conventional socket. The patients were blind to the type of socket and then asked to express preference regarding the comfort and fit of each socket. Only 3 of 10 patients preferred the CAD-CAM socket to the conventional socket.

Kohler et al.[73] compared sockets made by the CAD-CAM process and conventional handmade sockets. Ten unilateral, mature, below-knee amputees were fitted with two types of sockets and asked to grade each socket on a VAS regarding comfort, pressure, and pain. Patients were not aware of the type of socket they were using at any given time. Patients evaluated the sockets seven times from the day of delivery for 2 weeks after the initial fitting. The ratios of two VAS scores for two sockets at each of the seven measurements were calculated, and means of each type of socket were compared for statistical analysis. Valid data were obtained from 8 of 10 patients. All but one CAD-CAM socket had to be changed once compared to only two of the hand-made sockets. Statistical analysis did not show any significant difference between the sockets regarding comfort.

Topper et al.[74] carried out a single-blind, controlled trial involving 48 mature unilateral below-knee amputees who were fitted with conventional hand-casted and CAD-CAM sockets. Four prosthetists formed two teams and fitted all the patients. The two prosthetists in each team were of comparable experience and alternated for fitting with conventional or CAD-CAM socket for each new patient. The prosthetists were allowed two attempts for the conventional and five attempts for the CAD-CAM socket fitting. The patient were blinded regarding the type of socket, as both sockets appeared identical. Patients were asked to express their preference regarding each socket. Prosthetists were asked to fill out a questionnaire regarding their experience with the CAD-CAM system. A jury panel consisting of physicians, prosthetists, and an amputee was asked to make a detailed assessment of the CAD-CAM system.

After two attempts with each system, only 21 percent of the patients tested preferred the CAD-CAM sockets, and 54 percent preferred the CAD-CAM sockets after five attempts. Three prosthetists thought that the CAD-CAM system, in its present form, was clinically useful in a few patients, and the fourth prosthetist did not feel that the system was useful.

Ruder[75] studied the application of the CAD-CAM system in the production of a temporary transtibial prosthesis for dysvascular amputees. Thirty dysvascular amputees were randomly assigned to the study or control groups. The study group was fitted with a CAD-CAM and the control group with a conventional hand-casted socket. The total rehabilitation time was significantly less ($P \leq .05$) for the control group, and the control group also required significantly fewer appointments with the prosthetist ($P \leq .01$). The control group needed on average 2.9 ± 1.1 appointments and the study group 5.1 ± 1.8 appointments with the prosthetist during their inpatient stay.

Oberg et al.[76] carried out a single-blind, crossover trial involving 22 unilateral below-knee amputees. Each amputee was fitted with a CAD-CAM and conventional socket. The patients were divided into two groups. One group started with the conventional socket and the other group with the CAD-CAM socket. After 1 month, the patients switched to the other group. Patients were not aware of the type of socket they were using. All patients were interviewed at the beginning of the study and after 1 and 2 months, according to a protocol consisting of data regarding patient preference of socket, evaluation by the prosthetist and physiotherapist, gait analysis data, and degree of usage.

Statistical analysis of the data did not demonstrate any significant difference between the two types of socket regarding patient preference, gait parameters, and professional evaluation of the prosthesis. The authors concluded that the CAD-CAM system is capable of achieving the same results with socket fitting as the conventional system. The lack of difference in patient preference is consistent with other previously published studies.

Conclusion

These five controlled trials demonstrated that the CAD-CAM system socket design can achieve a comfortable fit in most transtibial amputees, but requires more time by the prosthetist because of the need for repeated socket fittings and modifications. It will require further improvement in software and experience of the prosthetist before the CAD-CAM system can provide a high-quality prosthesis at a cost comparable to the conventional system.

FINAL REMARKS

Lower extremity amputee rehabilitation underwent major changes after World War II. New surgical techniques and postoperative care have resulted in an increased healing rate at the below-knee level in dysvascular patients. New sockets and components have made a significant contribution toward improving the quality of life of all amputees. Many accepted methods of management require rigorous reevaluation through controlled trials to establish their efficacy. Introduction of new components should be preceded by appropriate controlled clinical trials regarding their efficacy and superiority over existing components.

REFERENCES

1. Berlmont M, Weber R, Willot JP et al: Ten years of experience with the immediate application of prosthetic devices to amputees of lower extremities on the operating table. Prosthet Orthot Int 3:8, 1969
2. Weiss M: Physiologic amputation, immediate prosthesis and early ambulation. Prosthet Orthot Int 3:38, 1969
3. Burgess EM, Romano RL, Zettl JH: Amputation management utilizing immediate post surgical prosthetic fitting. Prosthet Orthot Int 3:28, 1969
4. Burgess EM, Romano RL, Zettl JH et al: Amputation of the leg for peripheral vascular insufficiency. J Bone Joint Surg 53A:874, 1971
5. Sarmiento A, Bella JM, Sinclair WF et al: Lower extremity amputations: the impact of immediate post surgical prosthetic fitting. Clin Orthop 68:22, 1970
6. Mooney V, Harvey JP, McBride E et al: Comparison of post-operative stump management: plaster vs soft dressings. J Bone Joint Surg 53(A):241, 1971
7. Moore WS, Hale AD, Lim RC: Below the knee amputation for ischaemic gangrene: comparative results of conventional operation and immediate post-operative fitting technique. Am J Surg 124:127, 1972
8. Warren R, James RC, Banks HH et al: The Boston Interhospital Amputation Study: experience with a community service in immediate post-operative amputation. Arch Surg 107:861, 1973

9. Cohen SI et al: The deleterious effect of immediate post-operative prosthesis in below knee amputation for ischemic disease. Surgery 76:992, 1974

10. Mooney V et al: The below knee amputation for vascular disease. J Bone Joint Surg 58A:365, 1976

11. Nicholas G, DeMuth W: Evaluation of use of the rigid dressing in amputation of the lower extremity. Surg Gynecol Obstet 143:398, 1976

12. Baker W, Barnes RW, Shurr DG: The healing of below knee amputations: comparison of soft and plaster dressings. Am J Surg 133:716, 1977

13. Malone M, Moore WS, Goldstone J: Therapeutic and economic impact of a modern amputation program. Ann Surg 189:798, 1979

14. Kane TJ, Pollack EW: The rigid versus soft postoperative dressing controversy: a controlled study in vascular below knee amputees. Am Surg 46:244, 1980

15. Thorpe W, Gerber LH, Lampert M et al: A prospective study of the rehabilitation of the above knee amputee with rigid dressings: comparison of immediate and delayed ambulation and the role of physical therapists and prosthetists. Clin Orthop 143:133, 1979

16. Redhead RG, Snowdon C: A new approach to the management of wounds of the extremities. CET and its derivatives. Prosth Orthot Int 2:148, 1978

17. Burgess EM: Wound healing after amputation: effect of controlled environment treatment: a preliminary study. J Bone Joint Surg 59A:245, 1978

18. Troup IM: Controlled environment treatment. Prosthet Orthot Int 4:15, 1980

19. Ruckley CV, Rae A, Prescott RJ: Controlled environment unit in the treatment of the below knee amputation stump. Br J Surg 73:11, 1986

20. Little JM: A pneumatic weight bearing prosthesis for below knee amputees. Lancet 1:271, 1971

21. Barraclough GA et al: Airsplint used as immediate post-operative prosthesis after long posterior flap below knee amputation. Med J Aust 2:764, 1972

22. Kerstein MD: Utilization of an airsplint after below knee amputation. Am J Phys Med 53:119, 1974

23. Redhead RG, Davis BC, Robinson KP: Post amputation pneumatic walking aid. Br J Surg 65:611, 1978

24. Monga TN, Symington DC: The airsplint as a pneumatic prosthesis in management of the elderly amputee. Physiother Cana 36:61, 1984

25. Robbs JV, Kritzinger NA, Mogotlane KA et al: A clinical trial of a combination of amoxycillin and flucloxacillin in amputations for septic ischemic lower limb lesions. S Afr Med J 60:932, 1981

26. Huizinga WKJ, Robbs JV, Kritzinger NA: Prevention of wound sepsis in amputations by perioperative antibiotics cover with amoxycillin: clavulanic acid combination. S Afr Med J 63:71, 1983

27. Moller BN, Krebs B: Antibiotic prophylaxis in lower limb amputation. Acta Orthop Scand 56:327, 1985

28. Sonne Holm S, Boeckstyn M, Merek H et al: Prophylactic antibiotics in amputation of lower extremity for ischemia: a placebo controlled, randomized trial of cetokitin. J Bone Joint Surg 67A:800, 1985

29. Friss H: Penicillin G versus cefuroxime for prophylaxis in lower limb amputation. Acta Orthop Scand 58:666, 1987

30. Norlin R et al: Short term cefotaxime prophylaxis reduces the failure rate in lower limb amputations. Acta Orthop Scand 61:460, 1990

31. Dickhaut SC, DeLee J, Page CP et al: Nutritional status: importance in predicting wound healing after amputation. J Bone Joint Surg 66A:71, 1984

32. Kay SP et al: Nutritional status and wound healing in lower extremity amputations. Clin Orthop 217:252, 1987

33. Pedersen NW, Pederson D: Nutrition as a prognostic indicator in amputation: a prospective study of 47 cases. Acta Orthop Scand 63:675, 1992

34. Rayner HC et al: Relief of local stump pain by capsaicin (letter). Lancet 2:276, 1989

35. Weintraub M et al: Capsaicin for treatment of post traumatic stump pain (letter). Lancet 336:1003, 1990

36. Steinbach TV et al: A five year follow-up study of phantom limb pain in post traumatic amputees. Scand J Rehabil Med 14:203, 1982

37. Sherman RA, Sherman CJ, Parker L: Chronic phantom and stump pain amongst American veterans: results of a survey. Pain 18:83, 1984

38. Jensen TS, Krebs B, Nielson J et al: Immediate and long term phantom pain in amputees: incidence, clinical characteristics, and relationship to pre-amputation pain. Pain 21:267, 1985

39. Sherman RA: Special review: published treatments of phantom limb pain. Am J Phys Med 59:232, 1980

40. Davis RW: Phantom sensation, phantom pain and stump pain. Arch Phys Med Rehabil 74:79, 1993

41. Bach S, Noreng MF, Jellden T: Phantom limb pain in amputees during the first twelve months following limb amputation, after pre-operative lumbar epidural blockade. Pain, 33:397, 1988

42. Jaeger H, Maier C: Calcitonin in phantom limb pain: a double blind study. Pain 48:21, 1992

43. Davis RW: Successful treatment of phantom pain. Orthopaedics, 16:691, 1993

44. Oille WA: Beta adrenergic blockade and phantom limb (letter). Ann Intern Med L 73:1044, 1970

45. Ahmad S: Phantom limb and propranolol. BMJ 415, 1979

46. Marsland AR, Weekes JW, Atkinson RL et al: Phantom limb pain: a case for beta blockers. Pain 12:295, 1982

47. Elliott F et al: Carbamazepine for phantom limb phenomena (letter). N Engl J Med 295:678, 1976
48. Patterson JF: Carbamazepine in the treatment of phantom limb pain. South Med J 81:1100, 1988
49. Panerai AE, Morilia P, Bianchi M et al: A randomized with inpatient cross over, placebo controlled trial on the efficacy and tolerability of the tricyclic antidepressant chlorimipramine and nortriptyline in central pain. Acta Neurol Scand 82:34, 1990
50. Winnem MF: Treatment of phantom limb pain with TENS (letter). Pain 12:299, 1982
51. Lundeberg T: Relief of pain from a phantom limb by peripheral stimulation. J Neurol 232:79, 1985
52. Finsen V, Person L, Lovlien M et al: Transcutaneous electrical nerve stimulation after major amputation. Journal Bone Joint Surg 70B:109, 1988
52a. Shealy CN, Mortimer JT, Reswick JB: Electrical inhibition of pain by stimulation of dorsal column, preliminary report. Anaesth Analg Carr Res 67:489, 1967
53. Nielson KD et al: Phantom limb pain: treatment with dorsal column stimulation. Neurosurgery 42:301, 1975
54. Wester K: Dorsal column stimulation in pain treatment. Acta Neurol Scand 75:151, 1987
55. Kumar K, Nath R, Wyant G: Treatment of chronic pain by epidural spinal cord simulation: a 10 year experience. J Neurosurg 75:402, 1991
56. Saris SC et al: Dorsal root entry zone lesions for post amputation pain. J Neurosurg 62:72, 1985
57. Sherman R et al: Treatment of phantom limb pain with muscular relaxation training to disrupt the pain, anxiety, tension cycle. Pain 6:47, 1979
58. Manella K: Comparing effectiveness of elastic bandages and shrinker socks for lower extremity amputees. Phys Ther 61:3, 334, 1981
59. Mueller M: Comparison of removable rigid dressings and elastic bandages in prosthetic management of patients with below knee amputation. Phys Ther 62:1438, 1982
60. Kavanagh T et al: Application of exercise testing to elderly amputee. Can Med Assoc J 108:314, 1973
61. Cruts HEP, de Vries J, Zilvold G et al: Lower extremity amputees with peripheral vascular disease graded exercise testing and results of prosthetic training. Arch Phys Med Rehabil 68:14, 1987
62. Roth EJ, Wiesner SL, Green D et al: Dysvascular amputee rehabilitation: the role of continuous noninvasive cardiovascular monitoring during physical therapy. Am J Phys Med Rehabil 69:16, 1990
63. Miller LS, Naso F: Conditioning program for amputees with significant heart disease. Arch Phys Med Rehabil 57:238, 1976
64. Pitetti KH et al: Aerobic training exercises for individuals who had amputation of lower limbs. J Bone Joint Surg 69A:914, 1987
65. Klingenstierna U, Renstorm P, Grimby G et al: Isokinetic strength training in below knee amputees. Scand J Rehabil Med 22:39, 1990
66. Isakov E, Susak Z, Becker E: Energy expenditure and cardiac response in above knee amputees while using open and locked knee mechanism. Scand J Rehabil Med 12(S):108, 1985
66a. Long IA: Normal shape normal alignment (NSNA) above knee prosthesis. Clin Prosthet Orthot 9:9, 1985
66b. J Sablich: Contoured Adducted Drochametric Controlled Alignment Method (CAT-CAM): Introduction and Basic Principles. Clin Prosthet Orthot 9:15, 1985
67. Flandry F, Beskin J, Chambers RB: The Effect of CAT CAM above knee prosthesis on functional rehabilitation. Clin Orthopa 239:249, 1989
68. Gailey RS et al: The CAT CAM socket and quadrilateral socket: a comparison of energy cost during ambulation. Prosthet Orthot Int 17:95, 1993
69. Ehara Y, Beppu M, Nomuru S et al: Energy storing property of so called energy storing prosthetic feet. Arch Phys Med Rehabil 74:68, 1993
70. Menard MR, McBride ME, Sanderson DJ et al: Comparative biomechanical analysis of energy storing prosthetic feet. Arch Phys Med Rehabil 73:451, 1992
71. Lehman JF, Price R, Boswell-Bessettes R et al: Comprehensive analysis of energy storing prosthetic feet: flex foot and Seattle foot versus standard SACH foot. Arch Phys Med Rehabil 74:1225, 1993
72. Holden JM et al: Results of the pilot phase of a clinical evaluation of computer aided design of transtibial prosthesis sockets. Prosthet Orthot Int 10:142, 1986
73. Kohler P, Lindl L, Netz P: Comparison of CAD CAM and hand made sockets for PTB prosthesis. Prosthet Ortho Int 13:19, 1989
74. Topper AK, Fernie GR: An evaluation of computer aided design of below knee prosthetic sockets. Prosthet Orthot Int 14:136, 1990
75. Ruder AK: CAD CAM transtibial temporary prosthesis: analysis and comparison with an established technique. Prosth Orthot Int 16:189, 1992
76. Oberg T, Lilja M, Johansson T et al: Clinical evaluation of transtibial prosthesis sockets: a comparison between CAD CAM and conventionally produced sockets. Prosthet Orthot Int 17:164, 1993

10

Muscle Disease

Exercise and Orthotics

Barbara J. de Lateur

Logical choice making involves correct diagnosis and functional assessment to select the correct treatment modality. For this reason, it is important to distinguish inflammatory myopathies from hereditary muscle diseases. In this chapter, polymyositis has been selected as the prototype of inflammatory muscle disease. Duchenne muscular dystrophy (DMD) and facioscapulohumeral (FSH) dystrophy have been selected to represent the hereditary muscle diseases. It is also important to distinguish muscular weakness caused by peripheral neuropathy from that caused by motor neuron diseases such as poliomyelitis or amyotrophic lateral sclerosis. Furthermore, the weakness seen in multiple sclerosis is complicated by spasticity and impairment of motor control. Application of various types of exercise and orthoses are discussed here. In the second part of this chapter, drug treatment is discussed.

No attempt has been made to provide an exhaustive treatment of the various forms of myopathies, neuropathies, or neuromuscular disorders. The principles given can be tailored for application to these other disorders. With the exception of polymytositis, our ability to treat the disease process itself is limited, and we are faced with having to prevent or treat the consequences of the disease.

INFLAMMATORY VERSUS HEREDITARY MUSCLE DISEASE

Polymyositis as the Prototype of Inflammatory Muscle Disease

Polymyositis and dermatomyositis are diseases of uncertain origin that are generally considered with the rheumatic diseases. Along with such disorders as rheumatoid arthritis, systemic lupus erythematosus, progressive systemic sclerosis, and necrotizing vasculitis, polymyositis and dermatomyositis are classified as diffuse connective tissue diseases.[1] The *Primer on the Rheumatic Diseases*[1] gives the following groupings:

Group 1: Primary idiopathic polymyositis
Group 2: Primary idiopathic dermatomyositis
Group 3: Dermatomyositis (or polymyositis) associated with neoplasia
Group 4: Childhood dermatomyositis (or polymyositis) associated with vasculitis
Group 5: Polymyositis or dermatomyositis associated with collagen-vascular disease (overlap group)

As noted in the *Primer*, polymyositis causes symmetric weakness of striated muscles, especially of the limb girdle, neck, and pharynx. Females are affected twice as often as males, and the disorder may occur at any age. It is varied not only in its mode of onset, but also in rate of progression of symptoms.

As the *Primer* points out, "This variability makes it difficult to provide a unified clinical portrait of the disease." One may add that this variability also makes it difficult to assess the effects of treatment. One way to decrease measurement variability is to perform true quantitative measurements of strength. These measurements should be carried out daily during early recovery and twice a week in mid-recovery phase. Such measurements would include strain gauge or isokinetic dynamometry.

Measures of the functional consequences of strength loss or gain, such as the Functional Independence Measure (FIM) can be carried out every 1 to 2 weeks. The pelvic girdle weakness will manifest itself by difficulty in climbing a high bus step, arising from a low chair, getting out of the bathtub, and climbing stairs. When shoulder girdle muscles become involved, patients will have difficulty combing their hair or performing any activities involving keeping their arms elevated. Some patients will have muscular pain, tenderness, and induration.[2]

Malignancies coexist with dermatomyositis and polymyositis more frequently than in the general population, but especially in patients over the age of 40.[3] Callen et al.[3] reported that internal malignancies were found in 27 percent of adults over 35 years with polymyositis or dermatomyositis. Search for an occult malignancy, therefore, is warranted.

Enzymes such as transaminase, creatine kinase (CK), and aldolase are sensitive indicators of muscle injury. CK is usually elevated in advance of clinical worsening, whereas clinical improvement usually occurs in advance of enzymatic return toward normal. Thus, as one evaluates response to exercise, one should look at what is happening with CK *before* possible worsening and at muscle strength increase (rather than decreased CK) as evidence of muscle improvement in response to exercise.

Rest

Because polymyositis and dermatomyositis are systemic diseases, rest (as well as medication) will have a role in management. However, one must balance the need for rest against the deleterious effects of disuse and prolonged bed rest. Such deleterious effects happen faster (even in normal subjects) than recovery and improvement in response to exercise training.

Muscular Dystrophies

DMD and FSH dystrophy are featured here as representative dystrophies, the former being the most common X-linked recessive dystrophy, and the latter, the most common dominantly inherited dystrophy. For this reason, and because the clinical manifestations are sometimes amenable to exercise and orthotic interventions, these two forms of dystrophy are selected for discussion in this chapter. The dystrophies are frequently classified according to mode of inheritance and patterns of clinical manifestations. Table 10-1 gives such a classification and shows how DMD and FSH dystrophy fit in the classification.

Duchenne Muscular Dystrophy

The incidence of DMD is about 1 per 3,500 live male births.[4] It is found almost exclusively in boys, although it is occasionally expressed in girls with Turner's syndrome or Turner's mosaic syndrome. DMD is carried by females who are usually relatively normal clinically. The mutation rate for DMD is higher than in any other X-linked recessive disease (approximately 1 per 10,000 per gene per generation).

A classic clinical manifestation of hip extensor and quadriceps weakness is Gower's sign, in which the child "climbs up his legs" (Figs. 10-1 through 10-3). With respect to laboratory findings, CK is elevated at birth and is especially high while the child is still walking, but falls as the overall muscle mass declines later in the disease. Thus, in contrast to the case in polymyositis and dermatomyositis, the CK is not a good way to follow the patient's clinical status.

Table 10-1. Types of Muscular Dystrophies

X-linked recessive
Defects of dystrophin
DMD
BMD
Congenital
Quadriceps
Myalgia and cramps
Defects unknown
Emery-Dreiffus
Scapuloperoneal
Autosomal recessive
Limb-girdle
Scapulohumeral
Pelvifemoral
Childhood
Congenital
Autosomal dominant
Facioscapulohumeral
Limb-girdle
Scapuloperoneal
Distal
Oculopharyngeal

(From Morgan-Hughes,[25] with permission.)

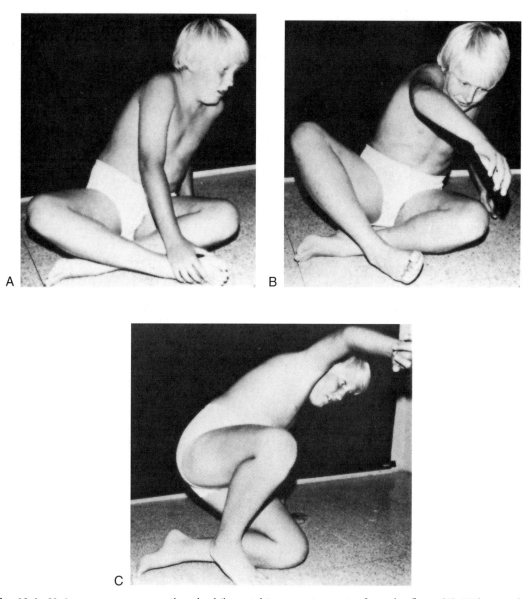

Fig. 10-1. Various components analyzed while watching a patient arise from the floor. (**A**) With a moderate degree of weakness, the first movement is a quarter turn of the body toward the weak side (**B,C**). Supporting himself with one hand on the floor, he rolls over, bringing his knees and feet under him. (*Figure continues.*)

The child may or may not have normal early developmental milestones. As many as 50 percent of boys may still be unable to walk by the age of 18 months.

Most textbooks indicate early weakness of the pelvic girdle musculature with a waddling, lordotic gait. In my experience abdominal muscle weakness is also an early finding that contributes to the lordosis and to the frequently seen protuberant abdomen (Fig. 10-4). This downward tilt of the pelvis causes the tensor fasciae latae (TFL) to remain in a chroni-

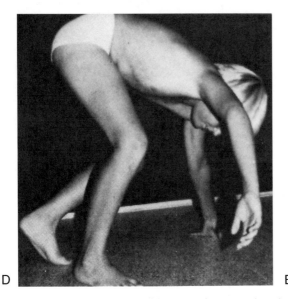
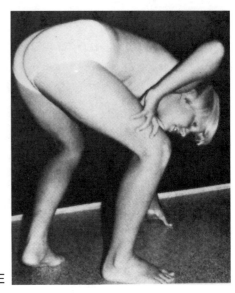

Fig. 10-1. (*Continued*) (**D**) The hips are then raised in the air while maintaining the support with one hand, the "butt first" maneuver. (**E**) Finally, one hand is placed on the thigh to provide the additional support needed in straightening the body from this position. Nonprogressive congenital myopathy, undiagnosed. (From Brooke,[6] with permission.)

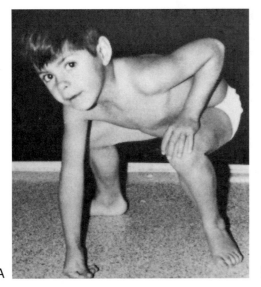
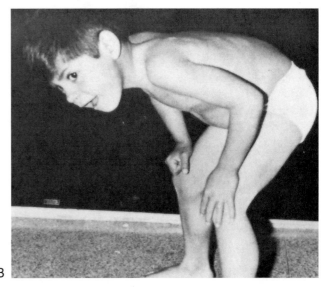

Fig. 10-2. (**A,B**) This patient with DMD arises from the floor with unilateral hand support on the floor, but then requires bilateral hand support on the thighs to attain the upright position. (From Brooke,[6] with permission.)

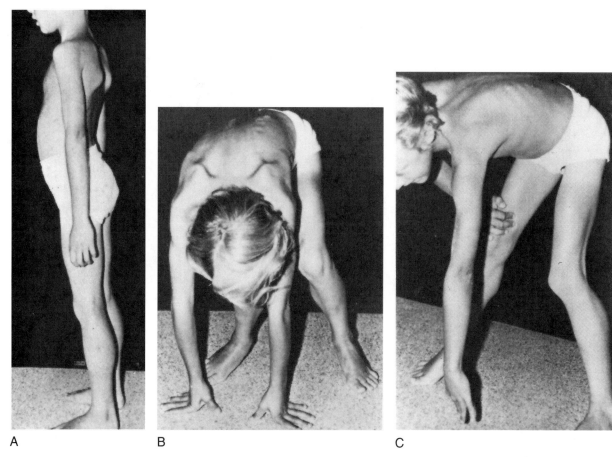

A   B   C

Fig. 10-3. In this child with DMD, the degree of weakness is sufficient to produce a moderate degree of lumbar lordosis. **(A)** The shoulder weakness is also apparent in the way in which the scapulae jut backwards. **(B)** When the child tries to arise from the floor, he needs bilateral hand support on the floor in the "butt first" maneuver. **(C)** He then transfers his hand to his thigh and stands by using bilateral hand support on the thighs. (From Brooke,[6] with permission.)

cally shortened position, which adds to the difficulty of extending the hip and contributes to an abducted stance. Lordosis becomes progressively more exaggerated as the child attempts to stabilize the hips in extension. It results from throwing the center of gravity posteriorly to maintain the weight line behind the hips.

As Johnson and Kennedy[5] point out, at the same time the child must maintain the weight line in front of the knees to stabilize the knee in extension (Fig. 10-5). This is particularly difficult to accomplish as the quadriceps become weaker. During gait, the child carries out this maneuver by walking on the toes. Gait instability is further contributed to by an imbalance between foot/ankle inverters and everters. The tibialis posterior is relatively stronger and becomes shortened, as it is no longer counterbalanced by the weakened peroneals.

Early on, the children are generally able to stand with their heels on the floor, but cannot walk with a heel strike. This toe-walking and subsequent heel-cord shortening are thus due to hip extensor weakness and tightness of the tensor fasciae latae rather than to weakness of the tibialis anterior muscles. The latter will subsequently become weak and contribute to the accelerating muscle strength imbalance and gastrocnemius-soleus contracture. These children are rarely able to run in a normal fashion, even

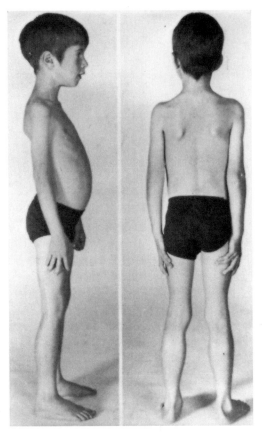

Fig. 10-4. DMD in a 6-year-old boy. Note the typical lordotic posture, enlargement of the calves, and early winging of the scapulae. (From Morgan-Hughes,[25] with permission.)

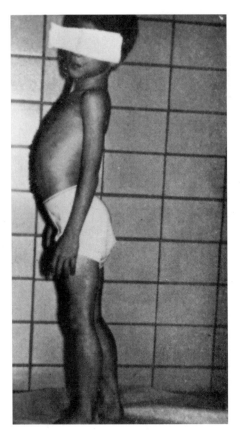

Fig. 10-5. Child with early DMD. Note the weight line behind the hips. (From Johnson and Kennedy,[5] with permission.)

early in the disorder. Likewise, difficulty climbing stairs is an early manifestation.

Proximal upper limb involvement is typical, with relative sparing of the hand and forearm muscles. Imbalance between biceps and triceps contributes to shortening of the biceps with flexion contracture at the elbow.

When the child requires a wheelchair for mobility, hip and knee flexion contractures and ankle plantarflexion and inversion contractures progress rapidly. Kyphoscoliosis is also common once the wheelchair stage is reached. A restrictive type of respiratory involvement is typical as the weakness advances. As the deformities progress, it may become progressively more difficult to find a position of comfort. The adolescent or young adult may achieve comfort only in the sitting and side-lying positions.

FSH Dystrophy

The incidence of FSH dystrophy is approximately 0.5 to 5.0 per 100,000. Although penetrance is virtually complete, the clinical manifestations vary quite widely, even within the same family. The disorder most commonly presents in the teenage years or in the early twenties, although the patient may always have had difficulty blowing a balloon or whistling.

A typical pattern of limb muscle involvement is shown in Fig. 10-6. The weakness may spread to the pelvic girdle and even to the anterior tibial and peroneal muscles. Weakness and atrophy of the biceps and triceps with relative preservation of the forearm lead to the Popeye arm (Fig. 10-7).[6]

NEUROGENIC MUSCLE WEAKNESS: PERIPHERAL NEUROPATHY AND POLIOMYELITIS

Peripheral Neuropathy

The peripheral neuropathies may be hereditary or acquired. An example of a genetically determined polyneuropathy is hereditary motor and sensory neuropathy type I (Charcot-Marie-Tooth disease).[7] This disease is also called peroneal or neuromuscular atrophy and has a prevalence of about 2 per 100,000. It is usually inherited as an autosomal dominant trait. The early signs of the disease appear in childhood or adolescence and are manifest by foot deformities, often as a true club foot.

As the disorder progresses, the anterior and lateral compartment muscles of the leg become weak, causing a steppage gait. The strength of the gastrocnemius and soleus muscles is relatively preserved. If toe walking does occur it is different from that seen in DMD. The atrophy of the leg muscles is in marked contrast to the preservation of the thigh muscles, which leads to an appearance sometimes called "stork legs" or an "inverted flask deformity."

Although the upper limb is involved later, the distal muscles (i.e., the small muscles of the hand) are

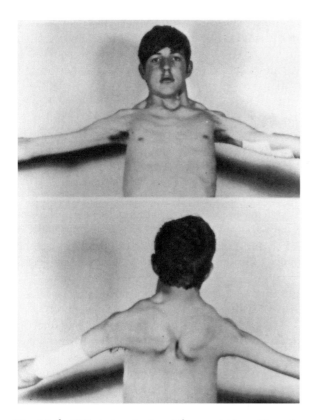

Fig. 10-6. FSH dystrophy in a 16-year-old boy. Note the myopathic facies and elevation of the scapulae on abduction of the arms. (From Morgan-Hughes,[25] with permission.)

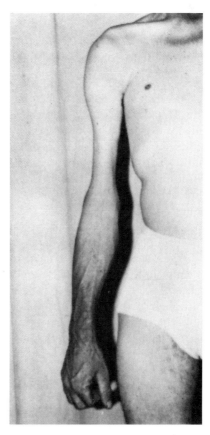

Fig. 10-7. Preservation of the deltoid muscle with marked atrophy of the biceps and triceps. (From Brooke,[6] with permission.)

the first to become involved, leading to a picture referred to by some as an "intrinsic minus hand" with extension or hyperextension at the metacarpophalangeal joints of digits 2 through 5 and flexion or hyperflexion at the proximal and distal interphalangeal joints.

Acquired polyneuropathies are often seen in metabolic disorders, although there may be a genetic predisposition. One example of an acquired neuropathy is diabetic polyneuropathy. It is difficult to obtain accurate statistics regarding this neurologic complication because the reported incidence varies with the thoroughness of clinical assessment. Nerve conduction slowing may be present before clinically recognized motor deficits. The sensory nerve fibers are frequently affected before the motor nerve fibers and may manifest their involvement as paresthesias, pain, and absent reflexes. As many as 40 percent of diabetic patients[8] have shown abnormal tendon jerks or sensory disturbances.

Acute Anterior Poliomyelitis

Acute anterior poliomyelitis is a viral disorder that affects the gray matter, particularly the anterior horn cells of the spinal cord. In those countries where active immunization has been carried out, the "wild" form of the disorder has become rare. Before such immunization was available, many persons probably had a mild form which they thought was "the flu." The weakness that occurred was mild and would have required subtle tests of strength to demonstrate. When clinically apparent, the residual weakness was usually asymmetric and most commonly involved the peroneals or anterior tibial muscles in the lower limb and less commonly various upper limb muscles. Asymmetry can be considered a characteristic feature of the wild forms of polio.

Because of preservation of sensory function, the gait seen in poliomyelitis generally differed from that seen in polyneuropathies such as Charcot-Marie-Tooth disease, even though both might typically have anterior compartment leg muscle weakness. Thus, a patient with Charcot-Marie-Tooth disease would typically have a steppage gait, whereas the polio patient would fling the foot in such a way as to provide minimal but adequate toe clearance and would strike with the foot flat rather

than with a toe strike. When the imbalance between anterior (weak) and posterior (preserved) compartment muscles of the leg were combined with quadriceps weakness, the patient typically would develop genu recurvatum because of the powerful toe-lever-arm used to stabilize the knee in extension. If the quadriceps weakness were severe enough, the patient would place the center of gravity firmly in front of the knee joint.

Post-polio Syndrome

In recent years, a post-polio syndrome has been recognized. Nearly a one-third of the 1.6 million polio survivors have developed symptoms such as fatigue, new muscle atrophy, and difficulty breathing.[9] At this time the syndrome is still poorly understood. Some manifestations, such as increasing difficulty with balance or progressive genu recurvatum, can be explained on a biomechanical basis. As patients age, they may gain weight while gradually decreasing their muscle strength. Thus, the relative strength (strength/weight ratio) may have decreased below the threshold required for ordinary activities such as standing balance.

An excellent discussion of the biomechanical aspects of the post-polio syndrome is provided by Perry and associates.[10] However, not all secondary weakness seen in the post-polio syndrome can be explained by their hypothesis, and some may well be due to a secondary pathologic process.

Sharief et al.[11] reported immunoglobin M antibodies specific to polio in patients with post-polio syndrome. It is possible that either a resurgent attack or a new infection may occur. Muir et al.[12] stated that "people who had polio in the past may be subject to infection from other enteroviruses. These new infections might trigger post-polio syndrome."

In 1958, Bennett and Knowlton[13] described "overwork weakness." Their article is essentially anecdotal; four of the five patients had polio. It is not clear whether any of the secondary weakness seen in polio is due to overwork, but prudence must be used (see later).

Weight Training and Exercise Effects

Milner-Brown and Miller[14] studied the effect of high-resistance weight training in patients with neuromuscular disorders. Muscle strength of these patients ranged from 2 to 75 percent of normal before the program. Fig. 10-8 illustrates the mean effect of the program on the maximum strength of knee extensors and elbow flexors, both of which increase significantly in their strength. Fig. 10-9 shows the effect of exercise on markedly weak elbow flexors and knee extensors of seven patients before and after 2 to 48 months of weight training. The improvement of the four patients with FSH dystrophy seems to contradict Johnson and Braddom,[15] who concluded that exercise has an adverse effect on FSH dystrophy. However, the two reports are not strictly comparable because one is an intervention and the other is the report of a family of affected subjects, all of whom had greater weakness of the more heavily used upper limb.

MULTIPLE SCLEROSIS

The central nervous system disorder of multiple sclerosis is most commonly seen in temperate climates with the greatest prevalence in northern and middle Europe, including Switzerland, Russia, Canada, the northern United States, New Zealand, and the southwestern part of Australia, where multiple sclerosis is present in 30 to 80 per 100,000 of the population.[16] This demyelinating disease of the central nervous system in its classic form is characterized by dissemination in time and space; that is to say, the clinical manifestations cannot be explained by one lesion occurring at one time. Again in a classic presentation, the disorder is characterized by attacks with exacerbations and remission, although there may be benign forms with mild disabilities and

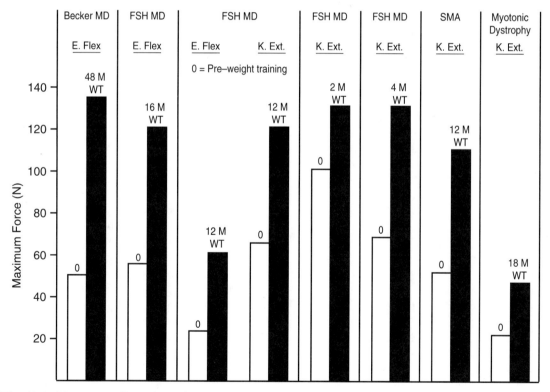

Fig. 10-8. The mean effect of weight training on the maximum force of knee extensors and elbow flexors. The open block, designated zero (0), represents the pre-weight-training maximum force. Blocks with diagonal lines represent the mean (±SD) maximum forces expressed relative to the pre-exercise value (100 percent). (From Milner-Brown and Miller,[14] with permission.)

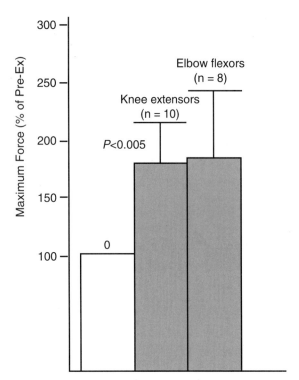

Fig. 10-9. The muscle strength of markedly weak (15 to 25 percent normal) elbow flexors (E. Flex) and knee extensors (K. Ext.) of seven patients compared before and after 2 to 48 months of weight training. Open blocks, designated zero (0), represent the maximum force before weight training. Blocks that are shaded represent the maximum force after specific months (M) of weight training (WT), indicated above each block. (From Milner-Brown and Miller,[14] with permission.)

a more severe form with a progressive course from the outset.

The neurologic impairment and resulting disabilities can be quantified by the expanded disability status scale (EDSS) of Kurtzke.[17] This variability is an important factor in the decision-making process for the management of multiple sclerosis. The upper motor neuron manifestations, especially spasticity, often make motor control and use of the otherwise available muscle strength difficult. The spasticity must be managed before exercise strengthening programs or orthotic management can be used effectively.

PASSIVE AND ACTIVE EXERCISE

The three types of exercise that theoretically may be beneficial in the aforementioned disorders include flexibility (stretching), strengthening (resistance), and aerobic or metabolic training.

Flexibility

Flexibility exercise is of greatest importance in DMD. In DMD, functional loss, especially loss of the ability to walk, is more a consequence of fixed muscle shortening (i.e., contracture) than a direct result of muscle weakness. Subjects with severe hip extensor weakness can stabilize the hip in extension by placing the center of gravity and weight line posterior to the hip and leaning against the iliofemoral ligament *if* there is no flexion contracture of the hip. Likewise, subjects with extremely weak quadriceps can stabilize the knee in extension by placing the weight line anterior to the knee, *if* there is no flexion contracture of the knee.

Tightness (contracture) of the tensor fasciae latae (TFL) and iliotibial band (ITB) is a culprit at both the hip and knee joints. Early in the disorder, this tightness may be quite subtle, and a special test (Ober test) is required for detection. The Ober test for tightness of the TFL and ITB is performed by placing the patient on the side, with the side to be tested in the superior position. The examiner stabilizes the pelvis by placing one hand firmly on the pelvis, just below the iliac crest. The examiner places his or her other hand just below the knee and grasps the leg firmly. The examiner then flexes the patient's hip to 90 degrees. From the flexed position, the patient's hip is abducted and then extended.

These maneuvers should place the TFL and ITB directly over the greater trochanter. Keeping the hip extended, the examiner then allows the thigh to drop (adduct) toward the examination table. In the normal child, the side examined should reach the examination table, or, at least, the opposite thigh. If the thigh remains abducted, tightness of the TFL and/or ITB is present. This position becomes the appropriate position for stretching the structures in question.

Because the number of interventions by a therapist will necessarily be limited, the family must be instructed in appropriate technique for stretching these and other structures such as the hamstrings and gastrocnemius muscles. These stretching exercises should become part of a daily exercise routine throughout the child's life, although it is difficult to convince patients and their families about the importance of this aspect of anticipatory management.

The muscular dystrophy clinic provides an environment in which patients and families can see other patients at more advanced stages of the disease and may encourage them to be faithful about exercise. It is also recognized, however, that this environment may have the unintended effect of suggesting that the deformities are inevitable regardless of the regularity with which patients exercise. It is important for the managing physician and therapist to maintain an optimistic attitude and positively reinforce the efforts of patient and family. Berating them for lack of performance is never productive and will only discourage their efforts.

Stretching is also important in the management of spasticity associated with multiple sclerosis. Spasticity, a rate- or velocity-dependent increase in resistance to passive stretching of muscle, typically affects the two-joint muscles such as the rectus femoris or gastrocnemius muscles. Prolonged static stretching to these muscles, particularly if preceded by a 20-minute application of an ice pack, will make ambulation and self-care management easier. To be effective, such stretching should be part of a daily routine.

Strengthening

Strengthening exercise (i.e., resistance training), has been controversial in all of the muscle and neuromuscular disorders described previously. Some clinicians and authors have asserted that resistance training is not only ineffective in such disorders, but also may actually be harmful. I believe the preponderance of evidence strongly suggests that judiciously used resistance exercise may indeed be helpful in these disorders and does not cause harm.

Isokinetic Exerciser

de Lateur and Giaconi[18] studied four children with DMD who had quadriceps of antigravity strength or better. Only one quadriceps was exercised, the side being determined randomly. The exercise, directly supervised, was submaximal isokinetic exercise using a Cybex isokinetic exerciser and recorder. The subjects trained for 6 months and were followed for 24 months. The absolute torque values of the exercised side were equal to or stronger than the control side during all months except month 24 when the control side averaged 3.3 foot pounds compared to the exercise side, which averaged 3.0 foot pounds. In two subjects who were also studied at 30 months, both sides were so weak that the subjects could not accelerate the mass of the limb and the lever arm of the dynamometer (Fig. 10-10).

Barbiroli et al.[19] showed that heavy eccentric contractions induced subjective perception of muscle pain and soreness, which started several hours after lengthening exercise and occurred to various degrees in each individual 48 hours after exercise in DMD/Becker's muscular dystrophy (BMD) carriers (*not* dystrophics). However, utilizing 31P-nuclear magnetic resonance (NMR) spectroscopy, they found that lengthening exercises cause less muscle injury in carriers than in noncarriers, although there was a slower than baseline rate of recovery of inorganic phosphate (Pi). This study by itself does not suggest any adverse effect of eccentric exercise in dystrophy.

Electrical Stimulation

Milner-Brown and Miller[20] also studied 10 patients with gradually progressive neuromuscular disorders, using unilateral electrical stimulation of the tibialis anterior muscles and unilateral stimulation of the quadriceps femoris muscles, in combination with voluntary knee extension against ankle weights. After electrical stimulation 2 h/day 5 days/week, for 2 to 14 months, the mean maximum force (muscle strength) of knee extension increased significantly by 108 ± 56 percent. The contralateral nonexercised knee extensors also showed some increase in strength.

The authors point out that electrical stimulation of the ankle dorsiflexors was not effective and that in general severely weak muscles (i.e., less than 10 percent of normal strength) did not improve. They concluded that electrical neuromuscular stimulation,

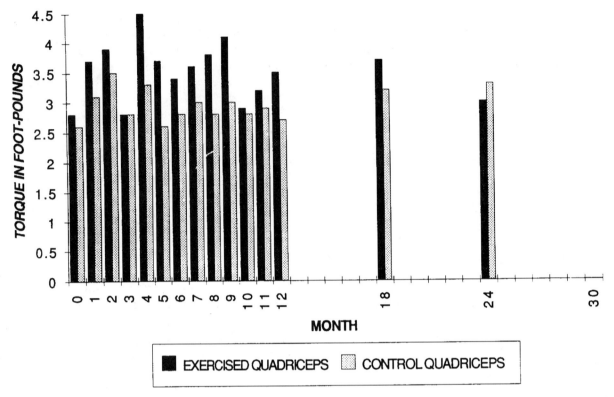

Fig. 10-10. All subjects. Maximal torques for exercised and control quadriceps. Pre-Ex, pre-exercise level. (From de Lateur et al.,[24] with permission.)

combined with low-resistance weights, can significantly increase muscle strength in patients with neuromuscular disorders if disease progression is gradual and initial muscle strength is greater than 15 percent of normal. The 10 subjects they referred to as having muscular dystrophy included two with FSH dystrophy, one with myotonic dystrophy, two with BMD, and two with limb-girdle muscular dystrophy, as well as three with spinal muscular atrophy.

Active Strengthening Exercises

Erwin et al.[21] studied a patient with hereditary distal myopathy. After a 3-week course of twice a day exercise, the patient's hand and wrist manual muscle testing score, hand grasp and pinch strength, and nine-hole peg test times had all improved to a modest degree.

In a pilot study of multiple sclerosis, Kraft et al.[22,23] studied eight subjects, four with mild disease

and four with severe disease. The subjects received progressive-resistance training 3 days a week for 3 months. We concluded that paretic muscles can be strengthened in patients with multiple sclerosis with upper motor neuron weakness. Our hypothesis that mildly affected muscles respond better to exercise was not disproved. We also evaluated the subjects' physical function and concluded that progressive resistance exercise training among persons with multiple sclerosis: (1) improves their ability to perform common daily activities; (2) has a significantly positive impact on the psychosocial, physical, and overall well-being in persons mildly and severely affected by multiple sclerosis; and (3) poses minimal risk of adverse effects compared to the benefits.

Decision Making

In the decision-making process regarding whether to use resistance exercise on patients with any of the previously mentioned neuromuscular disorders, we have used the following technique. Where the exercise appears to be symmetric, we put the patient on a unilateral program of exercise (side determined by the flip of a coin) and carefully monitor the strength of the two sides. If there is any sign of deterioration of strength of the exercised side, the resistance training is stopped immediately. If strength is constantly increasing, the program is continued and the comparison side is also started on an exercise program.

This technique is not applicable to subjects with asymmetric disorders. As noted by Johnson and Braddom[15] patients with FSH dystrophy often have greater weakness on the dominant side; we do not attempt to strengthen these muscles, in which overwork may have been added to genetically preprogrammed weakness.

Aerobic or Metabolic Training

Available data are so scant that it is difficult to make a firm recommendation regarding aerobic or metabolic training in these disorders. In a pilot study, de Lateur et al.[24] found that aerobic exercise was subjectively beneficial to patients with multiple sclerosis who were still ambulatory. Greater ease in performing ordinary activities of daily living was reported. We strongly urge adequate cooling if aerobic exercise is carried out in multiple sclerosis patients who are well known to have deterioration if their core temperatures are allowed to rise. For this reason, some patients have found devices such as the Schwinn Airdyne, which generate a breeze as they are operated, to be comfortable and useful.

ORTHOTICS

Bracing to Prevent or Correct Deformities

Anticipatory management is the key to effective use of orthotic devices, just as it is the key to the correct usage of exercise. The earliest deformities in DMD result from the imbalance of muscle strength between the weakened hip extensors and abdominal muscles on the one hand and the relatively strong hip flexors (including the iliopsoas and the

TFL) on the other. This imbalance causes early tightness of the TFL and the ITB, which, in turn, causes the patient to compensate by walking on the toes. Although the gastrocnemius muscles are generally stronger than the anterior tibial, this imbalance is not the cause of toe walking.

Unfortunately, bracing cannot prevent tightness of the TFL and ITB. Tightness must be prevented by stretching exercise and avoidance of prolonged positioning in hip flexion. The toe walking and the imbalance between the gastrocnemius and anterior tibial strength, however, will lead secondarily to plantarflexion and inversion contractures.

Various orthotic devices (bracing) can be useful in preventing secondary plantarflexion contractures at the ankle if the braces are properly designed and applied. Resting foot and ankle splints can be used at night to prevent acceleration of plantarflexion contractures. Here the key is comfort. If they are uncomfortable, the patient simply will not wear them.

The splints should be positioned, designed, and fabricated in such a fashion to *maintain* the range gained by stretching exercise. Do not attempt to *correct* deformities with these splints. For example, if the patient has a 12-degree plantarflexion contracture, the ankle angle of the splint should be 12 degrees, not 0 degrees plantarflexion.

In my unpublished study (Lehmann, de Lateur, and Stonebridge, personal communication) my associates and I found that patients with DMD who came in daily for stretching of plantarflexion contractures did not maintain the corrections unless they wore resting splints at night. Those who did wear them made modest gains over a period of weeks. Those who did not or could not tolerate the resting splints at night made several degrees progress throughout a session of stretching with weights and pulleys, but overnight they reverted to their baseline deformity.

As the patient begins to have more difficulty walking, one might consider use of a "standing chimney" or other standing device that maintains the upright posture by use of a three-point pressure principle. Such a device requires good padding over the extensor surface of the knee, a pelvic sling, and a stationary device to hold a firm shoe or boot in place. This device, if used at all, is appropriate when there is no more than 20 degrees flexion contracture at the hip or knee. It cannot be used effectively to *correct* contractures but only to prevent their occurrence or acceleration.

Spinal Orthoses

Because of their weak trunk, most patients with DMD will develop some degree of scoliosis with loss of the normal degree of spinal kyphosis. In contrast to idiopathic scoliosis, in which the discomfort produced by the brace prompts the patient to use the musculature to pull away from the pressure points to actively correct the deformity, bracing for spinal deformities in DMD must be comfortable because the patient cannot pull away from the pressure points. Therefore, three-point pressure braces such as the Milwaukee brace are not appropriate for use in DMD. Molded body jackets (thoracolumbosacral orthoses) are more appropriate.

It is unlikely that any off-the-shelf braces would be satisfactory, because no two patients are alike or even similar. Therefore, the body wrap must be undertaken by an experienced orthotist. It is also important to follow the patient's vital capacity (lung capacity) both in and out of the brace, and in sitting as well as supine positions. If there is undue restriction, particularly in patients with baseline lung capacity restriction, the brace will not be tolerated.

Bracing for Weakness

For ambulatory patients, particularly those with proximal muscle weakness, the key to acceptance is the weight and comfort of the device, particularly for DMD patients. Furthermore, as shown earlier, the toe walking of these patients results not so much from weakness of the anterior compartment as from tightness of the TFL and ITB. Thus, if one were to position the foot and ankle in a neutral position with an ankle-foot orthosis (AFO) the patient may be unable to walk at all.

Polio

Patients with polio rarely need or accept an AFO for isolated anterior compartment weakness. Likewise, if there is quadriceps weakness and minimal genu recurvatum, the patient is satisfied with his or her ability to stabilize the knee in extension by plan-tarflexing the foot at the ankle. When the genu recurvatum has progressed to the point of pain and swelling, the patient is likely to accept the temporary use of a knee-ankle-foot orthosis (KAFO) with a locked knee that positions the knee in 5 degrees of flexion. The knee is positioned by making the distal thigh band slightly more shallow than usual, as the position of the knee is determined by the relative depths of the thigh bands. If a molded polypropylene orthosis is used, the angle of tilt of the socket can be used in the same fashion to produce 5 degrees flexion of the knee.

Multiple Sclerosis

Patients with multiple sclerosis may accept lower limb bracing if bracing allows the patient to walk. An AFO is likely to be accepted if the spasticity of the powerful gastrocnemius makes it difficult or impossible to clear the foot in swing phase.

FSH Dystrophy

Bracing for patients with FSH dystrophy has not proved satisfactory. Our group has not seen patients with FSH dystrophy who accept any orthotic devices. In contrast to cervical spinal cord-injured patients who have preserved proximal muscle function but need help with prehension, patients with FSH dystrophy have good to excellent peripheral function (grasp and pinch) but poor ability to position their arms in space. No device is both portable and effective for positioning the upper limbs in space.

Inflammatory Myopathies

Patients with inflammatory myopathies have muscle weakness, with the worst weakness proximal. As mentioned earlier, there is no effective brace for proximal muscle weakness, although the hips can be stabilized in extension if the patient has sufficient quadriceps strength to tolerate throwing the center of mass (the trunk) behind the axis of motion of the hip joint. Thus, if the hip extensors are weak and the quadriceps and more distal muscles are marginal, one could consider using a lightweight KAFO to permit the patient to use alignment to stabilize the hips in extension. The KAFO must be lightweight because the hip flexors will also be weak and it will be difficult to accelerate a braced limb in swing phase. Furthermore, this weakness is usually transient and resolves with adequate steroid medication.

Peripheral Neurophathies

Orthotic management is more useful in peripheral neuropathies because the weakness tends to be peripheral. Thus, an AFO or KAFO may be highly effective and well tolerated. Plastic AFOs and KAFOs are generally preferred because of weight and cosmesis; however, if there is a sensory component to the neuropathy, observation of the skin for pressure must be meticulous.

Summary

Stretching exercise is almost always useful in the muscular and neuromuscular disorders described here. Strengthening and aerobic exercise and selected orthotic devices may be useful when judiciously applied.

REFERENCES

1. Rodnan GP, Schumacher HR (eds), Zyaifler NJ (associate ed): Primer on the Rheumatic Diseases, 8th Ed. The Arthritis Foundation, Atlanta, 1983
2. Williams RC Jr: Dermatomyositis and malignancy: a review of the literature. Ann Intern Med 50:1174, 1959
3. Callen JP, Hyla JF, Bole GG et al: The relationship of dermatomyositis and polymyositis to internal malignancy. Arch Dermatol 116:295, 1980
4. Moser H: Duchenne muscular dystrophy: pathogenetic aspects and genetic prevention. Hum Genet 66:17, 1984
5. Johnson EW, Kennedy JH: Comprehensive management of Duchenne muscular dystrophy. Arch Phys Med Rehabil 52:110, 1971
6. Brooke MH: A Clinician's View of Neuromuscular Diseases. Williams & Wilkins, Baltimore, 1977
7. Mumenthaler M: Neurology. p. 303ff. Translated by Edmund H. Burrows, 3rd Rev Ed. George Thieme Verlag, Stuttgart, 1990
8. Mumenthaler M: Neurology. Translated by Edmund H. Burrows, 3rd Rev Ed. George Thieme Verlag, Stuttgart, 1990
9. Stone R: Post polio syndrome: remembrance of viruses past. Science 264:909, 1994
10. Perry J, Mulroy SJ, Renwick SE: The relationship of lower extremity strength and gait parameters in patients with post-polio syndrome. Arch Phys Med Rehabil 74:165, 1993
11. Sharief M, Hentges R, Ciardi M: Intrathecal immune response in patients with post-polio syndrome. N Engl J Med 325:749, 1991
12. Muir P, Nicholson F, Sharief MK et al: Evidence for persistent enterovirus infection of the central nervous system in patients with previous paralytic poliomyelitis. Ann NY Acad Sci 753:219, 1995
13. Bennett RL, Knowlton GC: Overwork weakness in partially denervated skeletal muscle. Clin Orthop 12:22, 1958
14. Milner-Brown HS, Miller RG: Muscle strengthening through high-resistance weight training in patients with neuromuscular disorders. Arch Phys Med Rehabil 69:13, 1988
15. Johnson EW, Braddom R: Over-work weakness in facioscapulohumeral muscular dystrophy. Arch Phys Med Rehabil 52:333, 1971
16. Mumenthaler M: Neurology. p. 243. Translated by Edmund H. Burrows, 3rd Rev Ed. George Thieme Verlag, Stuttgart, New York, 1990
17. Kurtzke JF: Rating neurologic impairment in multiple sclerosis: an expanded disability status scale (EDSS). Neurol 33:1444, 1983
18. de Lateur BJ, Giaconi RM: Effect on maximal strength of submaximal exercise in Duchenne muscular dystrophy. Am J Phys Med 58:26, 1979
19. Barbiroli B, McCully KK, Iotti S et al: Further impairment of muscle phosphate kinetics by lengthening exercise in DMD/BMD carriers. J Neurol Sci 119:65, 1993
20. Milner-Brown HS, Miller RG: Muscle strengthening through electric stimulation combined with low-resistance weights in patients with neuromuscular disorders. Arch Phys Med Rehabil 69:20, 1988
21. Erwin JH, Keller C, Anderson S, Costa J: Hand and wrist strengthening exercises during rehabilitation of a patient with hereditary distal myopathy. Arch Phys Med Rehabil 72:701, 1991
22. Kraft GH, Alquist AD, de Lateur BJ: Effect of resistive exercise on function in multiple sclerosis. Poster presented to the Consortium of Multiple Sclerosis Centers, Portland, OR, 1995
23. Kraft GH, Alquist AD, de Lateur BJ: Effect of resistive exercise on strength in patients with multiple sclerosis. Poster presented to the Consortium of Multiple Sclerosis Centers, Portland, OR, 1995
24. de Lateur BJ, Giaconi RM, Alquist AD: Fatigue and performance data from normal adults and patients

with several neuromuscular and musculoskeletal syndromes: response to training. 1988 AAEE Didactic Program: Muscle Fatigue. Thirty-Fifth AAEE Annual Meeting, 1988

25. Morgan-Hughes JA: Diseases of striated muscle. In Asbury AK, McKhann GM, McDonald WI (eds): Diseases of the Nervous System, Clinical Neurobiology. Vol. 1. WB Saunders, Philadelphia, 1992

Pharmacologic Treatment

Scott E. Brown

Both primary muscle diseases and disorders that manifest primarily with muscle dysfunction are commonly encountered in rehabilitation medicine. For most of these conditions, treatment with medications has been disappointing. For others, controversy surrounds some treatments that have become part of common practice. This controversy may seem surprising because medication trials lend themselves well to randomized, double-blind, placebo-controlled studies, which provide the best evidence of clinical efficacy. The expanding pharmacopeia demands even more attention from researchers who must undertake well-designed studies.[1] Although internal design variations may cast doubt on reported results,[2] treatment recommendations can be gleaned from the currently available literature. Unless otherwise noted, all studies referred to are Level I evidence as defined by Sackett (See Ch. 1).

MUSCLE SPASM

Although not a muscle disease per se, muscle spasm is frequently seen as a manifestation of direct musculoligamentous injury and other peripheral injuries or disorders (e.g., radiculopathy and arthritis). Tonic skeletal muscle hyperactivity causes local pain, tenderness, palpable changes in muscle, reduced range of motion, and disabling limitations of activities of daily living, including work.

Most studies have used a 3- or 4-point scale to rate these subjective factors in assessing outcome. Only one has applied more objective study of the inhibitory effects of muscle spasm on muscle function.[3] Not included in this category is spasticity resulting from upper motor neuron injury.

The most commonly used agents to treat muscle spasm of local origin are centrally acting muscle relaxants, so called because of their ability to suppress polysynaptic reflexes in subcortical, brain stem, and spinal pathways in animals. Criticism of these drugs includes the following:

1. In humans, safe doses are far short of that necessary to produce direct skeletal muscle relaxation.
2. Sedation is a common concurrent effect (probably because of the effect on the reticular system), which may account for the muscle relaxant properties.
3. The conditions for which these drugs are used are predominantly self-limited.
4. There is little distinction clinically between analgesic effect and true relaxation.
5. Comparative studies between agents are difficult to perform.[2]

Muscle Relaxants

Metaxalone

Metaxalone is more closely related to mephenoxalone, a tranquilizer, than to the other muscle relaxants. Few studies about this drug are available. In an initial unblinded study, Fathie[4] found an 80 percent response in uncomplicated low back pain. In two later studies, he showed a 75 and 70 percent moderate to marked improvement with the drug, and only 17 and 28 percent improvement with placebo.[5] Diamond[6] found no difference, but described few details of the study protocol.

Methocarbamol

Methocarbamol is the closest analog of mephenesin, the first centrally acting muscle relaxant (no longer available). Valtonen[7] found 60 percent improvement in patients receiving the drug and 30 percent with placebo. Tisdale and Ervin[8] found statistically significant improvement using the drug versus placebo, especially within the first 48 hours. Feinberg et al.[9] found the drug to be more effective than placebo in producing marked or complete relief (70 percent compared to 41 percent). All of these studies used a diagnostically heterogeneous patient population.

In assessing the analgesic activity of methocarbamol, Feinberg et al.[9] found that the drug relieved

72 percent of those with severe pain, compared to 50 percent with aspirin (descriptive statistics only). In a small randomized, double-blind, crossover study of elderly patients with chronic lower extremity pain of nonmuscular origin, the drug demonstrated pain relief in 19 of 50 patients, compared to 1 of 50 patients with placebo.[10] Tisdale and Ervin[8] found the drug to be more effective than aspirin, with the combination of methocarbamol and aspirin more effective than aspirin alone ($P < .05$), but not statistically better than the drug alone.

Chlorzoxazone

Chlorzoxazone is a benzoxazolinone, a chemically distinct class from the other muscle relaxants. Using low back pain patients only, Scheiner[11] found significant improvement with the drug treatment versus placebo.

Vernon[12] found 97 percent of drug-treated patients to be symptom free by 9 days compared to 39 percent of patients treated with placebo. By day 4 of treatment in a heterogeneous group of patients, Walker[13] found 63 percent of drug-treated patients to have a good to excellent result compared to only 30 percent of patients receiving placebo. In all studies, sedation/drowsiness was rarely reported as a side effect.

Chlorzoxazone had equal analgesic effect compared to acetaminophen at day 4, but the combination was twice as effective as either agent alone (descriptive statistics only).[12] Walker[13] reported that 90 percent of patients who received the same combination had good or excellent results compared to 63 percent of those treated with chlorzoxazone alone. Scheiner[11] found the combination to be significantly more effective than either drug alone for both pain and spasm relief.

In a comparison with diazepam, chlorzoxazone was statistically superior for reduction of pain, spasm, and tenderness. Only one-third of patients treated with chlorzoxazone suffered mild drowsiness, compared to nearly all patients treated with diazepam.[14]

Cyclobenzaprine

Cyclobenzaprine is closely related to the tricyclic antidepressants. Bercel[15] found statistically significant improvement in pain, spasm, and motion in patients with chronic muscle spasm resulting from osteoarthritis. Similar results were noted by Brown and Womble[16] in patients with chronic soft tissue pain.

Nibbelink et al.[17] reported combined results of 20 studies showing statistically significant relief using the drug compared to placebo. Baratta[18] also found statistically significant improvement in an acute population with low back pain. In the only controlled study to utilize an objective measurement of muscle function, Basmajian[3] found the drug to be significantly superior than placebo. Basmajian[19] later found in a multicentered, controlled trial a combination of cyclobenzaprine and the nonsteroidal antiinflammatory drug (NSAID) diflunisal was more effective than either agent individually. In a smaller open label trial of acute patients, Borenstein et al.[20] also found a drug-NSAID combination to be more effective than NSAID alone.

Cyclobenzaprine can cause significant sedation and other anticholinergic side effects. Brown and Womble[16] found no difference in efficacy between cyclobenzaprine and diazepam; both produced drowsiness. Basmajian[3] noted an objective improvement in muscle function as measured by integrated electromyography with cyclobenzaprine, but not diazepam. Nibbelink et al.[17] found the drug to be statistically better than diazepam. They also demonstrated significantly better efficacy in patients who did not experience sedation when compared to those who received placebo.

Carisoprodol

Carisoprodol is a precursor of meprobamate, a schedule IV controlled substance, which is potentially addicting. In a diagnostically mixed patient group, including neurologic spasticity, the drug demonstrated overall statistically better effectiveness than placebo.[21] In a crossover study of diagnostically mixed patients, 71 percent showed moderate to marked improvement compared to 22 percent treated with placebo.[22] Lawrence and Forsyth[23] found the drug to be statistically better than placebo, and Hindle,[24] Baratta,[25] and Soyka and Maestripieri[26] determined carisoprodol to be statistically superior to placebo for the treatment of acute lumbar spasm.

Analgesic action in pain of nonmuscular origin was fair, with 30 of 50 patients achieving good or excellent relief[10]; 71 percent showed moderate to marked improvement compared to 34 percent given aspirin,[22] but there was no difference when compared to propoxyphene.[25] A combination of the drug plus analgesic proved more effective than any individual component.

In assessing the contribution of sedation to its muscle relaxing effect, carisoprodol was equally as effective and sedating as diazepam, but better than phenobarbital[27] and butabarbitol,[24] which also produced sedation.

Orphenadrine

Orphenadrine is an analog of diphenhydramine, an antihistamine. Gold[28] found the drug to be statistically better than placebo for the treatment of back spasm. Cailliet[29] also noted clinical effectiveness, but Valtonen[30] found the drug scarcely better than placebo (with a high placebo response of 53 percent). Combinations of the drug with an analgesic were more effective than either drug alone for immediate relief[31] and after 1 week.[30]

Relative Efficacy

Comparison studies are difficult to interpret and inconclusive. Not all agents have been evaluated against each other in homogeneous patient populations (Fig. 10-11). Chlorzoxazone has been consistently better than or equal to all other agents, and has the least sedating effect. Carisoprodol and cyclobenzaprine have yielded mixed results.

Summary and Recommendations

The centrally acting skeletal muscle relaxants are a heterogeneous group of drugs. All provide more relief than placebo with short duration of use in a wide spectrum of disorders that cause muscle spasm. None have been evaluated for long-term use. The degree of clinical improvement is controversial, as measurement is based on subjective factors, and most acute conditions for which they are used are self-limited. Some evidence suggests that muscle relaxing effect is independent of sedation. None appears clearly superior to any other agent, but contraindications and side effect profiles are different. The least sedating is chlorzoxazone. Cyclobenza-

	Carisoprodol	Methocarbamol	Cyclobenzaprine	Chlorzoxazone	Orphenadrine
Carisoprodol		Carisoprodol[10]	Carisoprodol = Cyclobenzaprine[33]	Chlorzoxazone[34]	
Methocarbamol				Chlorzoxazone[35]	
Cyclobenzaprine				Chlorzoxazone + APAP[36]	
Chlorzoxazone					Orphenadrine[37] Orphenadrine = Chlorzoxazone[38]
Orphenadrine					

Fig. 10-11. Comparison studies of muscle relaxant drugs. The drug listed in each box is the more effective of the pair in the study.

prine has been the only drug evaluated using objective measures of physiologic improvement. Carisoprodol is potentially addicting and should be used cautiously.[39] Combinations of muscle relaxants and non-narcotic analgesics have provided the greatest and fastest clinical improvement. Considering the extent of disability caused by this extremely common problem, treatment with this combination of medications can be recommended for short-term use, as part of a comprehensive plan.

MUSCLE CRAMP

Usually localized to the legs, these involuntary muscular contractions are more common at night or in the presence of an underlying disorder. As opposed to muscle spasm, they are much shorter in duration (minutes compared to days).

Quinine

Treatment of nocturnal cramps with quinine dates back at least to the 1940 report of effectiveness in an open trial with placebo crossover in 15 patients.[40] Four decades passed before its use was further evaluated. Eight randomized blinded crossover studies with limited power (N = 27 max) have demonstrated conflicting results. Three revealed statistically significant improvement in at least one parameter of severity, duration, or number of cramps.[41–43] Connolly et al.[43] used a higher dose divided in the evening and at bedtime to achieve benefits. Three other studies showed no beneficial effect.[44–46] Warburton et al.[47] found no statistically significant difference in number or severity of cramps, but did note a positive trend toward attenuation of cramps with higher serum quinine concentration. Dunn[48] evaluated only the initial treatment phase (finding no significant benefit) because the crossover phase revealed a significant improvement, apparently because of a carryover effect in the quinine to placebo group. He postulated that quinine withdrawal may induce worse cramps.

Other Treatments

Mixed results also have been reported with vitamin E therapy. Connolly et al.[43] noted no benefits, but Ayres,[49] in an unblinded, noncontrolled study of 125 patients, noted excellent results in 82 percent of patients. The muscle relaxants orphenadrine[50] and carisoprodol[51] have both shown benefit. Cramps resolved in seven of eight patients given verapamil after failure on quinine.[52]

Calcium was of no benefit in cramps associated with pregnancy.[53] The amino acid taurine was openly given to 12 nonalcoholic patients with cirrhosis. Cramps resolved in eight of twelve patients, and improvement was noted in the other four.[54] Uremic leg cramps were treated successfully with clonidine in one case report,[55] and statistically significant improvement was found with both quinine and vitamin E.[56]

Summary and Recommendations

Despite the common use of quinine and its over-the-counter availability, its efficacy for leg cramps continues to be controversial,[57] and no clear recommendation can be made for its use. Potentially hazardous side effects must be considered (cinchonism, thrombocytopenia), especially given the evidence that the response may be dose related. Vitamin E, verapamil, taurine, and muscle relaxants may hold promise with fewer side effects; but current evidence is inconclusive.

FIBROMYALGIA

Fibromyalgia is currently categorized as a nonarticular rheumatic syndrome characterized by widespread muscular pain and aching, with reproducible tender points at specific sites.[58] Its etiology is unknown, but a relationship to nonrestorative sleep has been postulated.[59]

Like muscle spasm, fibromyalgia is not a "disease" of muscle (to the best of current knowledge), but its primary disabling manifestations are perceived as muscular (i.e., pain, weakness, and fatigue). Mood disturbances and nonorganic psychological overlay are also thought to play a role. Pharmacologic treatment, therefore, has focused on pain relief, sleep restoration, and mood/psychological improvement.

Amitriptyline

Amitriptyline is a tricyclic antidepressant with serotonergic and anticholinergic properties. It is currently considered the drug of choice for the treatment of fibromyalgia. In a 9-week trial, Carette et al.[60] found that 37 percent had improved morning stiffness and pain, but the percentage was not statistically significant. Tenderness, however, was statistically significantly reduced, but without clinical significance (less than 0.5 kg pressure threshold change). Sleep was statistically improved at 5 weeks, but not at 9 weeks. Goldenberg et al.[61] did find statistically significant improvement in all parameters in a 6-week trial, as did Scudds et al.[62] in a 10-week trial. One-third of patients treated in an open trial demonstrated clinical benefit and were then evaluated in N of 1 randomized controlled trials. Of 23 trials, only 7 patients demonstrated statistical improvement, but 15 were continued on the drug, based on general response.[63] Connolly[64] used a combination of amitriptyline and fluphenazine in nine patients with good results, eventually tapering the fluphenazine.[64]

Cyclobenzaprine

Cyclobenzaprine is a tricyclic muscle relaxant related to amitriptyline. Bennett et al.[65] showed a significant improvement in pain, sleep, and overall response compared to placebo; but only one-third of drug-treated patients attained moderate to marked improvement. Over a 6-week period, Quimby et al.[66] noted significant improvement in stiffness, sleep, and overall effect compared to placebo, but no change in pain or fatigue. In a small study of seven patients, Hamaty et al.[67] noted significant improvement only in sleep over 5 months. Biochemical markers were also examined, and no clear changes were found in β-endorphin, dopamine, norepinephrine, epinephrine, or prostaglandin E_2, except as are found in any chronic pain state. In nine patients, Reynolds et al.[68] found a significant improvement in fatigue and sleep time, but no change in pain, tenderness, mood, or sleep electroencephalography.

Other Antidepressant Compounds

Other antidepressant drugs also have been evaluated. Imipramine was not found effective in an open trial with 20 patients.[69] Bibolotti et al.[70] found that maprotiline significantly reduced depression and chlorimiprimine significantly reduced tender points after a 3-week crossover trial. Caruso et al.[71] found dothiepin (a tricyclic antidepressant similar to amitriptyline) produced significant improvement in tender points by 4 weeks, and overall pain by 8 weeks. Fluoxetine, a nontricyclic antidepressant serotonin reuptake inhibitor, has been successful in three case reports.[72,73] No controlled trials of this drug have been reported.

Other Psychoactive Medications

5-hydroxy-L-tryptophan produced significant improvement in a large open trial,[74] but produced no effect in a smaller, randomized study.[75] Chlorpromazine produced significant improvement in all parameters including stages of sleep.[75] No beneficial effect was noted using chlormezanone.[76] Three case reports describe improvement after adding lithium to a tricyclic antidepressant.[77] Zopiclone, a nonbenzodiazepine hypnotic not available in the United States, demonstrated some improvement in sleep, but had no effect on pain and tenderness in two trials.[78,79]

Anti-inflammatory Agents

Although it is now clear that inflammation is not part of the pathology of fibromyalgia, several anti-inflammatory agents have been studied. Prednisone, 15 mg/day for 14 days, seems to precipitate deterioration of most clinical parameters in a small crossover study of 20 patients.[80] Ibuprofen has demonstrated little[80,82] or no effect[83] on the condition, as has naproxen.[61] Donald and Molla[84] showed improvement in a group of patients with a variety of soft tissue pain syndromes using triaprofenic acid and aspirin. Of 100 patients treated, only 15 had fibromyalgia.

S-adenosylmethionine, a new anti-inflammatory drug with analgesic and antidepressant effects, is not available in the United States but has been studied in Europe. Tavoni et al.[85] noted statistically significant improvement in tender points and depression. Jacobsen et al.[86] found statistical improvement in fatigue, stiffness, and pain at rest, a trend toward a reduction in tender points, but no change in pain with activity. The combination of ibuprofen and alprazolam showed greater benefit than either agent alone.[81]

Summary and Recommendations

No medications have proven satisfactory in the treatment of fibromyalgia. Antidepressants, in particular, those with serotonergic properties, have the greatest effect on sleep, pain, fatigue, and tenderness in short-term use. Only 25 to 60 percent of patients appear to respond. Phenothiazines may hold promise, especially in combination with an antidepressant, but clear evidence is lacking. Anxiolytics and sedatives have little effect, although few studies have been published. NSAIDs appear to be of no benefit alone, and prednisone may exacerbate symptoms. There is no information regarding long-term use of any medication, an unfortunate situation, as most patients require extended treatment for this chronic, painful condition.

DUCHENNE MUSCULAR DYSTROPHY

Duchenne muscular dystrophy (DMD) is an X-linked inherited myopathic disease, resulting from a mutation in the gene coding for the structural protein dystrophin.

Many different medications have been examined for use in this disease based on various theories to account for the inevitable muscle damage and consequent disability.

Prednisone

Prednisone, an inactive corticosteroid precursor of the active prednisolone, has been studied extensively. Siegel et al.[87] reported no benefit from prednisone in a study of seven patients. In the same year, Drachman et al.[88] reported improved motor function and slowed progression in an open trial with 14 patients over 28 months. He also reinterpreted Siegel's results, noting evidence of effectiveness despite regression with drug withdrawal.[89] In a long-term trial, De Silva et al.[90] found a statistical benefit for the ability of treated patients to retain the ability to ambulate. Using natural history controls, Brooke et al.[91] used a high daily dose of 1.5 mg/kg for 6 months and found improvement in strength, functional tests, and pulmonary function tests. Contractures were not delayed. Mendell et al.[92] found similar results in a randomized trial, with equal efficacy demonstrated using 1.5 or 0.75 mg/kg per day.

Griggs et al.[93] tested 0.75 and 0.3 mg/kg and found the higher dose to be statistically better, although improvement was noted with both doses. In an extension of a previous trial,[92] Fenichel et al.[94] examined the effect of alternate-day dosing. Patients started on four times a day dosing improved at 3 months, but did not maintain the benefits at 6 months. Patients reduced from daily to alternate-day schedules regressed. In long-term treatment, treated patients demonstrated significantly slower decline over 3 years when compared to natural history controls.[95] Significant side effects from prednisone were noted in all of these studies. In a small trial of 14 patients, deflazacort was statistically better than placebo and produced fewer side effects than have been reported with prednisone (the two steroids were not compared).[96] Angelini et al.[97] further confirmed statistically significant improvement with deflazacort in functional tasks that were maintained for 2 years. Side effects were moderate.

Other Immunosuppresant Agents

Azathioprine was investigated in combination with prednisone by Griggs et al.,[98] who concluded the former drug added no benefit, and that the beneficial affect of prednisone was not due to immune suppression. Conversely, in an open 2-month trial of cyclosporine on 15 patients, this drug produced statistically significant improvement of muscular force.[99]

Other Agents

A variety of other agents have been evaluated, based on theoretical or nonhuman experimental enthusiasm for antidioxidant effects on cellular energetics and intracellular modulation.

Antioxidants

Penicillamine produced no benefit alone (in a small study)[100] or in combination with vitamin E.[101] Fitzgerald and McArdle[102] noted no benefit from vitamin E in five cases. In a small study using selenium (a component of the antioxidant enzyme glutathione peroxidase), no benefit was found.[103] Two trials, one uncontrolled[104] and one using historical controls,[105] noted no significant clinical benefit using selenium and vitamin E for 1 year. Stern et al.[106] investigated superoxide dismutase and found a trend toward slower deterioration over 18 months when compared to placebo, but the trend did not reach statistical significance.

Calcium Channel Blockers

No benefit was found using flunarizine for 1 year[107] or nifedipine for 18 months.[108] Chronic use of diltiazem for 2 to 2.5 years demonstrated a trend toward preserved lower extremity function and strength that did not reach statistical significance in eight matched pairs.[109] In an even smaller group verapamil preserved ergometric muscle strength after 1 year, but observable clinical improvement was small. Three of seven drug-treated boys developed PR interval increases on electrocardiogram.[110] Because of its inhibitory effect on calcium release from the sarcoplasmic reticulum, dantrolene has been studied in a small open trial. Creatine kinase was significantly reduced compared to a prior natural history phase, with only a trend toward less strength deterioration.[111]

Cellular Energetics

The branched-chain amino acid leucine,[112] with its experimental ability to improve muscle protein balance, the growth hormone secretion inhibitor mazindol,[113] and the antiserotonin agent methysergide[114] demonstrated no beneficial effect. Potential benefits of allopurinol led to controversy in the early 1980s after Thompson and Smith[115] reported significant functional improvement in 16 patients. Two other trials, one open and uncontrolled[116] and the other blinded and controlled,[117] confirmed their results. Six additional small randomized trials[118–123] and one larger trial (of possibly sufficient power)[124] found no benefit using allopurinol. (An additional study used an inappropriate adult patient population and claimed no benefit.)[125] No large trial has been undertaken and Thomson and Smith[115] maintain their hypothesis and results.[126]

Summary and Recommendations

Drug treatment of DMD remains disappointing. The best studied agent with the best results is prednisone. In daily doses of 0.75 mg/kg, the progression of disease is slowed for at least 3 years. The development of contractures is unaffected despite maintained strength and function. Unfortunately, significant side effects preclude the use of prednisone in many patients, and because it does not alter the ultimate course of the disease, it must be used selectively and cautiously.

There is no basis to recommend other immunosuppressants, antioxidants, calcium channel blockers, or allopurinol. Deflazacort, an oxazoline derivative of prednisone, which is not available in the United States, may be as effective as prednisone with fewer side effects.

MYOTONIA

Myotonia is a clinical phenomenon of slow relaxation after a muscle contraction and is seen in several disorders including myotonic dystrophy, paramyotonia congenita, and myotonia congenita. These myopathies are also frequently accompanied by weakness. A wide variety of drugs have been utilized, but few controlled studies have been undertaken.

Antiarrhythmics

These agents have been the best studied over many years, beginning with four case reports of effectiveness using quinine in 1936.[127] Leyburn and Walton[128] compared quinine to procaine amide, prednisone, and placebo, and noted 50 percent improvement in 6 of 20, 15 of 20, and 15 of 19, in the active drug groups (no statistics given). There was no improvement in grip strength. A small open trial found better relief of active myotonia using procaine amide compared to placebo.[129] In two randomized small crossover studies, procaine amide was equivalent to disopyramide with highly variable overall responses in one,[130] but demonstrated statistically significant grip relaxation in the other.[131]

Tocainide prevented cold-induced stiffness and weakness in paramyotonia congenita in a small open trial[132] and was statistically beneficial in a randomized study.[133] Mexiletine has been effective in two case reports,[134,135] and Kwiecinski et al.[133] found it to be statistically beneficial in relieving myotonia. Diphenylhydantoin (Phenytoin) has shown statistically significant benefit reducing myotonia in three studies.[131,133,136] Myotonic symptoms were well controlled with serum levels above and below the standard therapeutic range of 10 to 20 µg/ml.

No benefit was found with diazepam.[137] Adrenocortitrophic hormone (ACTH) produced some benefit in several early case reports, with improvement in myotonia noted early,[138] but strength affected with longer treatment.[139] Leyburn and Walton[128] confirmed the delayed benefit of prednisone. The tricyclic antidepressants imipramine and amitriptyline benefitted 34 patients in an open trial, decreasing myotonia and increasing strength.[140] Lithium carbonate required a sedating blood level for effectiveness in one case report.[141] A small open trial with verapamil reduced cold-induced stiffness,[142] and Grant et al.[143] demonstrated a statistically significant reduction in myotonia with nifedipine, 20 mg. In a small, open noncontrolled long-term (1 year) trial, selenium and vitamin E produced benefit in strength and myotonia,[144] but a subsequent study showed no benefit.[145]

Durelli et al.[146] noted statistically significant improvement in myotonia after 6 months of oral taurine with no worrisome side effects. They speculate on its use as the drug of choice for myotonia.

Summary and Recommendations

The agents found to be most effective in randomized trials have been the antiarrhythmics, particularly phenytoin, mexiletine, and procaine amide. Dosing appears to be individualized. Because myotonic disorders are chronic, these drugs are best used sparingly during winter months and in cold climates to control symptoms. Side effects must be monitored. More severe side effects limit the use of quinine, tocainide, and prednisone. Calcium channel blockers, tricyclic antidepressants, selenium plus vitamin E, and the amino acid taurine may hold promise; but there is insufficient information to recommend their use. Diazepam and disopyramide are ineffective.

INFLAMMATORY MYOPATHIES

Understanding of the pathogenesis of these heterogeneous disorders, which include polymyositis, dermatomyositis, and inclusion body myositis, has advanced considerably; but in most cases, the underlying triggers remain unknown. Because the natural history is somewhat variable and pathologic changes may be the result of acute or chronic processes, questions have been raised regarding treatment response.[147]

Few studies have proven efficacy, and empiric treatment predominates focusing on nonselective immunosuppression.

Prednisone in Polymyositis/Dermatomyositis

Walton[148] points out that treatment with steroids have been so obviously successful since the 1950s that it has been impossible to undertake a double-blind, controlled trial. Dalakas[149] believes nearly all patients with true polymyositis or dermatomyositis will "respond to steroids to some degree and for some period of time." In an early series review, however, 24 of 66 steroid-treated patients deteriorated, whereas half of the 39 patients who attained complete remission received no steroids.[150] This series did elucidate prognostic factors for steroid treatment including better outcome with early treatment after onset, less severe disease, and higher dose. Similar factors were noted by Vignos et al.[151] 1 year later.

In a series of 89 patients, 84 percent obtained a good result with prednisone. More relapses occurred if treatment was tapered or stopped within 1 year.[152] Bohan et al.,[153] who criticized earlier results for imprecise diagnostic assessment, reviewed 124 steroid and immunosuppressant treatment patients. Serum enzymes returned to normal by 4 months, and strength increased by 5 months in the responders. On alternate day dosing after an initial period of large daily doses 76 percent improved, with improvement correlated to dose.

Henriksson and Sandstedt[154] also found a marginal response to prednisone, with only 50 percent improving. They confirmed a statistically significant correlation of improvement with younger age, earlier treatment, and larger dose in the first 3 months. In a much smaller series, Baron and Small[155] noted that 42 percent of treated patients had discontinued prednisone by the third year of treatment and maintained benefits. Uchino et al.[156] noted a better response (70 percent) with fewer side effects with alternate day dosing, compared to daily dosing (53 percent).

Immunosuppressants

Malaviya et al.[157] described four steroid-resistant cases successfully treated with intravenous methotrexate in 1968. Five of seven were successfully treated by Sokoloff et al.,[158] and Metzger et al.[159] reported 77 percent improvement in a larger series. He also noted the steroid-sparing effect. Wallace et al.[160] reported two successful cases combining prednisone, methotrexate, and chlorambucil. Bohan et al.[153] obtained a good result in 77 percent of steroid-resistant patients treated with methotrexate, compared to 35 and 33 percent with azathioprine and cyclophosphamide, respectively, (retrospective series review). The steroid-sparing effect was 40 to 50 percent for all three immunosuppressants. They further defined steroid resistance as no benefit with a minimum dose of 40 mg/day for at least 4 months.

Benson and Aldo[161] described four successful cases using azathioprine. Bunch et al.[162] performed one of the few blinded controlled trials comparing prednisone alone with combination prednisone-azathioprine. At 3 months, both groups improved without a significant difference between them, but at 3 years, the combination treatment was statistically significantly better, with a clear steroid-sparing effect.[163] In a complex retrospective review of 113 patients, Joffe et al.[164] compared prednisone, methotrexate, and azathioprine. Good response was noted with all three, but methotrexate was more effective than azathioprine. Certain immunologic subsets responded differently. Walton[148] and Dalakas[149] believe azathioprine is the preferred immunosuppressant.

Intravenous immune globulin was beneficial in several small series.[165,166] In a randomized, double-blind study comparing patients on prednisone receiving immune globulin versus placebo, a statistically significant improvement in strength was noted with immune globulin after 3 months. After crossover, 9 of 12 treated patients showed major improvement, whereas 11 placebo trials showed no major improvement.[167]

Inclusion Body Myositis

Response to treatment of inclusion body myositis has been poor. Cohen et al.[168] reported an excellent response in only two of 10 patients, all of whom were treated with prednisone and a variety of other drugs and interventions. In 28 patients treated with prednisone and various immunosuppressants, 68 percent worsened, but 12 demonstrated delayed progression.[169] Leff et al.[170] reviewed 25 patients and noted that 40 percent benefitted somewhat with prednisone, but only 20 to 25 percent of resistant cases benefitted with azathioprine and methotrexate. They also undertook a prospective, open randomized crossover trial comparing oral azathioprine plus methotrexate with intravenous methotrexate and leucovorin. None produced any complete responses. Some patients demonstrated laboratory improvement but clinical stagnation. The worse the disease, however, the better the response. Joffe et al.[164] found no complete responders to prednisone, methotrexate, or azathioprine.

Summary and Recommendations for Inflammatory Myopathies

Although no randomized, blinded, controlled trials demonstrate efficacy, prednisone continues to be the first-line drug of choice for polymyositis/dermatomyositis. Initial doses should be high (greater than 40 mg/day) and should be continued for at least 3 months. Tapering is empiric and based on maintenance of clinical response with the lowest possible dose. Steroid-resistant cases will likely benefit from prednisone plus azathioprine or methotrexate. There is some evidence that a combination may be preferable at the outset because of the steroid-sparing effect. Intravenous immune globulin may hold great promise because it produces fewer side effects, but the cost is significant. Inclusion body myositis may be treated similarly, but response is less favorable. Stabilization rather than improvement may be the reasonable treatment goal.

REFERENCES

1. Basmajian JV: Special considerations for research with pharmacologic agents. Am J Phys Med Rehabil 70:101, 1991

2. Deyo RA: Conservative therapy for low back pain—distinguishing useful from useless therapy. JAMA 250:1057, 1983

3. Basmajian JV: Cyclobenzaprine hydrochloride effect on skeletal muscle spasm in the lumbar region and neck; two double-blind controlled clinical and laboratory studies. Arch Phys Med Rehabil 59:58, 1978

4. Fathie K: AHR-438 Metaxalone (Skelaxin) and clinical effects on muscular rigidity and spasm. Electroencephalogr Clin Neurophysiol 14:953, 1962

5. Fathie K: A second look at a skeletal muscle relaxant: double-blind study of metaxalone. Curr Ther Res 6:677, 1964

6. Diamond S: Double-blind study of Metaxalone. JAMA 195:479, 1966

7. Valtonen EJ: A double-blind trial of methocarbamol versus placebo in painful muscle spasm. Curr Med Res Opin 3:382, 1975

8. Tisdale SA, Ervin DK: Controlled clinical trial of roboxisal. Curr Ther Res 23:166, 1978

9. Feinberg I, Carey J, Hussussian J et al: Treatment of painful skeletal muscle disorders: a report of a double-blind study of methocarbamol, aspirin and placebo. Am J Orthop 4:280, 1962

10. Stern FH: A controlled comparison of three muscle relaxant agents. Clin Med 71:367, 1964

11. Scheiner JJ: Evaluation of a combined muscle relaxant—analgesic as an effective therapy for painful skeletal muscle spasm. Curr Ther Res 14:168, 1972

12. Vernon WG: A double-blind evaluation of Parafon Forte in the treatment of musculoskeletal back conditions. Curr Ther Res 14:801, 1972

13. Walker JM: Value of an acetaminophen—chlorzoxazone combination (Parafon Forte) in the treatment of acute musculoskeletal disorders. Curr Ther Res 15:248, 1973

14. Scheiner JJ: Muscle relaxants: chlorzoxazone compared with diazepam (a double-blind study). Curr Ther Res 19:51, 1976

15. Bercel NA: Cyclobenzaprine in the treatment of skeletal muscle spasm in osteoarthritis of the cervical and lumbar spine. Curr Ther Res 22:462, 1977

16. Brown BR, Womble J: Cyclobenzaprine in intractable pain syndromes with muscle spasm. JAMA 240:1151, 1978

17. Nibbelink DW, Strickland MD, McLean LF et al: Cyclobenzaprine, diazepam and placebo in the treatment of skeletal muscle spasm of local origin. Clin Ther 1:409, 1978

18. Baratta RR: A double-blind study of cyclobenzaprine and placebo in the treatment of acute musculoskeletal conditions of the low back. Curr Ther Res 32:646, 1982

19. Basmajian JV: Acute back pain and spasm—a controlled multicenter trial of combined analgesic and antispasm agents. Spine 14:438, 1989

20. Borenstein DG, Lacks S, Wiesel SW: Cyclobenzaprine and naproxen versus naproxen alone in the treatment of acute low back pain and muscle spasm. Clin Ther 12:125, 1990

21. Cowan IC, Mapes RE: Carisoprodol in the management of musculoskeletal disorders—a controlled trial. Ann Phys Med 7:140, 1963

22. Balch HW, Bain LS: Evaluation of carisoprodol in the management of musculoskeletal disorders—a controlled clinical trial. Ann Phys Med 7:159, 1963

23. Lawrence GB, Forsyth JI: Carisoprodol in the management of musculoskeletal disorders in a general practice. Br J Clin Pract 18:603, 1964

24. Hindle TH: Comparison of carisoprodol, butabarbital and placebo in treatment of the low back syndrome. Calif Med 117:7, 1972

25. Baratta RR: A double-blind comparative study of carisoprodol, propoxyphene, and placebo in the management of low back syndrome. Curr Ther Res 20:233, 1976

26. Soyka JP, Maestripieri LR: Soma compound (carisoprodol plus phenacetin and caffeine) in the treatment of acute, painful musculoskeletal conditions. Curr Ther Res 26:165, 1979

27. Snell W, Corrigan RF, Zimmerman RC: Comparative drug evaluation in treatment of skeletal muscle spasm. Clin Med 72:957, 1965

28. Gold RH: Treatment of low back syndrome with oral orphenadrine citrate. Curr Ther Res 23:271, 1978

29. Cailliet R: Clinical value of orphenadrine citrate as a skeletal muscle relaxant. Clin Med 7:1581, 1960

30. Valtonen EJ: A controlled clinical trial of chlormezanone, orphenadrine, orphenadrine/paracetamol and placebo in the treatment of painful skeletal muscle spasms. Ann Clin Res 7:85, 1975

31. Birkeland IW, Clawson DK: Drug combinations with orphenadrine for pain relief associated with muscle spasm. Clin Pharmacol Ther 9:639, 1968

32. Elenbaas JK: Centrally acting oral skeletal muscle relaxants. Drug Ther Rev 37:1313, 1980

33. Rollings HE, Glassman JM, Soyka JP: Management of acute musculoskeletal conditions—thoracolumbar strain or sprain: a double-blind evaluation comparing the efficacy and safety of carisoprodol with

cyclobenzaprine hydrochloride. Curr Ther Res 34:917, 1983

34. Miller AR: A comparative study of Parafon Forte tablets and Soma compounds in the treatment of painful skeletal muscle conditions. Curr Ther Res 19:444, 1976

35. Gready DM: Parafon Forte versus Roboxisal in skeletal muscle disorders; a double-blind study. Curr Ther Res 20:666, 1976

36. Azoury, FJ: Double-blind comparison of Parafon Forte and Flexeril in the treatment of acute musculoskeletal disorders. Curr Ther Res 26:189, 1979

37. Mok MS, Lippmann M, Steen SN: Pain relief with two combination analgesics. Curr Ther Res 22:361, 1977

38. Cranston JP: Double-blind comparison of Parafon Forte tablets versus Norgesic Forte for the relief of pain and spasm of musculoskeletal disorders. Curr Ther Res 21:809, 1977

39. Littrell RA, Hayes LR, Stillner V: Carisoprodol (Soma): a new and cautious perspective on an old agent. South Med J 86:753, 1993

40. Moss HK, Herrmann LG: Use of quinine for relief of 'night cramps' in the extremities. JAMA 115:1358, 1940

41. Jones K, Castleden CM: A double-blind comparison of Quinine sulphate and placebo in muscle cramps. Age Aging 12:155, 1983

42. Fung MC, Holbrook JH: Placebo-controlled trial of quinine therapy for nocturnal leg cramps. West J Med 151:42, 1989

43. Connolly PS, Shirley EA, Wasson JH: Treatment of nocturnal leg cramps—a crossover trial of quinine versus vitamin E. Arch Intern Med 152:1877, 1992

44. Smith C, Jee R, O'Neill C et al: Double-blind, placebo controlled, cross-over study of maintenance treatment with quinine bisulfate for night cramps. Br J Clin Pharmacol 21:108P, 1986

45. Lim SH: Randomized double-blind trial of quinine sulphate for nocturnal leg cramps. Br J Clin Pract 40:462, 1986

46. Sidorov J: Quinine sulfate for leg cramps: does it work? J Am Geriatr Soc 41:498, 1993

47. Warburton A, Royston JP, O'Neill CJA et al: A quinine a day keeps the leg cramps away? Br J Clin Pharmacol 23:459, 1987

48. Dunn NR: Effectiveness of quinine for night cramps. Br J Gen Pract 43:127, 1993

49. Ayres S, Mihan R: Nocturnal leg cramps (systremma): a progress report on response to vitamin E. South Med J 67:1308, 1974

50. LaHa D, Turner E: An alternative to quinine in nocturnal leg cramps. Curr Ther Res 45:833, 1989

51. Chesrow EJ, Kaplitz SE, Breme JT et al: Use of carisoprodol for treatment of leg cramps associated with vascular, neurologic or arthritic disease. J Am Geriatr Soc 11:1014, 1963

52. Baltodano N, Gal BV, Weidler DJ: Verapamil versus quinine in recumbent nocturnal leg cramps in the elderly. Arch Intern Med 148:1969, 1988

53. Hammer M, Berg G, Solheim F et al: Calcium and magnesium status in pregnant women: a comparison between treatment with calcium and Vitamin C in pregnant women with leg cramps. Int J Vitam Nutr Res 57:179, 1987

54. Matsuzaki Y, Tanaka N, Osuga T: Is taurine effective for treatment of painful muscle cramps in liver cirrhosis. Am J Gastroenterol 88:1466, 1993

55. Schwartz J: Clonidine for painful diabetic—uremic leg cramps and pruritus: a case report. Angiology 44:985, 1993

56. Roca AO, Jarjoura D, Blend D et al: Dialysis leg cramps—efficacy of quinine versus vitamin E. ASAIO J 38:481, 1992

57. Walton T, Kolb KW: Treatment of nocturnal leg cramps and restless leg syndrome. Clin Pharmacol 10:427, 1991

58. Wolfe F, Smythe HA, Yunus MD et al: The American College of Rheumatology 1990 Criteria for the Classification of Fibromyalgia; report of the multicenter criteria Committee Arthritis Rheum 33:160, 1990

59. Moldofsky M, Scarisbrick P, England R et al: Musculoskeletal symptoms and non-REM sleep disturbance in patients with 'fibrositis syndrome' and healthy subjects. Psychosom Med 37:341, 1975

60. Carette S, McCain GA, Bell DA et al: Evaluation of amitriptyline in primary fibrositis—a double-blind, placebo controlled study. Arthritis Rheum 29:655, 1986

61. Goldenberg DL, Felson DT, Dinerman M: A randomized, controlled trial of amitriptyline and naproxen in the treatment of patients with fibromyalgia. Arthritis Rheum 29:1371, 1986

62. Scudds RA, McCain GA, Rollman GB et al: Improvements in pain responsiveness in patients with fibrositis after successful treatment with amitriptyline. J Rheumatol, suppl. 1a, 16:98, 1989

63. Jaeschke R, Adachi J, Guyathi G et al: Clinical usefulness of amitriptyline in fibromyalgia: the results of 23 N—1 randomized controlled trials. J Rheumatol 18:447, 1991

64. Connolly RG: Treatment of fibromyositis with fluphenazine and amitriptyline: a preliminary report. Del Med J 53:189, 1981

65. Bennett RM, Gatler RA, Campbell SM et al: A combination of cyclobenzaprine and placebo in the management of fibrositis. Arthritis Rheum 31:1535, 1988

66. Quimby LG, Gratwick GM, Whitney CD et al: A randomized trial of cyclobenzaprine for the treatment

of fibromyalgia. J Rheumatol, suppl. 19. 16:140, 1989

67. Hamaty D, Valentine JL, Howard R et al: The plasma endorphin, prostaglandin and catecholamine profile of patients with fibrositis treated with Cyclobenzaprine and placebo: a five month study. J Rheumatol, suppl. 19, 16:164, 1989

68. Reynolds WJ, Moldofsky H, Saskin P et al: The effects of cyclobenzaprine on sleep physiology and symptoms in patients with fibromyalgia. J Rheumatol 18:452, 1991

69. Wysenbeck AJ, Mor F, Lurie Y et al: Imipramine for the treatment of fibrositis: a therapeutic trial. Ann Rheum Dis 44:752, 1985

70. Bibolotti E, Borghi C, Pasculli E et al: The management of fibrositis: a double-blind comparison of maprotiline (Ludiomilo), chlorimipramine and placebo. Clin Trial J 23:269, 1986

71. Caruso I, Sarzi Puttini PC, Bosccassini L et al: Double-blind study of dothiepin versus placebo in the treatment of primary fibromyalgia syndrome. J Int Med Res 15:154, 1987

72. Geller SA: Treatment of fibrositis with fluoxetine hydrochloride (Prozac). Am J Med 87:594, 1989

73. Finestone DH: Fluoxetine and fibromyalgia. JAMA 264:2869, 1990

74. Sarzi Puttini P, Caruso I: Primary fibromyalgia syndrome and 5-Hydroxy-L-Tryptophan: a 90 day open study. J Int Med Res 20:182, 1992

75. Moldofsky H, Lve FA: The relationship of alpha and delta EEG frequencies to pain and mood in 'fibrositis' patients treated with chlorpromazine and L-tryptophan. Electroencephalogr Clin Neurophysiol 50:71, 1980

76. Pattrick M, Swannell A, Doherty M: Chlormezanone in primary fibromyalgia syndrome: a double-blind placebo controlled study. Br J Rheumatol 32:55, 1993

77. Tyber MA: Lithium carbonate augmentation therapy in fibromyalgia. Can Med Assoc J 143:902, 1990

78. Gronblad M, Nykanen J, Kontlineny et al: Effect of zopiclone on sleep quality, morning stiffness, widespread tenderness and pain, and general discomfort in primary fibromyalgia patients. A double-blind randomized trial. Clin Rheumatol 12:186, 1993

79. Drewes AM, Andreasen A, Jennum P et al: Zopiclone in the treatment of sleep abnormalities in fibromyalgia. Scand J Rheumatol 20:288, 1991

80. Clark S, Tindall E, Bennett RM: A double-blind crossover trial of prednisone versus placebo in the treatment of fibrositis. J Rheumatol 12:980, 1985

81. Russell IJ, Fletcher EM, Michalekj JE et al: Treatment of primary fibrositis/fibromyalgia syndrome with ibu-

profen and alprazolam: a double-blind placebo controlled study. Arthritis Rheum 34:552, 1991

82. Le Gallez P, Reeve FB, Crawley MA et al: A double-blind comparison of ibuprofen, placebo and ibuprofen with meptazinol. Med Res Opin 10:663, 1988

83. Yunus MB, Masi AT, Aldeg JC: Short term effects of ibuprofen in primary fibromyalgia syndrome: a double-blind, placebo controlled trial. J Rheumatol 16:527, 1989

84. Donald JF, Molla AL: A comparative double-blind study of tiaprofenic acid and aspirin in the treatment of muscular rheumatism, fibrositis, sprains and soft tissue injuries in general practice. J Int Med Res 8:382, 1980

85. Tavoni A, Vitali C, Bombardieri S et al: Evaluation of S-adenosylmethionine in primary fibromyalgia. Am J Med, suppl. SA, 83:107, 1987

86. Jacobsen S, Danneskiold—Samsoe B, Andersen RB: Oral S-adenosylmethionine in primary fibromyalgia. Double-blind clinical evaluation. Scand J Rheumatol 20:294, 1991

87. Siegel IM, Miller JE, Ray RD: Failure of corticosteroids in the treatment of Duchenne (pseudohypertrophic muscular dystrophy). Illinois Med J 145:32, 1974

88. Drachman DB, Toyka KV, Meyer E: Prednisone in Duchenne muscular dystrophy. Lancet 2:1409, 1974

89. Drachman DB, Toyka KV, Meyer E: Letter to the editor. Lancet 1:94, 1975

90. De Silva S, Drachman DB, Mellits D: Prednisone treatment in Duchenne muscular dystrophy: long-term benefit. Arch Neurol 44:818, 1987

91. Brooke MH, Fenichel GM, Griggs RC et al: Clinical investigation of Duchenne muscular dystrophy. Arch Neurol 44:812, 1987

92. Mendell JR, Moxley RT, Griggs RC et al: Randomized, double-blind six month trial of prednisone in Duchenne's muscular dystrophy. N Engl J Med 320: 1592, 1989

93. Griggs RC, Moxley RT, Mendell JR et al: Prednisone in Duchenne dystrophy: a randomized, controlled trial defining the time course and dose response. Arch Neurol 48:383, 1991

94. Fenichel GM, Mendell JR, Moxley RT et al: A comparison of daily and alternate-day prednisone therapy in the treatment of Duchenne muscular dystrophy. Arch Neurol 48:575, 1991

95. Fenichel GM, Florence JM, Pestronk A et al: Long-term benefit from prednisone therapy in Duchenne muscular dystrophy. Neurology 41:1874, 1991

96. Dubrovsky AL, Mesa L, Marco P et al: Deflazacort treatment in Duchenne muscular dystrophy (DMD). Neurology, suppl. 1, 41:136, 1991

97. Angelini C, Pegoraro E, Turella E et al: Deflazacort in Duchenne dystrophy: study of long-term effect. Muscle Nerve 17:386, 1994

98. Griggs RC, Moxley RT, Mendell JR et al: Duchenne dystrophy: randomized, controlled trial of prednisone (18 months) and azathioprine (12 months). Neurology 43:520, 1993

99. Sharm KR, Munhier MA, Miller RG: Cyclosporine increases muscular force generation in Duchenne muscular dystrophy. Neurology 43:527, 1993

100. Roelots RI, Saavedra de Arango G, Law PK et al: Treatment of Duchenne's muscular dystrophy with penicillamine—results of a double-blind trial. Arch Neurol 36:266, 1979

101. Fenichel GM, Brooke MM, Griggs RC et al: Clinical investigation in Duchenne muscular dystrophy: penicillamine and vitamin E. Muscle Nerve 11:1164, 1988

102. Fitzgerald G, McArdle B: Vitamin E and B6 in the treatment of muscular dystrophy and motor neuron disease. Brain 64:19, 1941

103. Jackson MJ, Coakley J, Stokes M et al: Selenium metabolism and supplementation in patients with muscular dystrophy. Neurology 39:655, 1989

104. Gamstorp I, Gustavson KH, Hellstrom O et al: A trial of selenium and vitamin E in boys with muscular dystrophy. J Child Neurol 1:211, 1986

105. Backman E, Nylander E, Johansson I et al: Selenium and vitamin E treatment of Duchenne muscular dystrophy: no effect on muscle function. Acta Neurol Scand 78:429, 1988

106. Stern LZ, Ringel SP, Ziter FA et al: Drug trial of superoxide dismutase in Duchenne's muscular dystrophy. Arch Neurol 39:342, 1982

107. Dick DJ, Gardner-Medwin D, Gates PG et al: A trial of flunarizine in the treatment of Duchenne muscular dystrophy. Muscle Nerve 9:349, 1986

108. Moxley RT, Brooke MH, Fenichel GM et al: Clinical investigation in Duchenne dystrophy. VI. Double-blind controlled trial of Nifedipine. Muscle Nerve 10:22, 1987

109. Bertorini TE, Palmiei GMA, Griffin JW et al: Effect of chronic treatment with the calcium antagonist diltiazem in Duchenne muscular dystrophy. Neurology 38:609, 1988

110. Emery AEM, Skinner R, Howden LC et al: Verapamil in Duchenne muscular dystrophy. Lancet 1:5559, 1982

111. Bertorini TE, Palmieri GMA, Griffin J et al: Effect of dantrolene in Duchenne muscular dystrophy. Muscle Nerve 14:503, 1991

112. Mendell JR, Griggs RC, Moxley RT et al: Clinical investigation in Duchenne muscular dystrophy IV.
Double-blind controlled trial of leucine. Muscle Nerve 7:535, 1984

113. Griggs RC, Moxley RT, Mendell JR et al: Randomized, double-blind trial of mazindol in Duchenne dystrophy. Muscle Nerve 13:1169, 1990

114. Patlen BM, Zeller RS: Clinical trials of vasoactive and antiserotonin drugs in Duchenne muscular dystrophy. Ann Clin Res 15:164, 1983

115. Thomson WHS, Smith I: X-linked recessive (Duchenne) muscular dystrophy (OMD) and purine metabolism: effects of oral allopurinol and adenylate. Metabolism 27:151, 1978

116. Castro-Gago M, Jimenez Jr, Pombo M et al: Allopurinol in Duchenne muscular dystrophy. Lancet 1:1358, 1980

117. Tamari H, Ohtaini Y, Higashi A et al: Xanthine oxidase inhibitor in Duchenne muscular dystrophy. Brain Dev 4:137, 1982

118. Mendell JR, Wiechers DO: Lack of benefit of allopurinol in Duchenne dystrophy. Muscle Nerve 2:53, 1979

119. Stern LM, Fenwings JD, Breteg AH et al: The progression of Duchenne muscular dystrophy: clinical trial of allopurinol therapy. Neurology 31:422, 1981

120. Doriguzzi C, Bertolotto A, Ganzit GP et al: Ineffectiveness of allopurinol in Duchenne muscular dystrophy. Muscle Nerve 4:176, 1981

121. Pergament E, Christiansen N, De Berry M et al: Inefficacy of allopurinol in treatment of Duchenne muscular dystrophy. Curr Ther Res 34:832, 1983

122. Bertorini TE, Palmieri GMA, Griffin J et al: Chronic allopurinol and adenine therapy in Duchenne muscular dystrophy. Neurology 35:61, 1985

123. Griffiths RD, Cady EB, Edwards RMT et al: Muscular energy metabolism in Duchenne dystrophy studied by 31 P-NMR: controlled trials show no effect of allopurinol or ribose. Muscle Nerve 8:760, 1985

124. Hunter JR, Galloway JR, Brooke MM et al: Effects of allopurinol in Duchenne's muscular dystrophy. Arch Neurol 40:294, 1983

125. Backouche P, Chaouat D, Nick J et al: Allopurinol not effective in muscular dystrophy. N Engl J Med 301:785, 1979

126. Thomson WHS: Clinical trials of allopurinol in Duchenne muscular dystrophy. Med Hypotheses 17:175, 1985

127. Wolf A: Quinine: an effective form of treatment for myotonia. Preliminary report of four cases. Arch Neurol Psychiatry 36:382, 1936

128. Leyburn P, Walton JN: The treatment of myotonia. A controlled clinical trial. Brain 82:81, 1959

129. Geschwind N, Simpson JA: Procaine amide in the treatment of myotonia. Brain 78:81, 1955

130. Finlay W: A comparative study of disopyramide and procaine amide in the treatment of myotonia in myotonic dystrophy. J Neurol Neurosurg Psychiatry 45:461, 1982

131. Munsat TL: Therapy of myotonia—a double-blind evaluation of diphenylhydantoin, procaine amide and placebo. Neurology 17:359, 1967

132. Ricker K, Haass A, Rudel R et al: Successful treatment of paramyotonia congenita (Eulenburg), muscle stiffness and weakness prevented by tocainide. J Neurol Neurosurg Psychiatry 43:268, 1980

133. Kwiecinski H, Ryniewicz B, Ostrzyck A: Treatment of myotonia with antiarrhythmic drugs. Acta Neurol Scand 86:371, 1992

134. Ceccarelli M, Rossi B, Siciliano G et al: Clinical and electrophysiological reports in a case of early onset myotonia congenita (Thomsen's disease) successfully treated with Mexiletine. Acta Pediatr 81:453, 1992

135. Jackson CE, Barohn RJ, Ptacek LJ: Paramyotonia congenita: abnormal short exercise test, and improvement after mexiletine therapy. Muscle Nerve 17:763, 1994

136. Kwiecinski H, Ryniewicz B: A comparative study of disopyramide and diphenylhydantoin in the treatment of myotonia. Eur J Clin Invest 15:A36, 1985

137. Lewis I: Trial of Diazepam in myotonia—a double-blind, single crossover study. Neurology 16:831, 1966

138. Garai O: The treatment of dystrophia myotonia with ACTH. J Neurol Neurosurg Psychiatry 17:83, 1954

139. Reese HH, Peters HA: Therapeutic effects of ACTH in myotonia dystrophica. Dis Nerv Syst 13:99, 1952

140. Brumback RA, Carlson KM: Treatment of myotonic dystrophy with tricyclics. Muscle Nerve 6:233, 1983

141. Gerst JW, Brumback RA, Staton RD: Lithium induced improvement of myotonia. J Neurol Neurosurg Psychiatry 47:1044, 1984

142. Cook JD, Henderson-Tilton AC, Daigh JD et al: Beneficial response to a Ca Channel antagonist in myotonic syndromes. Neurology, suppl. 34:193, 1984

143. Grant R, Sutton DL, Behan PO: Nifedipine in the treatment of myotonia in myotonic dystrophy. J Neurol Neurosurg Psychiatry 50:199, 1987

144. Orndahl G, Sellden V, Hallin S et al: Myotonic dystrophy treated with selenium and vitamin E. Acta Med Scand 219:407, 1986

145. Orndahl G, Grimby G, Grimby A et al: Functional deterioration and selenium-vitamin E treatment in myotonic dystrophy: a placebo-controlled study. J Intern Med 235:205, 1994

146. Durelli L, Mutani R, Fassio F: The treatment of myotonia: evaluation of chronic oral taurine therapy. Neurology 33:599, 1983

147. Mader R, Keystone EC: Inflammatory myopathy—do we have adequate measures of the treatment response? J Rheumatol 20:1105, 1993

148. Walton J: The idiopathic inflammatory myopathies and their treatment. J Neurol Neurosurg Psychiatry 54:285, 1991

149. Dalakas MC: Clinical, immunopathologic, and therapeutic considerations of inflammatory myopathies. Clin Neuropharmacol 15:327, 1992

150. Mulder DW, Winkelman RK, Lambert EH et al: Steroid therapy in patients with polymyositis and dermatomyositis. Ann Intern Med 58:969, 1963

151. Vignos PJ, Bowling GF, Watkins MP: Polymyositis—effect of corticosteroids on final result. Arch Intern Med 114:263, 1964

152. Rose AL, Walton JN: Polymyositis: a survey of 59 cases with particular reference to treatment and prognosis. Brain 89:747, 1966

153. Bohan A, Peter JB, Bowman RL et al: A computer-assisted analysis of 153 patients with polymyositis and dermatomyositis. Medicine 56:255, 1977

154. Henriksson KG, Sandstedt P: Polymyositis—treatment and prognosis: a study of 107 patients. Acta Neurol Scand 65:280, 1982

155. Baron M, Small P: Polymyositis/dermatomyositis: clinical features and outcome in 22 patients. J Rheumatol 12:283, 1985

156. Uchino M, Araki S, Yoshida O et al: High single-dose alternate day corticosteroid regimens in treatment of polymyositis. J Neurol 232:175, 175

157. Malaviya AN, Many A, Schwartz RS: Treatment of dermatomyositis with methotrexate. Lancet 2:485, 1968

158. Sokoloff MC, Goldberg LS, Pearson CM: Treatment of corticosteroid-resistant polymyositis with methotrexate. Lancet 1:14, 1971

159. Metzger AL, Bohan A, Goldberg LS et al: Polymyositis and dermatomyositis: combined methotrexate and corticosteroid therapy. Ann Intern Med 81:182, 1974

160. Wallace DJ, Metzger AL, White KK: Combination immunosuppressive treatment of steroid-resistant dermatomyositis/polymyositis. Arthritis Rheum 28:590, 1985

161. Benson MD, Aldo MA: Azathioprine therapy in polymyositis. Arch Intern Med 132:547, 1973

162. Bunch TW, Worthington JW, Combs JJ et al: Azathioprine and prednisone for polymyositis: a controlled clinical trial. Ann Intern Med 92:365, 1980

163. Bunch TW: Prednisone and azathioprine for polymyositis: a long-term follow-up. Arthritis Rheum 24:45, 1981

164. Joffe MM, Lore LA, Leff RL et al: Drug therapy of the idiopathic inflammatory myopathies: predictors of

response to prednisone, azathioprine, and methotrexate, and a comparison of their efficacy. Am J Med 94:379, 1993

165. Roifman CM, Schaffer FM, Wachsmuth SE et al: Reversal of chronic polymyositis following intravenous immune serum globulin therapy. JAMA 258:513, 1987

166. Cherin P, Herson S, Wechsler B et al: Efficacy of intravenous gamma globulin therapy in chronic refractory polymyositis and dermatomyositis: an open study with 20 adult patients: Am J Med 91:162, 1991

167. Dalakas MC, Illa I, Dambrosia JM et al: A controlled trial of high-dose intravenous immune globulin infu-

sions as treatment for dermatomyositis. N Engl J Med 329:1993, 1993

168. Cohen MR, Sulaiman AR, Garancis JC et al: Clinical heterogeneity and treatment response in inclusion body myositis. Arthritis Rheum 32:734, 1989

169. Sayers ME, Chou SM, Calabrese LH: Inclusion body myositis: analysis of 32 cases. J Rheumatol 19:1385, 1992

170. Leff RL, Miller FW, Hicks J et al: The treatment of inclusion body myositis: a retrospective review and a randomized, prospective trial of immunosuppressive therapy. Medicine 72:225, 1993

11
Arthritis

Lawrence E. Hart

Arthritis, in its broadest sense, encompasses a varied array of progressive musculoskeletal disorders that differ in their pathogenesis and outcome. Effective management of many of these conditions is often empiric and may depend more on immune modulation than on the traditional concepts of controlling pain, suppressing inflammation, and restoring function. Most rheumatic diseases are chronic and their fluctuations over time usually require frequent changes in both the type and extent of specific interventions. Moreover, there is a complex relationship between functional impairment and the severity of arthritis that depends on both intrinsic disease characteristics at any given time and a variety of external factors that determines how individual patients cope with their disease.

It is beyond the scope of this chapter to explore the management of all, or even most, forms of arthritis. Instead, the intended focus is on the two most commonly occurring of the joint diseases: osteoarthritis and rheumatoid arthritis. Osteoarthritis (OA) or degenerative arthritis is characterized by progressive loss of articular cartilage, appositional new bone formation in the subchondral trabeculae, and formation of new cartilage and new bone at the joint margins (osteophytes). Low-grade synovitis is often seen and is considered to be secondary to the changes in the hard tissues within the joint.[1,2] Rheumatoid arthritis (RA), by contrast, is a systemic autoimmune disease that causes chronic, symmetric, and erosive synovitis of peripheral joints.[1,2] Over time, and depending on severity, both conditions can cause joint destruction, disfigurement, and disability.

In their analysis of the National Health Interview Survey and a review of more than 50 studies on the effects of musculoskeletal conditions (in the United States), Felts and Yelin[3,4] found that of the more than 16 million persons with a diagnosed musculoskeletal condition, 62 percent were unable to perform one or more of their usual daily activities. Both OA and RA were common causes of disability: 60 percent of persons with OA but no comorbid conditions experienced some form of activity limitation, and this number increased to 82 percent when comorbidity was included in the calculations. For persons with RA and no comorbidity, 70 percent experienced activity limitation, whereas such limitations were reported in 89 percent of those who had both RA and a comorbid condition. The economic impact of both conditions has been enormous and with the increasing prevalence of morbidity from both conditions as the population ages, the provision of rehabilitation services will need to be carefully rationalized to adequately address demands.

METHODOLOGY

As in other segments of the biomedical literature, the quality of studies that have guided, and continue to guide, the management of both OA and RA vary greatly. When defining *optimal treatment* it is important to make rational judgments on only the best available evidence. The randomized controlled trial (RCT) is generally regarded as the most robust method for assessing the efficacy of treatment. Even the RCT, however, needs to meet certain criteria before its reliability can be accepted.[5] Regardless of whether the result of such a study reaches statistical significance, its design, conduct, and published report should be of high quality.

Methodologically, robust trials and their reports should lead to better and more realistic estimates of treatment effects, more accurate and reproducible predictions of treatment efficacy, and greater acceptance of these results within the health care community.[5] In some instances, where RCTs have not been performed for various reasons, inferences must be drawn from observational studies (that have usually relied on cohort or case control designs). Given that such studies tend to overestimate efficacy[6,7] and are much more prone to bias, their results should be interpreted with caution.[8]

To retrieve the relevant literature on the management of OA and RA, a MEDLINE search was conducted on the available English language literature for the period between 1984 and 1995. Additional studies were identified through reference lists in some of the searched reports and those contained in textbooks of rheumatic diseases. Treatment studies, accumulated in this way, were then categorized under the headings of *drugs, exercise and rest (including splinting), modalities, and nutrition.* Surgical interventions, although important in the overall management of advanced arthritis, are not included in this chapter.

The quality of evidence in published research can be assessed according to various critical appraisal criteria, but for the specific purposes of this overview, the general guidelines developed by Sackett et al.[9] (on the effectiveness of therapy) provided the basis for judging the merits of particular studies. In evaluating each report, the following questions were addressed:

1. (In RCTs) was the assignment of patients *really* randomized?
2. Were clinically important outcomes assessed objectively?
3. Was there at least 80 percent follow-up of subjects?
4. Were both statistical and clinical significance considered?
5. If the study was negative, was power assessed?

As a further stage in the "quality filter," a level of evidence was assigned to the selected studies, and a hierarchy for grading recommendations (for applica-

tion of the research conclusions) was assigned. The relationship between the levels of evidence and grades of recommendation is summarized in Table 11-1.[10] This framework, although less rigorous than a precursor advocated by Sackett,[7] is a useful medium for categorizing treatment recommendations.

In addition to drawing inferences on the conclusions of individual studies, this chapter also includes the recommendations based on suitably designed and executed overviews and meta-analyses. The set of guidelines proposed by Oxman and Guyatt[11] were used in the selection of such reports. These criteria addressed the following issues:

1. Were the questions and methods used clearly stated?
2. Were the search methods used to locate relevant studies comprehensive?
3. Were explicit methods used to determine which articles to include in the review?
4. Was the methodologic quality of the primary studies assessed?
5. Were the selection and assessment of the primary studies reproducible and free from bias?
6. Were differences in individual study results adequately explained?
7. Were the results of the primary studies combined appropriately?
8. Were the reviewers' conclusions supported by the data cited?

The rigid application of critical appraisal guidelines across all segments of this overview would

Table 11-1. Categories for Quality of Evidence on Which Treatment Recommendations Are Made

Grade	Definition
I	Evidence from at least one properly randomized, controlled trial.
II	Evidence from at least one well-designed clinical trial without randomization, from cohort or case-controlled analytic studies, preferably from more than one center, from multiple time series, or from dramatic results in uncontrolled experiments.
III	Evidence from opinions of respected authorities on the basis of clinical experience, descriptive studies, or reports of expert committees.

(Adapted from MacPherson,[10] with permission.)

have resulted in the exclusion of studies which, although imperfect, are the "best available" and have had a demonstrable impact on clinical practice patterns. In such instances, the studies in question nonetheless have been included but, where applicable, attention is drawn to their relative lack of methodologic rigor.

The optimal management of RA and OA requires an integrated and comprehensive approach that combines drug therapy with ancillary, nonpharmacologic measures. For both conditions, the primary objectives are to control pain, preserve joint and muscle function, and enable the patient to maintain a satisfactory quality of life.

RHEUMATOID ARTHRITIS

A pyramidal, or stepped care, approach (Fig. 11-1) has traditionally been used in the treatment of RA. According to this paradigm, patients with properly diagnosed RA are started on one or another of the nonsteroidal anti-inflammatory drugs (NSAIDs) and then graduated to a disease-modifying antirheumatic drug (DMARD) once it becomes evident that the NSAID is not adequately controlling either the patient's symptoms or objective indicators of disease activity and progression. In addition to pharmacologic agents, the treatment pyramid also invokes the use of mechanical measures such as physiotherapy

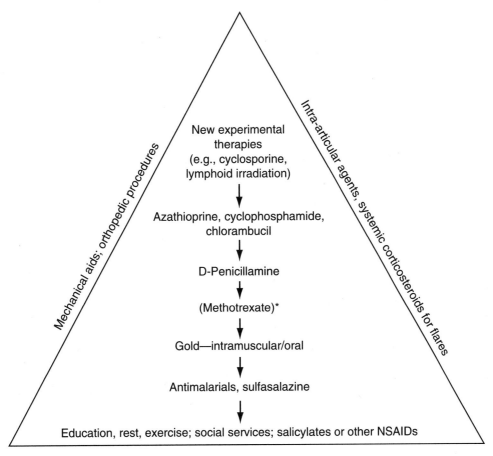

Fig. 11-1. The treatment pyramid: an example of the stepped care approach to managing rheumatoid arthritis. *Definitive position in sequence has yet to be determined. (Modified from Schumacher et al,[1] with permission.)

and occupational therapy and an early emphasis on education, counseling, and advice on rest and exercise.[1,12]

Nonsteroidal Anti-inflammatory Drugs

Although aspirin remains the prototypical NSAID, many newer preparations have been introduced over the last several years and are widely prescribed in the management of RA. Table 11-2 provides a partial listing of the categories and subtypes of NSAIDs currently available in Canada and most other western nations. Except for the enteric-coated or sustained-release forms, all NSAIDs are almost completely absorbed after oral administration. They are metabolized in the liver and excreted in the

Table 11-2. Nonsteroidal Anti-inflammatory Drugs and Dose Ranges

Drug	Dose range (mg)	Half-life (hours)	Doses per day
Carboxylic acids			
Aspirin (acetylsalicylic acid)	1000–6000	4–15	2–4
Magnesium choline salicylate	1500–4000	4–15	2–4
Salsalate	1500–5000	4–15	2–4
Diflunisal	500–1500	7–15	2
Meclofenamate sodium	200–400	2–34	
Phenylacetic acids			
Ibuprofen	1200–3200	2	3–6
Fenoprofen	1200–3200	2	3–4
Ketoprofen	100–400	2	3–4
Diclofenac	75–150	1–2	2–3
Flurbiprofen	100–300	3–4	2–3
Naphthaleneacetic acids			
Naproxen	250–1500	13	2
Indoleacetic acids			
Indomethacin	50–200	3–11	2–4
Sulindac	300–400	16	2
Etodolac	600–1200	7	3–4
Pyrrolealkanoic acids			
Tolmetin	800–1600	1	4–6
Pyrazolidinediones			
Phenylbutazone	200–800	40–80	1–4
Oxicams			
Piroxicam	20	30–86	1
Pyrrolo-pyrrole			
Ketorolac	15–150	4–6	4
Naphthylalkanone			
Nabumetone	1000–2000	3–4	1–2
Oxazolepropionic acid			
Oxaprozin	600–1200	21–25	1

(Adapted from Schumacher et al,[1] with permission.)

urine. NSAIDs inhibit the activity of various natural mediators of inflammation, such as bradykinins, prostaglandins, and oxygen radicals, thereby partially impairing the final expression of inflammation. Because they act on terminal events in the inflammatory cascade, their benefits are quickly evident, but because they do not fully prevent tissue injury, joint damage may nonetheless progress during therapy. Sustained drug-induced remissions are not known to occur with these short-acting antirheumatic agents, and there is no evidence to suggest that they have a major effect on the underlying disease process in patients with RA. Moreover, although the presence of drug in the blood is associated with a rapid onset of benefit, exacerbations of disease activity usually occur soon after its metabolism or excretion.[2]

Although NSAIDs share a common spectrum of clinical toxicities, the frequency of particular side effects varies among compounds. Potential beneficial effects and adverse effects tend to be dose related, necessitating careful consideration of benefit/risk ratios. Important toxicities occur in the gastrointestinal tract, central nervous system, hematopoietic system, kidney, skin, and liver.[13] It is evident that differences in toxicity may exist between NSAIDs.[14] At one end of the spectrum it has been demonstrated that indomethacin may be associated with more side effects than some of the other NSAIDs[15,16]; at the other end, ibuprofen appears to have a relatively lower toxicity profile.[17] With regard to efficacy, there is little evidence to suggest superiority of one NSAID over another.[13] Given the vagaries of both efficacy and toxicity of these drugs, it is often difficult to predict outcomes in particular patients.

When prescribing an NSAID, attention must be given to the presence of possible complicating illnesses and concurrent drug therapy.[13] Even in cases where drug selection has been carefully rationalized, however, the need for subsequent changes is not uncommon (because of lack of efficacy or drug toxicity). Although the cumulative experiences of individual physicians seem to determine specific treatment preferences,[18] there is as yet no generally accepted rank order for the prescription of individual NSAIDs for particular patients,[19] and most of those with RA are still likely to try three or more of these agents before an optimal selection is made.[2]

Many practitioners will opt for (usually enteric coated) salicylate as their drug of first choice, whereas others will immediately initiate treatment with one of the nonsalicylate NSAIDs. Although occasionally salicylate can be combined with one of the nonsalicylate compounds,[13] there is no defensible reason to administer combinations of the nonsalicylate NSAIDs (which tend not to improve efficacy but may augment potential toxicity).

To acquire endorsement by the US Food and Drug Administration or its equivalent in Canada and elsewhere, NSAIDs and other prescription drugs for arthritis must demonstrate efficacy and an acceptable benefit/risk profile. To meet such requirements, most of the NSAIDs currently marketed in North America have been subjected to the rigors of RCTs, and there is adequate Grade I evidence to promote their use in the management of RA.

Disease Modifying Antirheumatic Drugs

The DMARDs play an essential role in the comprehensive drug treatment of progressive RA. These drugs suppress the clinical sequelae of disease activity and are known to promote symptomatic relief and an improved quality of life in patients with RA.[12]

There are no clear-cut guidelines for timing the introduction of DMARD therapy. In general, it is difficult to estimate the amount of joint destruction at any given time and, as a result, physicians tend to underestimate the extent of disease progression that may occur even early in the course of the disease. To combat this tendency, DMARD therapy is being prescribed earlier than was previously considered optimal. For those who still adhere to the "stepped care" paradigm (i.e., the treatment pyramid), it would now be commonplace to start DMARD therapy within the first 6 months after a definitive diagnosis of RA. Judgments in this regard may be reinforced by the following guidelines:[20]

1. *Impressions of the patient.* The rheumatoid patient with active, progressive, disease almost always complains of tiredness, easy fatiguability, and loss of functional capacity. When such patients give up pleasurable activities, no matter what the excuse, disease is usually active and

earlier aggressive interventions (with DMARDs) are justified.

2. *Examination of the Patient.* Joint destruction rarely occurs in the absence of significant periarticular soft tissue swelling. Joint counts for simultaneous swelling and tenderness are useful quantitative measures, and signs of synovitis in a joint or set of joints not previously involved is a good indicator of progressive disease, as is enlargement of already existing rheumatoid nodules. Warm joints and the prominence of superficial veins over involved joints are confirmation of continued aggressive synovitis.

3. *Radiographic Findings.* Periarticular osteopenia can develop before joint space narrowing or erosions in subchondral intracapsular bone and reflects active inflammation and release by synovial cells of cytokines that mediate bone loss. The earliest signs are usually evident in the wrists and the small joints of the hands and feet.

4. *Laboratory Tests.* Several laboratory tests have been used in the ongoing assessments of patients with RA. The acute phase reactants are routinely measured to assess progression of disease activity. Sequential assessments of the erythrocyte sedimentation rate (ESR) in a given patient can provide a useful index of disease intensity, whereas quantitation of the C-reactive protein, usually in combination with the ESR, may correlate with the development of erosive disease. A falling hemoglobin level, thrombocytosis, and eosinophilia are other indicators of disease activity that may be used to determine whether earlier DMARD use is warranted. Synovial fluid analysis may also be helpful in this regard. A joint fluid leucocyte count greater than 50,000/L in RA indicates a joint at risk for rapid destruction.

When introducing a DMARD, it is not necessary to decrease or withdraw NSAID therapy. Although there is often concern that side effects might increase when such drugs are administered concurrently, there are, in effect, few documented examples of cumulative toxicity between NSAIDs and DMARDs.[20] The more commonly used DMARDs, their recommended dosages, and some of their recognized side effects are listed in Table 11-3. It is usually prudent to begin with a DMARD that is known to have the least toxicity. The antimalarials (of which hydroxychloroquine is the most widely used) and sulfasalazine are the best examples. The antimalarials have been associated with various gastrointestinal, dermatologic, neurologic, and hematologic side effects. Although their ophthalmologic toxicity has received the most attention, retinal damage is actually very uncommon in patients taking no more than the usually prescribed dosage of 400 mg/day.[20–23]

Initially used for the treatment of RA in 1941, sulfasalazine then fell into disuse and only reemerged as a credible addition to the DMARD armamentarium during the 1970s. Several studies have indicated that the rate of discontinuation of sulfasalazine is comparable to (or better than) that of other DMARDs. One study has shown a continuation rate at 5 years of 22 percent (compared with a 5-year gold continuation rate of 8 percent, for example).[2]

If an antimalarial or sulfasalazine is not effective, one of the gold preparations should be considered as the next line of treatment. Aurothiomalate and aurothioglucose are the intramuscular preparations in common use; an oral preparation, auranofin, also has been introduced over the last several years.[20,21,24–28] Unfortunately, toxicity to the intramuscular preparations occurs in a high percentage of patients, and the oral compound is less efficacious than other DMARDs.[12]

D-Penicillamine has been used for many years in the treatment of RA and is as efficacious as injectable gold. Because of its varied and unpredictable toxicity, however, it should probably be introduced only after a trial of gold has failed, or when, for other reasons, gold salts are contraindicated.[20,21,29–31]

Methotrexate has become a popular choice for the management of RA in recent years.[2,32–35] Its place in the treatment pyramid has not yet been completely established, but many rheumatologists now use it as the "DMARD of first choice" despite the fact that it is generally regarded as potentially more toxic than at least hydroxychloroquine and sulfasalazine. Some evidence suggests that the efficacy of low dose (i.e., usually 7.5 mg) weekly methotrexate can be sustained for 5 years or more.[20]

Drugs such as azathioprine, cyclophosphamide, and chlorambucil are also used in the management of RA,[12] but are usually reserved for cases that have been unresponsive to treatment with other DMARDs. Trials on the use of cyclosporine in RA have demonstrated efficacy, but (especially renal) toxicity has been a source of persisting concern for those prescribing it.[36–39] Combining DMARDs (e.g., methotrexate + sulfasalazine, methotrexate + sulfasalazine + hydroxychloroquine, or methotrexate + azathioprine) has also been tried, but the benefits of this approach, compared to more conventional

Table 11-3. Commonly Used Disease Modifying Antirheumatic Drugs, Dose Ranges, and Selected Side Effects

Drug	Dose	Side Effects
Hydroxychloroquine	400 mg/day PO	Indigestion; skin rash; visual disturbance, retinopathy
Sulfasalazine	500–3000 mg/day PO	Fever, malaise, headache, amnesia, nausea, abdominal pain; pruritic rash, oral ulcers, alopecia; bone marrow suppression; hepatic enzyme changes; reversible infertility, oligospermia
Gold sodium thiomalate	Start with 10, 25, and then 50 mg/week IM	Pruritis, rash, mucous membrane ulcers; leukopenia, thromboctopenia; proteinuria; diarrhea, enterocolitis; polyneuropathy; nitritoid reaction; pneumonitis
Auranofin	3 mg PO bid	Diarrhea; others similar to intramuscular gold, but usually less severe
D-Penicillamine	250 mg/day PO for 4–6weeks, then 500–750 mg/day	Skin rash; proteinuria; neutropenia, aplastic anemia, thrombocytopenia; obliterative bronchiolits; polymyositis
Methotrexate	7.5–15 mg PO or IM once weekly	Abdominal pain, nausea, stomatitis; abnormal hepatic enzymes, hepatic fibrosis; bone marrow suppression; alopecia; proteinuria; pneumonitis
Azathioprine	2–2.5 mg/kg/day (100–150 mg/day)	Nausea, vomiting, diarrhea; bone marrow suppression; hepatitis; increased incidence of lymphoproliferative malignancies

single-drug treatment, has yet to be firmly established.[20,38]

Newer (mostly experimental) therapies for the management of RA include biologic response modifiers (e.g., cytokines), immunosuppressors, immunomodulators, arachidonic acid metabolite modifiers, antioxidants (e.g., vitamin E and fish oil), inhibitors of cartilage catabolism, and antibiotics (e.g., minocycline).[2]

Corticosteroids

The therapeutic administration of oral corticosteroids rapidly and effectively suppresses inflammation. Because of their excellent short-term benefits, corticosteroids are generally regarded as an integral component in the management of RA and several other rheumatic diseases.[2] The most common application of oral corticosteroid is to provide "bridge therapy" between the time that individual patients are started on a DMARD and the time when the latter begins to exert its effect. Prednisone, usually 5 to 15 mg/day, is commonly used for this purpose. When the DMARD is not successful, it is likely that more prolonged therapy with the corticosteroid is required. The risk of accelerated osteopenia is an obvious concern in patients with RA who require corticosteroid therapy (even in relatively modest doses) for extended time periods.[2,20]

In addition to their role in bridge therapy, corticosteroids have been commonly used intravenously to suppress inflammation in severely ill patients with RA who are not responsive to other treatment strategies. In this context, pulsed doses of methylprednisolone, 1 g/day for 1 to 3 days, have been efficacious.[2,20] Moreover, intra-articular corticosteroid injections are used routinely to treat acutely inflamed joints and are invariably effective in providing short-term symptomatic relief.

Remodeling the Pyramid

Based on the premise that optimal management of RA requires prompt suppression of inflammation, consideration has been giving to modifying the traditional treatment pyramid (Fig. 1-1). According to the new paradigm, prednisone, 10 mg/day, becomes the drug of first choice and is introduced soon after

a new diagnosis of RA has been confirmed. If inflammation is not controlled within 1 month of starting this regimen, it is inferred that the patient in question has persistent synovitis and is at risk for accelerated joint destruction. At this point, a combination of DMARDs is recommended (e.g., methotrexate + hydroxychloroquine + oral and injectable gold). A "step-down bridge" follows, in which prednisone, and the DMARDs are sequentially withdrawn, one at a time over a period of months, until maintenance can be achieved on the least toxic drug, usually hydroxychloroquine.[40] This basic approach has its proponents and detractors[40,41] and awaits further clarification before being endorsed as the preferred protocol for managing RA.

In addition to meeting the stringent requirements of government agencies, studies on the DMARDs are unlikely to be supported by traditional funding agencies unless they evaluate a comprehensive set of outcomes recommended by the American College of Rheumatology (ACR). As a result, a majority of studies[12,42-55] that have addressed efficacy and safety issues in individual DMARDs have been relatively well-designed RCTs that have provided Grade I evidence favoring the use of these agents.

Prognosis in RA

Even optimal doses of NSAIDs do not completely suppress all evidence of inflammation. These drugs, as a group, are not known to definitively alter the natural history of RA. When considering prognosis, after the introduction of DMARD therapy, clinical outcomes and radiologic end points have been examined. In perhaps the most comprehensive longterm study of RA, Scott et al.[56] found that patients tended to deteriorate more rapidly during the second decade of their disease than during the first 10 years after their diagnosis. All of the 112 patients who were followed during the 20-year study were aggressively treated with DMARDs. Falls in ESR and improvements in functional capacity were noted in a majority of patients during the first 10 years, but this trend was reversed during the second 10-year period. Similar deteriorations in functional capacity have been demonstrated in two other longitudinal studies that followed patients for 16 years[57] and 15 years,[58] respectively.

Debate has continued regarding whether DMARDs actually slow the progression of joint erosions. Several studies have addressed this issue,[56] but, to date, there has been little agreement on the impact of these drugs. Luukkanian et al.[59] have suggested that gold therapy is effective in slowing the rate of radiologic deterioration, but their study groups were not comparable and the observed differences were small. Although other studies have suggested that disease severity, assessed clinically or by acute phase responses at a specified point in time, is related to the extent of radiologic progression, they fail to show that such progression is favorably influenced by DMARDs over time.[60–62]

In a study by Sharp,[63] mean radiographic scores, when plotted against years after diagnosis of RA, showed no deviation from the straight line determined by a regression equation, implying that when RA is fairly well established, progression of joint deterioration is irrevocable and inevitable.[63] In another study, 50 patients with RA were followed for a minimum of 10 years.[64] In 48 cases, the total joint score deteriorated (with a mean increase in maximal damage of 13 percent) regardless of treatment.

Evidence supporting an improved outcome in shorter-term studies has been similarly disappointing. Pullar et al.[65] followed 47 patients on gold and D-penicillamine for 24 months. Hand radiographs of all patients showed a statistically significant deterioration (when compared to controls), and although there was a trend toward slowing of the rate of erosions in the DMARD-treated groups, healing of erosions was unusual.

In an overview of controlled trials since 1960, it was inferred that gold and cyclophosphamide were the only agents where the weight of evidence indicated some retardation of radiographic progression.[66] On balance, however, the ability of DMARDs to meaningfully delay joint destruction has not been demonstrated.

OSTEOARTHRITIS

OA is characterized by intermittent exacerbations of disease that often settle without intervention. The natural history of the condition makes it difficult to demonstrate differences between investigational drugs and placebos in clinical trials. In addition, no recognized histologic or radiographic end points can provide definitively reliable and valid indicators of disease progression. Moreover, without standardized disease definitions and study designs, it is difficult to assess the effectiveness of different therapeutic interventions.[2,67]

After a definitive diagnosis of OA, therapeutic decisions are made on the basis of the patient's pain, discomfort, level of disability, and, to some extent, degree of radiologic damage. Simple, noninvasive, measures provide the first line of treatment in OA. If there is evidence of a "mechanical" problem, such as pain developing during the day or after activity, management should be directed toward improving biomechanical alignment by promoting joint protection and improving muscle strength. If an optimal physical therapy program does not relieve pain or lessen disability, other approaches need to be introduced. These approaches might include analgesics, NSAIDs, and intra-articular glucocorticoids (or viscosupplementation)[2] and measures to avoid further mechanical damage (such as the use of assistive devices and avoidance of activities that previously aggravated the joint pain).

The selection of a specific therapeutic program must be individualized. In some instances, however, patients may require no more than the reassurance that they do not have a rapidly debilitating and inevitably crippling form of rheumatic disease such as RA.[1]

Analgesics

Pain relief is the primary goal in the treatment of patients with symptomatic OA. The patient's degree of pain, extent of functional disability, and lack of improvement with nonpharmacologic therapies are the major reasons for considering the introduction of an analgesic or NSAID. Although there is little consensus among clinicians on the optimal way to begin drug management in OA,[68] analgesics are being increasingly prescribed as the initial, and often, only agent used for this purpose. Acetaminophen is usually the analgesic of choice and is regarded as relatively safe if intake is kept under 4000 mg/day (eight tablets of 500 mg/day or 12 tablets of 325 mg/day), except for patients in whom preexisting liver disease may limit full therapeutic dosages.[2] Despite their popularity as drugs of first choice in OA, however, analgesics have not been proven efficacious in this condition. Most of the studies have focused on comparisons between analgesics and NSAIDs rather than examining actual efficacy of the analgesics themselves (by way of placebo-controlled trials).[69–74]

In 1981, Doyle et al.[73] compared ketoprofen with propoxyphene/acetaminophen in the treatment of OA. In this double-blind, crossover study of 44 patients, there were no observed differences in pain relief. However, the articular index score and the "patient preference" scale favored ketoprofen as the drug of choice. In a second RCT of 864 patients with OA of the hip, knee, wrist, or ankle, there was a significant decrease in pain with slow-release diclofenac as compared with propoxyphene/acetaminophen.[74]

Bradley et al.[71] compared two doses of ibuprofen with acetaminophen in the treatment of patients with exacerbations of knee pain. In this study, 195 subjects (with mild to moderate disease) were randomly assigned to one of three groups: low or analgesic dosage of ibuprofen (1200 mg/day), high or anti-inflammatory levels of ibuprofen (2400 mg/day), and acetaminophen (4000 mg/day). After 4 weeks of therapy, no significant changes among groups were evident in pain and disability scores, walking pain scores, walking distance, 50-foot walk time, and physician assessments of patient. These results suggest that high-dose acetaminophen may be as effective as high- and low-dose ibuprofen for a flare of knee OA. The absence of a placebo group was an identified weakness of this study.

The most recent study to assess the relative safety and efficacy of NSAIDs versus analgesics compared naproxen and acetaminophen in a 2-year, double-blind, multicentered parallel trial performed by the Cooperative Systematic Studies of Rheumatic Disease group.[72] In this study, 178 patients with OA of the knee were followed for up to 2 years. The primary end point was radiographic progression of OA and withdrawal of the drug because of lack of efficacy. The results indicated comparable efficacy for naproxen and acetaminophen, but this outcome needs to be viewed with great caution, given the study's high dropout rate. Only 62 patients actually completed the 2-year follow-up study. The reasons for withdrawal from the acetaminophen group were lack of response and noncompliance, whereas those randomized to the naproxen group withdrew from the study predominantly because of gastrointestinal side effects, lack of efficacy, and noncompliance. The toxicity rate of acetaminophen was slightly lower than that of naproxen and was reversible.

Nonsteroidal Anti-inflammatory Drugs

Despite a lack of compelling evidence to support their use, NSAIDs are widely prescribed for the treatment of OA.[68,75,76] In low doses, they are regarded as effective analgesics; in higher doses they exert anti-inflammatory activity. The range and availability of NSAIDs promoted for use in OA are almost identical to those commonly used in RA. However, dosage schedules differ and even when so-called anti-inflammatory doses are required, the recommended optimal schedule in OA is somewhat less than what is usually prescribed for RA. Although the potential chondroprotective effects of NSAIDs have been explored[75] and there has been some encouraging evidence, clinical studies have not yet convincingly demonstrated the ability of these agents to protect articular cartilage or slow the progression of OA.[2]

When considering analgesia in arthritis management, it is important to regard pain as a physiologic response. If an analgesic or NSAID effectively controls pain, patients are often tempted to "test" the joint and an overuse injury may then occur. Both clinicians and patients should be aware of this possibility, and the patient should be cautioned against undue exertion despite seeming remission of their arthritis pain. In 1989, Rashad et al.[77] randomized 105 subjects with hip OA to treatment with either indomethacin or azapropazone (a weak prostaglandin inhibitor) and followed the progression of OA to determine the need for surgical arthroplasty. The azapropazone-treated subjects took 5 months longer than the indomethacin group to reach the arthroplasty end point (15.6 versus 10.4 months). Moreover, less radiographic deterioration was demonstrated in the azapropazone group. These data suggest that potent inhibitors of prostaglandin synthesis, such as indomethacin, may accelerate OA of the hip. Although the actual mechanism responsible for this effect has not been determined, indomethacin may have created an "analgesic arthropathy" by effective pain relief and, in the process, worsened the course of OA of the humoral head.

Intra-articular Therapy

Corticosteroids

Although systemic corticosteroids are not recommended in the routine management of OA, intra-articular corticosteroid esters are commonly used in the management of selected (active) joints. Their use should still be considered as only palliative and temporary. Intra-articular therapy has been used to facilitate rehabilitation, to aid patients undergoing physical therapy, to decrease effusions, and to prevent stretching and laxity of the capsule and ligaments. The size of the joint, the volume of the effusion, the type and dose of corticosteroid preparation, the injection technique, and the severity of synovitis are factors that influence the efficacy of these injections.[2,78]

The clinical efficacy of intra-articular corticosteroid therapy was described by Hollander,[79] but was rigorously documented in only three clinical trials, all focusing on OA of the knee.[80–82] Although the study design of each was different, the results were surprisingly similar and entirely consistent with Hollander's uncontrolled findings (recorded 30 years earlier). Compared to placebo, corticosteroid injections were associated with definite but limited improvement, primarily decreased pain, with little if any alteration in function-related end points. Pain relief was usually short lived, with most dramatic relief at 1 to 2 weeks after treatment and loss of efficacy by 4 weeks.[78]

Early reports linking intra-articular corticosteroids to accelerated joint destruction have been a cause of some concern. Most reports have been anecdotal and uncontrolled, however, and no substantive evidence exists to support the notion that intra-articular corticosteroid treatment hastens joint deterioration.[78]

Viscosupplementation

Hyaluronic acid or hyaluranon is the major nonsulfated glycosaminoglycan component of synovial fluid and cartilage. It has been extracted from rooster combs for veterinary medical use. Intra-articular injection of this preparation has been used in race horses with OA since the 1970s in an attempt to limit corticosteroid injections. The material is viscous, but does not act effectively as an intra-articular lubricant because its half-life is less than 24 hours. It is thought to exert a local anti-inflammatory effect or may stimulate cartilage and synovial metabolism.

Hyaluranon exerts a positive effect in humans. Benefits have been recorded after 5 weekly intra-articular injections in several clinical trials in Japan.[83,84] and two North American trials, utilizing three weekly intra-articular injections, attest to its efficacy and safety.[85–87]

Other Intra-articular Therapies

Various other biologic compounds, such as Rumalon and Arteparon (glycosaminoglycans), Cartrofen (a semisynthetic polysaccharide), and Orgotein (a metalloprotein enzyme) have all been investigated for use as intra-articular preparations in humans with OA, but their efficacy and safety await further confirmation.[2,78]

Prognosis in OA

It is difficult to describe a uniform natural history for OA because disease progresion may differ from joint to joint and may vary according to whether clinical or radiologic end points are being considered.[88] In general, however, it seems apparent that patients with multiple joint arthritis have more rapid disease progression in their individual joints.[89–91] Although it may be compelling to assume that the potential chondroprotective effect attributed to certain NSAIDs could delay disease progresion, there is no definitive evidence to support this hypothesis. Moreover, by preventing the activation or synthesis of metalloproteases, it has been proposed that intra-articular corticosteroids may have an ameliorative effect on joint degeneration.[88,92,93] While OA is not usually associated with increased mortality, it has been reported that women with OA may have higher mortality rates than those without the condition.[94] Another study (of both men and women), however, found no differences in mortality rates between subjects with OA and the general population.[95]

THE NONPHARMACOLOGIC MANAGEMENT OF ARTHRITIS

As already inferred, both RA and OA are complex rheumatic diseases that follow unpredictable courses and require a multifaceted approach to management. Rehabilitative techniques and surgical interventions of various sorts are integral to the comprehensive management of a majority of patients with these conditions.

Specific rehabilitative measures include local therapies to maintain or improve strength, range of motion, stamina, joint stability, and efficiency of motion and to reduce pain and swelling. Optimal exercise routines, various modalities (within the broad categories of heat, cold, and electricity), traction, splints, environmental design modification, education, and counseling are among the spectrum of techniques that are usually incorporated into treatment programs for individual patients.[96] Single treatments or combinations of different techniques may be required in specific cases, and it is not unusual for patients and therapists to have to work through different options before a practical and effective regimen is implementable. In this regard, the approach strongly resembles the strategy used in optimizing NSAID or DMARD therapy, where frequent changes are often necessary before satisfactory drug management is achieved. The outcome measures used to evaluate the success of the rehabilitation effort are not unlike those used in drug trials, although in many instances studies of nonpharmacologic interventions in the rheumatic diseases have not been designed with the same robustness that has been demanded of the NSAID and DMARD studies.

REST AND EXERCISE

Rest

The notion that rest should provide a cornerstone for optimal arthritis care purportedly dates back to 1874, when James Sayre recommended the "application of rest in splint-like devices with the joint extended as a cure for a variety of joint diseases."[97] At around the same time, Dr. Hugh Owen Thomas designed a device, now known as the Thomas splint, which was used to immobilize lower extremity joints for extended periods (often up to 4 months).[96,98] This regimen was reported to relieve joint pain (although no mention was ever made of attendant stiffness), but testaments to its efficacy can be regarded as no more than anecdotal. Nonetheless, since 1874, the value of rest in patients with various forms of arthritis has been advocated.

Although no optimally designed RCTs have reported the value of bed rest in either RA or OA, some Grade II evidence supports the use of different "rest regimens," primarily in the management of RA. The studies in question, all of which proposed 4 weeks of immobility in a hospital setting, were all performed more than 20 years ago. With improved pharmacologic interventions and the impracticality of hospital admissions of this duration in our current climate of managed care and reengineering, such an "intervention" would be impossible to accomplish, even if desirable. Rest, in the current context of arthritis management, therefore, implies that patients with arthritis interrupt their physical activity with periods of rest and that they pace themselves to allow periodic recumbency during the daytime hours to offset the inevitable fatigue that is associated with activation of their arthritis. One pilot study (Grade II evidence) has, in fact, indicated that rest intervals during physical activity results in more total hours of activity over a 24-hour period.[99]

Splints, Casts, and Orthoses

A static splint or orthosis is commonly used to support a weak or unstable joint, promote pain relief by immobilizing and resting an active joint, or provide functional alignment for a specific body segment.[1] Despite the widespread marketing of a vast selection of such devices, however, evidence favoring their use has been largely empirical.

Grade II evidence has been demonstrated for the use of splints and casts in the management of RA.[96,100] Bilateral plaster casts were effective in the treatment of 18 patients with painful knees who were immobilized in plaster casts for 8 weeks,[101] fiberglass splints were shown to provide relief in 15 patients with knee pain, and plaster casts apparently relieved inflammation in the wrists and hands of seven patients with activation of small joint arthritis.[102] A further study has demonstrated that nocturnal resting splints can potentially relieve wrist and hand pain in patients with RA, but this strategy has no demonstrable benefit in slowing the progression of ulnar deviation (even when used for prolonged time periods).[100]

It is estimated that symptomatic and often debilitating foot involvement occurs in approximately 80 percent of patients with RA and 50 percent of those with OA.[1] Forefoot problems, such as painful callosities, cock-toe deformities, subluxations of the metatarsophalangeal joints and hallux valgus are common in RA, whereas OA patients may present with mallet toes, hallux valgus, or hallux rigidus. Common rearfoot problems include heel pain, Achilles tendonitis, collapse of the medial arch, and alignment changes emanating from overpronation.[1] Appropriately customized shoes or corrective inserts are routinely prescribed to correct obvious mechanical problems, but suitably designed prospective studies are awaited before any definitive conclusions can be drawn on the relative merits of the available devices.

The potential positive effects of therapeutic rest must be weighed against the inevitable local and systemic adverse responses to such treatment. Deconditioning is an all too common sequela to enforced rest, even in healthy subjects,[103] and can have even greater consequences in a patient already debilitated by chronic arthritis.

Local problems such as stiffness, contractures, and accelerated muscle atrophy also commonly occur after prolonged immobilization in patients with RA or OA. Therefore, when defending the potential benefits of rest, such rest programs should be balanced with appropriate therapeutic exercise that usually requires careful consideration of the individual patient's needs and capabilities.

Exercise

Fatigue, weakness, and decreased endurance are frequent concomitants in patients with rheumatic disease, and therapeutic exercise, therefore, has assumed a role of increasing importance in this population. The goals of an integrated exercise program are to increase muscle strength and joint range of motion, improve stamina, and provide patients with a sense of well-being and enhanced psychosocial function.[1,78] In general, exercise routines can be categorized as passive, active, or active-assisted. Active exercise is further classified as isotonic, isometric, or isokinetic. A usual regimen will be customized to a specific patient's needs and will include combinations of different types of exercises, performed either on land or in an aquatic medium (hydrotherapy). Stretching routines and recreational activity are also emphasized in such programs.

Ytterberg et al.[104] have alluded to some of the potential pitfalls in the methodology and interpretation of the existing literature on exercise for arthritis. Despite their concerns, however, an emerging body of knowledge, based on credible Grade I evidence, attests to the efficacy of therapeutic exercise in both RA and OA.

A low-intensity aerobic exercise protocol (three times a week for 12 weeks) was effective in patients with RA.[105] Subjects enrolled in the exercise arm demonstrated improvements in their activities of daily living and reduced joint pain and fatigue, compared to those in the nonexercising control group. Improvements in activities of daily living were also shown in a long-term follow-up of 23 patients with RA who were enrolled in a home-based aerobic exercise program.[106] Although this Scandanavian study met the requirements of an RCT and reported a positive outcome, results may not be generalizable to a North American population because of some apparent differences in management style and patient assessment. Minors et al.[107] have demonstrated the efficacy of physical conditioning exercises in patients with both RA and OA when compared with controls. Both aquatic and walking exercise improved aerobic capacity, 50-foot walking time, depression, anxiety, and physical activity (following a 12-week protocol). In patients with OA, a supervised walking program for 8 weeks was effective.[108]

Two RCTs have provided Grade I recommendations for the use of exercise programs in improving the grip strength of patients with RA of the hands.[109,110] Grade II and III evidence exists to support the use of the following:

1. Dynamic rather than static training techniques in RA affecting lower extremity joints[111]
2. Physical training in an elderly population of patients with RA on corticosteroid treatment[112]

3. Isokinetic knee extension training in RA[113]
4. Evening exercise to reduce morning stiffness in patients with RA[114]
5. Muscle strengthening to improve the exercise capacity and aerobic fitness in patients with OA[115]
6. Passive muscle stretching to increase abduction in OA of the hip[116]
7. A quantitative progressive rehabilitative program to increase muscle strength and endurance in patients with knee OA[117]
8. A customized range of motion dance program to increase joint range in patients with RA[118]

Hydrotherapy

Hydrotherapy is the external use of water for therapeutic purposes in which both the thermal and physical properties of the water are considered. As currently practiced, an exercise component is integral to these water-based programs. It is generally acknowledged that exercise in water provides the patient with an opportunity to perform movements in a medium that not only provides buoyancy to the body but also allows movement with much less effort so that seriously weakened limbs may be moved and exercised in a manner not possible without support.[119,120] First proposed by Hippocrates (c. 450 to 375 BC) and now commonly used in rheumatic disease units worldwide, hydrotherapy has not, until recently, been subjected to the rigors of an RCT.

In the one study that has been reported,[121] no differences in outcomes (including function, muscle power, joint tenderness and swelling, early morning stiffness, and grip strength) were demonstrated in 22 patients with RA who were enrolled in a standardized therapeutic exercise program in the pool versus matched controls who did not receive this intervention. Inferences based on these results need to be viewed with caution because a smaller than intended sample size may have reduced the power of the study. Nonetheless, this study would need to be regarded as Grade II evidence *against* the use of hydrotherapy in patients with RA. An additional study (that provides Grade I evidence) demonstrated that a home exercise regimen is as effective as hydrotherapy for OA of the hips.[122] In contrast to these two negative, though reasonably

well-designed trials, there are several studies with weaker designs (Grade II and III evidence) that support the use of hydrotherapy protocols of various sorts in the comprehensive management of RA[123–126] and low back pain.[127]

In summary, there is accumulating evidence that patients with either RA or OA are able to increase their strength and function with an appropriately planned and supervised exercise program. Pool-based programs require further exploration, by way of robust methodology before any conclusions on their efficacy can be reached.

PHYSICAL MODALITIES

Heat and Cold

Therapeutic heat or cold remain the cornerstones of physical therapy in the management of arthritis. The administration of heat can be either superficial (by way of hot packs, hydrotherapy, or infrared) or deep (using diathermy or ultrasound). Ice packs or topical sprays provide the mediums for cold application. Beginning with the work of Hollander in the 1940s,[128] a plethora of studies have examined the effects of heat and cold on inflamed joints and the impact of these modalities on patient outcome. However, the accumulated literature is remarkably lacking in robust RCTs that might help to determine the true worth of these approaches in the management of either RA or OA. Instead, treatment guidelines have been largely dictated by either Grade II or (more frequently) Grade III evidence.

Several of the earlier studies have been well synthesized in an overview by Nicholas,[128] while the more recent literature includes the following: (1) an investigation by Yung et al.[129] in which no difference in joint stiffness (the study's primary outcome measure) was found between patients with RA and controls following the application of short wave diathermy, wax baths, and ultrasound; (2) a study by Spiegel et al.,[130] which reported a decreased severity of arthritis in the knees of patients with RA after heat treatment; (3) a "negative" RCT in which ultrasound was not shown to be effective in the management of OA of the knees[131]; (4) an investigation of ultrasound, short wave, and galvanic stimulation in OA of the hip and knee, which showed only a marginal treatment effect[132]; and (5) a study by Mainardi et al.[133] in which an electric mitten failed to relieve tender, swollen joints or increase grip strength in patients with RA.

The evidence favoring the use of cold in the sustained suppression of inflammatory or degenerative arthritis is similarly equivocal.

Laser

Except for anecdotal reports of success in individual patients, there is no evidence to support the use of cold laser therapy in the management of acute or chronic RA or OA.

Electrical Current

Faradic stimulation, neuroprobes, microdyne machines, and medcosonolators have all been used in the treatment of arthritis[96]; but none has been subjected to the scrutiny of prospective study. Transcutaneous nerve stimulation (TENS), by contrast, has been investigated more extensively. An RCT, using Codetron, demonstrated pain improvement (but no change in functional outcome) in patients with OA of the knees.[134] Grade II and III evidence, based on various study designs and patient populations, has been reported,[135–139] but even the cumulative data have not been sufficiently persuasive to establish TENS as a proven modality in the treatment of arthritis.

Acupuncture

Although used more commonly in China than in North America, acupuncture is considered as a possible option in the management of arthritic pain. No placebo-controlled trials have been reported, but based on Grade II and III evidence, it has been suggested that the technique may be as effective as TENS in relieving musculoskeletal pain.[96]

Lack of Consensus

Physicians find it difficult to agree on the appropriateness of specific modalities in the management of musculoskeletal conditions. In a survey of 100 specialists in rehabilitation medicine and 100 rheumatologists, conducted by Rush and Shore,[140] significant differences were reported in the perceived benefits of modalities. Benefits varied by both modality and condition.

NUTRITION AND DIETARY PRACTICES

In the United States, it is estimated that more than 90 percent of arthritis patients spend nearly $1 billion annually on unproven remedies.[141] A report on an Australian population indicates that 82 percent of patients with RA had used more than one unproven remedy since the diagnosis of their condition. In total, 352 different remedies were being used, with a mean of four remedies per patient.[142]

Dietary manipulation is a popular alternate therapy among patients with arthritis. Particularly with RA, dietary modification has become part of the folklore of the disease.[143] Fish oils, evening primrose oil, New Zealand green-lipped mussel, selenium, copper, zinc, folic acid, and vitamins are among the more popular supplements.[143] Elemental (hypoallergenic)[144] or vegetarian diets[145] and even fasting[146,147] also have become part of the cornucopia of alternate therapy for arthritis.

Of the dietary supplements, the potential therapeutic role of fish oil has been investigated most intensively and, based on several RCTs, Grade I evidence is available to support its efficacy in RA.[148–153] Moreover, fish oil supplements can potentially reduce NSAID requirements in patients with RA without precipitating an exacerbation.[154]

To address some of the controversies and uncertainties surrounding the widespread use (and abuse) of diet therapy and arthritis, the ACR has issued a position statement on this topic.[155] In it, two inferences (based on available evidence) were drawn:

1. A type of allergic reaction to foods may occur in the joints of some patients. It is believed that the number of patients affected in this manner is small, but the ACR nonetheless urges continued research in this area.
2. Diets of certain nutritional content may alter inflammation. Studies are still needed to better

define which patients, if any, benefit and by how much.

The statement goes on to caution patients against "miraculous" claims and urges them to cultivate balanced and healthy eating habits and to avoid elimination diets and fad nutritional practices.

CONCLUSIONS

The management of RA and OA has been driven by variably robust research that has focused primarily on the development and clinical assessments of pharmacologic agents that may potentially alter the natural history of these conditions. To date, however, little convincing evidence demonstrates that one or another of these agents actually delays the progression of arthritis. Instead, current strategies emphasize the need for comprehensive, multifaceted programs that are directed toward symptomatic relief and the prevention (where possible) of mechanically mediated joint damage.

This chapter has weighed evidence supporting (or criticizing) the many interventions that are commonly used to treat inflammatory and degenerative arthritis. By endorsing a pragmatic framework that proposes recommendations based on the "best available evidence," clinicians may be able to better rationalize their management strategies in a way that has optimal benefit for individual patients under their care.

REFERENCES

1. Schumacher HR, Klippel JH, Koopman WJ: Primer on the Rheumatic Diseases. 10th Ed. Arthritis Foundation, Atlanta, 1993
2. Weisman MH, Weinblatt ME: Treatment of the Rheumatic Diseases. WB Saunders, Philadelphia, 1995
3. Felts W, Yelin E: The economic impact of the rheumatic diseases in the United States. J Rheumatol 16:867, 1989
4. Yelin EH, Felts WR: A summary of the impact of musculoskeletal conditions in the United States. Arthritis Rheum 33:750, 1990
5. Moher D, Jadad AR, Nichol G et al: Assessing the quality of randomized controlled trials: an annotated bibliography of scales and checklists. Control Clin Trials 16:62, 1995
6. Hart LE: The role of evidence in promoting consensus in the research literature on physical activity, fitness, and health. p. 89. In Bouchard C, Shepard RJ, Stephens T (eds): In Physical Activity, Fitness, and Health. 1st Ed. Human Kinetics Publishers, Champaign, IL, 1994
7. Sackett D: Rules of evidence and clinical recommendations. Can J Cardiol 9:487, 1993
8. Fletcher RH, Fletcher SW, Wagner EH: Clinical Epidemiology. The Essentials. 2nd Ed. Williams & Wilkins, Baltimore, 1988
9. Sackett DL, Haynes RB, Guyatt GH, Tugwell P: Clinical Epidemiology. A Basic Science for Clinical Medicine. 2nd Ed. Little, Brown, Boston, 1991
10. MacPherson DW: Evidence-based medicine. Can Commun Dis Rep 20:145, 1994
11. Oxman AD, Guyatt G: Guidelines for reading literature reviews. Can Med Assoc J 138:697, 1988
12. Hart LE, Tugwell P: The use of disease modifying antirheumatic drugs in the management of rheumatoid arthritis. Postgrad Med J 65:905, 1989
13. Clements PJ, Paulus HE: Nonsteroidal anti-inlammatory drugs (NSAIDs). p. 700. In Kelly WN, Harris ED, Ruddy S, Sledge CB (eds): Textbook of Rheumatology. 4th Ed. WB Saunders, Philadelphia, 1993
14. Singh G, Ramey DR, Morfeld D, Fries JF: Comparative toxicity of non-steroidal anti-inflammatory agents. Pharmacol Ther 62:175, 1994
15. Hardin JG, Longenecker GL: Handbook of Drug Therapy in Rheumatic Disease. Pharmacology and Clinical Aspects. Little, Brown, Boston, 1992
16. Wijnands M, van Riel P, van't Hof M et al: Longterm treatment with nonsteroidal antiinflammatory drugs in rheumatoid arthritis: a prospective drug survival study. J Rheumatol 18:184, 1991
17. Committee on Safety of Medicines: Non-steroidal anti-inflammatory drugs and serious gastrointestinal adverse reactions—2. BMJ 292:1190, 1986
18. Pincus T, Callahan LF: Clinical use of multiple nonsteroidal antiinflammatory drug preparations within individual rheumatology private practices. J Rheumatol 16:1253, 1989
19. Schlegel SI, Paulus HE: NSAIDs, use in rheumatic disease, side effects and interactions. Bull Rheum Dis 6:1, 1986
20. Harris ED: Treatment of rheumatoid arthritis. p. 912. In Kelley WN, Harris ED, Ruddy S, Sledge CB (eds): Textbook of Rheumatology. 4th Ed. WB Saunders, Philadelphia, 1993

21. Brooks P: Slow-acting antirheumatic drugs and cyto-toxic agents. p. 303. In Schumacher HR, Klippel JH, Koopman WJ (eds): Primer on the Rheumatic Diseases. 10th Ed. Arthritis Foundation, Atlanta, 1993

22. Maksymowych W, Russell AS: Antimalarials in rheumatology: efficacy and safety. Semin Arthritis Rheum 16:206, 1987

23. Bellamy N, Brooks PM: Current practice in antimalarial drug prescribing in rheumatoid arthritis. J Rheumatol 13:551, 1986

24. Rau R, Herborn G, Karger T et al: A double blind randomized parallel trial of intramuscular methotrexate and gold sodium thiomalate in early erosive rheumatoid arthritis. J Rheumatol 18:328, 1991

24. Champion GD: Gold compounds in rheumatic diseases—1. Med J Aust 140:73, 1984

25. Blodgett RC, Heuer MA, Pietrusko RG: Auranofin: a unique oral chrysotherapeutic agent. Semin Arthritis Rheum 13:255, 1984

26. Ward JR, Williams HJ, Egger MJ et al: Comparison of Auranofin, gold sodium thiomalate, and placebo in the treatment of rheumatoid arthritis. Arthritis Rheum 26:1303, 1983

27. Davis P, Menard H, Thompson JF et al: One-year comparative study of gold sodium thiomalate and auranofin in the treatment of rheumatoid arthritis. J Rheumatol 12:60, 1985

28. Abruzzo JL: Auranofin: a new drug for rheumatoid arthritis. Ann Intern Med 105:274, 1986

29. Howard-Lock H, Lock CJL, Mewa A, Kean WF: D-Penicillamine: chemistry and clinical use in rheumatic disease. Semin Arthritis Rheum 15:261, 1986

30. Lyle WH: Penicillamine. Clin Rheum Dis 5:569, 1979

31. Stein HB, Patterson AC, Offer RC et al: Adverse effects of D-penicillamine in rheumatoid arthritis. Ann Intern Med 92:24, 1980

32. Tugwell P, Bennett K, Gent M: Methotrexate in rheumatoid arthritis. Ann Intern Med 107:358, 1987

33. Tugwell P, Bennett K, Bell M, Gent M: Methotrexate in rheumatoid arthritis. Ann Intern Med 110:581, 1989

34. Kremer JM, Lee JK: The safety and efficacy of the use of methotrexate in long-term therapy for rheumatoid arthritis. Arthritis Rheum 29:822, 1986

35. Weinblatt ME, Coblyn JS, Fox DA et al: Efficacy of low-dose methotrexate in rheumatoid arthritis. N Engl J Med 312:818, 1985

36. Weinblatt ME, Coblyn JS, Fraser PA et al: Cyclosporin A treatment of refractory rheumatoid arthritis. Arthritis Rheum 30:11, 1987

37. Dougados M, Awada H, Amor B: Cyclosporin in rheumatoid arthritis: a double blind placebo controlled study in 52 patients. Ann Rheum Dis 7:127, 1988

38. Cash JM, Wilder RL: Refractory rheumatoid arthritis. Therapeutic options. Rheum Dis Clin N Am 21:1, 1995

39. Yocum DE, Torley H: Cyclosporine in rheumatoid arthritis. Rheum Dis Clin North Am 21:835, 1995

40. Wilske KR, Healey LA: Remodeling the pyramid—a concept whose time has come. J Rheumatol 16:565, 1989

41. Hess E, Luggen ME: Remodeling the pyramid—a concept whose time has not yet come. J Rheumatol 16:1175, 1989

42. Clark P, Casas E, Tugwell P et al: Hydroxychloroquine compared with placebo in rheumatoid arthritis. Ann Intern Med 119:1067, 1993

43. Capell HA, Porter DR, Madhok R, Hunter JA: Second line (disease modifying) treatment in rheumatoid arthritis: which drug for which patient? Ann Rheum Dis 52:423, 1993

44. Felson DT, Anderson JJ, Meenan RF: Use of short-term efficacy/toxicity tradeoffs to select second-line drugs in rheumatoid arthritis. Arthritis Rheum 10:1117, 1992

45. Carroll GJ, Will RK, Breidahl PD, Tinsley LM: Sulphasalazine versus penicillamine in the treatment of rheumatoid arthritis. Rheumatol Int 8:251, 1989

46. Faarvang KL, Egsmose C, Kryger P et al: Hydroxychloroquine and sulphasalazine alone and in combination in rheumatoid arthritis: a randomised double blind trial. Ann Rheum Dis 52:711, 1993

47. Hannonen P, Mottonen T, Hakola M, Oka M: Sulfasalazine in early rheumatoid arthritis. A 48-week double-blind, prospective, placebo-controlled study. Arthritis Rheum 36:1501, 1993

48. Williams HJ, Ward JR, Dahl SL et al: A controlled trial comparing sulfasalazine, gold sodium thiomalate, and placebo in rheumatoid arthritis. Arthritis Rheum 31:702, 1988

49. The Australian Multicentre Clinical Trial Group: Sulfasalazine in early rheumatoid arthritis. J Rheumatol 19:1672, 1992

50. Weinblatt ME, Weissman BN, Holdsworth DE et al: Long-term prospective study of methotrexate in the treatment of rheumatoid arthritis. 84-month update. Arthritis Rheum 35:129, 1992

51. Williams HJ, Ward JR, Reading JC et al: Comparison of auranofin, methotrexate, and the combination of both in the treatment of rheumatoid arthritis. A controlled clinical trial. Arthritis Rheum 35:259, 1992

52. Weinblatt ME, Kaplan H, Germain BF et al: Methotrexate in rheumatoid arthritis. A five-year prospective mulicenter study. Arthritis Rheum 37:1492, 1994

53. Wells G, Tugwell P: Cyclosporin A in rheumatoid arthritis: overview of efficacy. Br J Rheumatol, suppl. 1, 32:51, 1993

54. Tugwell P, Bombardier C, Gent M et al: Low-dose cyclosporin versus placebo in patients with rheumatoid arthritis. Lancet 335:1051, 1990

55. van Rijthoven AWAM, Dijkmans BAC, The HSG et al: Comparison of Cyclosporine and d-Penicillamine for rheumatoid arthritis: a randomized, double blind, multicenter study. J Rheumatol 18:815, 1991

56. Scott DL, Symmons DPM, Coulton BL, Popert AJ: Long-term outcome in treating rheumatoid arthritis: results after 20 years. Lancet 1:1108, 1987

57. Ragan CH, Farringdon E: The clinical features of rheumatoid arthritis. JAMA 181:663, 1962

58. Rasker JJ, Cosh JA: The natural history of rheumatoid arthritis: a fifteen year follow-up study. Clin Rheumatol 3:11, 1984

59. Luukkainen R, Isomaki H, Kajander A: Effect of gold treatment on progression of erosions in RA patients. Scand J Rheumatol 6:123, 1977

60. Scott DL, Coulton BL, Chapman JH et al: The long-term effects of treating rheumatoid arthritis. J R Coll Physicians Lond 17:79, 1983

61. Brook A, Fleming A, Corbett M: Relationship of radiological changes to clinical outcome in rheumatoid arthritis. Ann Rheum Dis 36:274, 1977

62. Amos RS, Constable TJ, Crockson RA et al: Rheumatoid arthritis: relation of C-reactive protein and erythrocyte sedimentation rates to radiographic changes. BMJ 1:195, 1977

63. Sharp JT: Radiographic evaluation of the course of particular disease. Clin Rheum Dis 9:541, 1983

64. Scott DL, Coulton BL, Popert AJ: Long term progression of joint damage in rheumatoid arthritis. Ann Rheum Dis 45:373, 1986

65. Pullar T, Hunter JA, Capell HA: Does second-line therapy affect the radiological progression of rheumatoid arthritis? Ann Rheum Dis 43:18, 1984

66. Iannuzi L, Dawson N, Zein N et al: Does drug therapy slow radiographic deterioration in rheumatoid arthritis? N Engl J Med 309:1023, 1983

67. Batchlor EE, Paulus HE: Principles of drug therapy. p. 465. In Moskowitz RW, Howell DS, Goldberg VN, Mankin HJ (eds): Osteoarthritis: Diagnosis and Management. 2nd Ed. WB Saunders, Philadelphia, 1992

68. Brandt KD: Should osteoarthritis be treated with non-steroidal anti-inflammatory drugs? Rheum Dis Clin North Am 19:697, 1993

69. March L, Irwig L, Schwarz J et al: n of 1 trials comparing a non-steroidal anti-inflammatory drug with paracetamol in osteoarthritis. BMJ 309:1041, 1994

70. Bradley JD, Brandt KD, Katz BP et al: Treatment of knee osteoarthritis: relationship of clinical features of joint inflammation to the response to a nonsteroidal antiinflammatory drug or pure analgesic. J Rheumatol 19:12, 1992

71. Bradley JD, Brandt KD, Katz BP et al: Comparison of an antiinflammatory dose of ibuprofen, an analgesic dose of ibuprofen, and acetaminophen in the treatment of patients with osteoarthritis of the knee. New Engl J Med 325:87, 1991

72. Williams HJ, Ward JR, Egger MJ et al: Comparison of naproxen and acetaminophen in a two-year study of treatment of osteoarthritis of the knee. Arthritis Rheum 36:1196, 1993

73. Doyle DV, Dieppe PA, Scott J, Huskisson EC: An articular index for the assessment of osteoarthritis. Ann Rheum Dis 40:75, 1981

74. Parr G, Darekar B, Fletcher A, Bulpitt AJ: Joint pain and quality of life: results of a randomised trial. Br J Clin Pharmacol 27:235, 1989

75. Paulus HE, Bulpitt KJ: Clinical trials of osteoarthritis therapies. Br J Rheumatol 32:529, 1993

76. Dieppe P, Cushnaghan J, Jasani MK et al: A two-year, placebo-controlled trial of nonsteroidal anti-inflammatory therapy in osteoarthritis of the knee joint. Br J Rheumatol 32:595, 1993

77. Rashad S, Hemingway A, Rainsford K et al: Effect of non-steroidal antiinflammatory drugs on the course of osteoarthritis. Lancet 2:519, 1989

78. Schnitzer TJ: Management of osteoarthritis. p. 1761. McCarty DJ, Koopman WJ (eds): Arthritis and Allied Conditions. 12th Ed. Lea & Febiger, Philadelphia, 1993

79. Hollander JL: Intra-articular hydrocortisone in arthritis and allied conditions. A summary of two years' clinical experience. J Bone Joint Surg 5A:983, 1953

80. Dieppe PA, Sathapatayavongs B, Jones HE et al: Intra-articular steroids in osteoarthritis. Rheumatol Rehabil 19:212, 1980

81. Wright V, Chandler GN, Morison RAH, Hartfall SJ: Intra-articular therapy in osteoarthritis. Comparison of hydrocortisone acetate and hydrocortisone tertiary-butylacetate. Ann Rheum Dis 19:257, 1960

82. Friedman DM, Moore ME: The efficacy of intraarticular steroids in osteoarthritis: a double-blind study. J Rheumatol 7:850, 1980

83. Oshima Y: Intraarticular injection therapy of high molecular weight sodium hyaluronate on osteoarthritis of the knee joint: phase II clinical study. Jpn Pharmacol Ther 11:2253, 1983

84. Honma T: Clinical effects of high molecular weight sodium hyaluronate (ARTZ) injected into osteoarthritis knee joints. Jpn Pharmacol Ther 17:5057, 1989

85. Moreland LW, Arnold WJ, Saway A et al: Efficacy and safety of intra-articular Hylan G-F (Synvisc), a viscoelastic derivative of hyaluronan, in patients with osteoarthritis of the knee. Arthritis Rheum 37:S165, 1993

86. Adams ME, Atkinson M, Lussler AJ et al: Comparison of intra-articular Hylan G-F (Synvisc), a viscoelastic derivative of hyaluronan and continuous NSAID therapy, in patients with osteoarthritis of the knee. Arthritis Rheum 37:S165, 1993

87. Adams ME, Atkinson MH, Lussier A et al: The role of viscosupplementation with hylan G-F 20 (Synvisc) in the treatment of osteoarthritis of the knee: a Canadian multicenter trial comparing hylan G-F 20 alone, hylan G-F 20 with non-steroidal anti-inflammatory drugs (NSAIDs) and NSAIDs alone. Osteoarthritis and Cartilage 3:1, 1995

88. Felson DT: The course of osteoarthritis and factors that affect it. Rheum Dis Clin North Am 19:607, 1993

89. Dougados M, Gueguen A, Nguyen M et al: Longitudinal radiologic evaluation of osteoarthritis of the knee. J Rheumatol 19:378, 1992

90. Spector TD, Dacre JE, Harris PA et al: Radiological progression of osteoarthritis: an 11 year follow up study of the knee. Ann Rheum Dis 51:1107, 1992

91. Schouten JSAG, van den Ouweland FA, Valkenburg HA: A 12 year follow up study in the general population on prognostic factors of cartilage loss in osteoarthritis of the knee. Ann Rheum Dis 51:932, 1992

92. Pelletier JP, Martel-Pelletier J: Protective effects of corticosteroids on cartilage lesions and osteophyte formation in the pond-nuki dog model of osteoarthritis. Arthritis Rheum 32:181, 1989

93. Pellettier JP, Martel-Pelletier J: The therapeutic effects of NSAID and corticosteroids in osteoarthritis: to be or not to be. J Rheumatol 16:266, 1989

94. Lawrence RC, Everett DF, Cornoni-Huntley J et al: Excess mortality and decreased survival in females with osteoarthritis (OA) of the knee. Arthritis Rheum, suppl. 4, 30:S130, 1987

95. Monson RR, Hall AP: Mortality among arthritics. J Chronic Dis 29:459, 1976

96. Hicks JE, Nicholas JJ: Treatments utilized in rehabilitative rheumatology. p. 32. In Hicks JE, Nicholas JJ, Swezey RL (eds): Handbook of Rehabilitative Rheumatology. 1st Ed. American Rheumatism Association, Atlanta, 1988

97. Sayre L: Orthopedic Surgery and Diseases of the Joints (Delivered at Bellevue Hospital Medical College during the Winter Session of 1985). D Appleton and Company, New York, 1876

98. Thomas HO: Diseases of the Hip, Knee and Ankle Joints with Their Deformities, Treated by a New and Efficient Method. 3rd Ed. Lewis, London, 1878

99. Gerber L, Furst G, Shulman B et al: Patient education program to teach energy conservation behaviors to patients with rheumatoid arthritis: a pilot study. Arch Phys Med Rehabil 68:442, 1987

100. Johnson PM, Savdkvist G, Eberhardt K et al: The usefulness of nocturnal resting splints in the treatment of ulnar deviation of the rheumatoid hand. Clin Rheumatol 11:72, 1992

101. Harris R, Copp EP: Immobilization of the knee joint in rheumatoid arthritis. Ann Rheum Dis 21:353, 1962

102. Nicholas JJ, Ziegler G: Cylinder splints: their use in the treatment of arthritis of the knee. Arch Phys Med Rehabil 58:264, 1977

103. Drinkwater BL, Horvath SM: Detraining effects on young women. Med Sci Sports 4:91, 1972

104. Ytterberg SR, Mahowald ML, Krug HE: Exercise for arthritis. Baillieres Clin Rheumatol 8(1):161, 1994

105. Harkcom TM, Lampman RM, Banwell BF, Castor CW: Therapeutic value of graded aerobic exercise training in rheumatoid arthritis. Arthritis Rheum 28:32, 1985

106. Nordemar R: Physical training in rheumatoid arthritis: a controlled long-term study. Scand J Rheumatol 10:25, 1981

107. Minors MA, Hewett JE, Webel RR et al: Efficacy of physical conditioning exercise in patients with rheumatoid arthritis. Arthritis Rheum 32:1396, 1989

108. Kovar PA, Allegrante JP, MacKenzie CR et al: Supervised fitness walking in patients with osteoarthritis of the knee: a randomized, controlled trial. Ann Intern Med 116:529, 1992

109. Brighton SW, Lubbe JE, van der Merwe CA: The effect of long-term exercise programme on the rheumatoid hand. Br J Rheumatol 32:392, 1993

110. Hoenig H, Groff G, Pratt K et al: A randomized controlled trial of home exercise on the rheumatoid hand. J Rheumatol 20:785, 1993

111. Ekdahl C, Andersson SI, Moritz U, Svensson B: Dynamic versus static training in patients with rheumatoid arthritis. Scand J Rheumatol 19:17, 1990

112. Lyngberg KK, Harreby M, Bentzen H et al: Elderly rheumatoid arthritis patients on steroid treatment tolerate physical training without an increase in disease activity. Arch Phys Med Rehabil 75:1189, 1994

113. Lyngberg KK, Ramsing BU, Nawrocki A et al: Safe and effective isokinetic knee extension training in rheumatoid arthritis. Arthritis Rheum 37:623, 1994

114. Byers PH: Effect of exercise on morning stiffness and mobility in patients with rheumatoid arthritis. Res Nurs Health 8:275, 1985

115. Fisher NM, Pendergast DR: Effects of a muscle exercise program on exercise capacity in subjects with osteoarthritis. Arch Phys Med Rehabil 75:792, 1994

116. Leivseth G, Torstensson J, Reikeras O: Effect of passive muscle stretching in osteoarthritis of the hip. Clin Sci 76:113, 1989

117. Fisher NM, Gresham G, Pendergast DR: Effects of quantitative progressive rehabilitation program applied unilaterally to the osteoarthritic knee. Arch Phys Med Rehabil 74:1319, 1993

118. Van Deusen J, Harlowe D: The efficacy of the ROM dance program for adults with rheumatoid arthritis. Am J Occup Ther 41:90, 1987

119. Banwell BF: Physical therapy in arthritis management. p. 264. In Ehrlich GE (ed): Rehabilitation Management of Rheumatic Conditions. Williams & Wilkins, Baltimore, 1986

120. Duffield MH: Exercise in Water. Balliere, Tindall, Cassell, London, 1969

121. Hart LE, Goldsmith CH, Churchill EM, Tugwell P: A randomized controlled trial to assess hydrotherapy in the management of patients with rheumatoid arthritis. Arthritis Rheum 37:S416, 1994

122. Green J, McKenna F, Redfern EF, Chamberlain MA: Home exercises are as effective as outpatient hydrotherapy for osteoarthritis of the hip. Br J Rheumatol 32:812, 1993

123. Goldby LJ, Scott DL: The way forward for hydrotherapy. Br J Rheumatol 32:771, 1993

124. Damneskiold-Samsoe B, Lyngberg K, Risum T, Telling M: The effect of water exercise therapy given to patients with rheumatoid arthritis. Scand J Rehabil Med 19:31, 1987

125. Dial C, Windsor RA: A formative evaluation of a health education-water exercise program for class II and class III adult rheumatoid arthritis patients. Patient Educ Couns 7:33, 1985

126. Langridge JC, Phillips D: Group hydrotherapy exercises for chronic back pain sufferers—introduction and monitoring. Physiotherapy 74:269, 1988

127. Smit TE, Harrison R: Hydrotherapy and chronic lower back pain: a pilot study. Aust J Physiotherapy 37:229, 1991

128. Nicholas JJ: Physical modalities in rheumatological rehabilitation. Arch Phys Med Rehabil 75:994, 1994

129. Yung P, Unsworth A, Haslock I: Measurement of stiffness in the metacarpophalangeal joint: the effects of physiotherapy. Physiol Meas 7:147, 1986

130. Spiegel TM, Hirschberg J, Taylor J, Paulus HE: Heating rheumatoid knees to an intra-articulare temperature of 42.1°C. Ann Rheum Dis 46:716, 1987

131. Flaconer J, Hayes KE, Chang RW: Effect of ultrasound on mobility in osteoarthritis of the knee. Arthritis Care Res 5:29, 1992

132. Svarcova J, Trnavsky K, Zvarova J: The influence of ultrasound, galvanic currents and short wave diathermy on pain intensity in patients with osteoarthritis. Scand J Rheumatol, suppl. 67:83, 1988

133. Mainardi C, Walter JM, Spiegel PK et al: Rheumatoid arthritis: failure of daily heat therapy to affect its progression. Arch Phys Med Rehabil 60:390, 1979

134. Babjak-Fargas A, Rooney P, Gerecz E: Randomized trial of codetron for pain control in osteoarthritis of the hip/knee. Clin J Pain 5:137, 1989

135. Mannheimer C, Carlsson C: The analgesic effect of transcutaneous electrical nerve stimmulation (TNS) in patients with rheumatoid arthritis. A comparative study of different pulse patterns. Pain 6:329, 1979

136. Kumar VN, Redford JB: Transcutaneous nerve stimulation in rheumatoid arthritis. Arch Phys Med Rehabil 63:595, 1982

137. Langley GB, Sheppeard H, Johnson M, Wigley RD: The analgesic effects of transcutaneous electrical nerve stimulation and placebo in chronic pain patients. Rheumatol Int 4:119, 1983

138. Lewis D, Lewis B, Sturrock RD: Transcutaneous electrical nerve stimulation in osteoarthritis: a therapeutic alternative? Ann Rheum Dis 43:47, 1984

139. Lewis B, Lewis D, Cumming G: The comparative analgesic efficacy of transcutaneous electrical nerve stimulation and a non-steroidal anti-inflammatory drug for painful osteoarthritis. Br J Rheumatol 33:455, 1994

140. Rush PJ, Shore A: Physician perceptions of the value of physical modalities in the treatment of musculoskeletal disease. Br J Rheumatol 33:566, 1994

141. Panush RS: Does food cause or cure arthritis? Rheum Dis Clin North Am 17:259, 1991

142. Kestin M, Miller L, Littlejohn G, Wahlqvist M: The use of unproven remedies for rheumatoid arthritis in Australia. Med J Aust 143:516, 1985

143. Darlington LG: Dietary therapy for arthritis. Rheum Dis Clin North Am 17:273, 1991

144. Haugen MA, Kjeldsen-Kragh J, Forre O: A pilot study of the effect of an elemental diet in the management of rheumatoid arthritis. Clin Exp Rheumatol 12:275, 1994

145. Kjeldsen-Kragh J, Haugen M, Foree O et al: Vegetarian diet for patients with rheumatoid arthritis: can the clinical effects be explained by the psychological characteristics of the patients? Br J Rheumatol 33:569, 1994

146. Skoldstam L, Magnusson KE: Fasting, intestinal permeability, and rheumatoid arthritis. Rheum Dis Clin North Am 17:363, 1991

147. Palmblad J, Hafstrom I, Ringertz B: Antirheumatic effects of fasting. Rheum Dis Clin North Am 17:351, 1991

148. Geusens P, Wouters C, Nijs J et al: Long-term effect of omega-3 fatty acid spplementation in active rheumatoid arthritis. Arthritis Rheum 37:824, 1994

149. Kremer JM, Lawrence DA, Jubiz W et al: Dietary fish oil and olive oil supplementation in patients with rheumatoid arthritis. Arthritis Rheum 33:810, 1990

150. Skoldstam L, Borjesson O, Kjallman A et al: Effect of six months of fish oil supplementation in stable rheumatoid arthritis. A double-blind, controlled study. Scand J Rheumatol 21:178, 1992

151. Nielsen GL, Faarvang KL, Thomsen BS et al: The effects of dietary supplementation with n-3 polyunsaturated fatty acids in patients with rheumatoid arthritis: a randomized, double blind trial. Eur J Clin Invest 22:687, 1992

152. Van der Tempel H, Tulleken JE, Limburg PC et al: Effects of fish oil supplementation in rheumatoid arthritis. Ann Rheum Dis 49:76, 1990

153. Belch J: Fish oil and rheumatoid arthritis: Does a herring a day keep rheumatologists away? Ann Rheum Dis 49:71, 1990

154. Lau CS, Morley KD, Belch JJF: Effects of fish oil supplementation on non-steroidal anti-inflammatory drug requirement in patients with mild rheumatoid arthritis—a double-blind placebo controlled study. Br J Rheumatol 32:982, 1993

155. American College of Rheumatology Position Statement: Diet and arthritis. Rheum Dis Clin North Am 17:443, 1991

12
Many Challenges Remain

John V. Basmajian

This book was never proposed or written as the "final word." In fact, its conception was a deliberate attempt to present the current unsettled state of the decision-making processes in medical rehabilitation. As each foregoing chapter clearly reveals, for whatever the reason, the general state of the art appears to be only moderately successful; however, the *primary* reason for success is rarely a solid base of scientific data and clear reasoning. Our hope is to promote and seek valid improvements, built at least in part by acknowledgment and consideration of the problems raised in this book.

The field is relatively new as far as organized health care in industrialized society is concerned, although it has been a part of healing efforts since the dawn of civilization in both the West and the East. The burden of ancient beliefs and practices, including a fantastic array of nostrums, have weighed as heavily on rehabilitation as they have on the etiology and pathophysiology of diseases and on their acute treatments.

We grimace and groan now about the physiologic ignorance of our predecessors, but as we do, we dare not look down at our own feet for they may be made of clay. Human ignorance is infinite in all fields and requires strenuous effort to reduce. Medical rehabilitation—nursing, physical and occupational therapies, psychology, medical specialties, and social services—is not exempt from this problem.

grams. The lack of these keys has not only prevented progress but has kept clinicians and their patients frustrated and in the dark. Recent efforts by physical therapists in North America in this area of study have begun to shed some light on problems.[1-3] Physical rehabilitation outcome measures have three purposes: discriminative, predictive, and evaluative.[3] The last is the most relevant in our context, both for clinicians and individual patients and for researchers seeking evidence of the efficacy of a procedure or program in the management of specific disabilities.

Outcome measures and their application themselves require validation and here progress is being made.[3] Clinicians must rely on evidence from investigators to select appropriate valid measures for a given population. Administrators, too, are involved and should actively promote the use of accurate outcome measures. To develop recommendations for needed initiatives in medical rehabilitation outcomes research, a conference was organized by the National Center for Medical Rehabilitation Research under the distinguished leadership of Marcus Fuhrer and cosponsored with the Agency for Health Care Policy and Research. The resulting recommendations are presented in four areas: philosophic issues, strategy and design issues, measurement of disability and handicap, and measurement of quality of life and of health status.

OUTCOME MEASURES

The keys to solving many (if not all) problems in health care are having valid and reproducible methods to measure outcomes of treatment/training pro-

PHILOSOPHIC ISSUES

Values

Outcomes are unavoidably value laden and may differ in importance depending on who is judging

223

them—consumer, payer, provider of services, or researchers. Exploratory research to identify the values of these groups and survey research to determine variations in values are recommended along with flexible approaches for weighing outcomes, promoting dialogue, and obtaining valid proxy judgments for people who cannot represent themselves.[4]

Cross-Domain Issues

A broad effort must be made to address (1) boundaries among domains, (2) terminology, and (3) how to consider people's abilities rather than their deficits.

Development of conceptual models of the disablement process and empirical testing of such models are needed. Provisions must be made to gather and relate data across multiple domains. Measurement and analytic tools appropriate to multidomain analysis that use collaborative and interdisciplinary methods are necessary.[4]

STRATEGY AND DESIGN ISSUES

Measures

The conference emphasized the importance of obtaining valid, reliable, and sensitive outcome measures for comparing the effectiveness of alternative rehabilitation interventions, systems of care, methods of financing, and consumers' satisfaction and preferences.

Controlled Studies

Much greater effort is needed to provide evidence for the effectiveness or efficacy of defined rehabilitative interventions by comparing them to practical service alternatives.

Medical rehabilitation interventions and the service delivery systems of which they are a part are poorly and inconsistently described in reports of outcome studies. Well-documented descriptions of services are also missing for most ongoing clinical databases. Work needs to be done, therefore, to develop theory-based models and classification systems of rehabilitation interventions and practice models that are uniformly applicable to a variety of services and that are related to the outcomes goals of medical rehabilitation.[4] There is a need for better

data elements, including more details about impairments, broader coverage of outcomes, more refined information about the severity of conditions, and more complete characterizations of interventions and service delivery systems.

MEASUREMENT OF DISABILITY AND HANDICAP

A uniformly useful measure of instrumental activities of daily living appears essential. Developing a measure that can be used for people with various disabling conditions was viewed as being a worthwhile objective. Developing a supplement to scales like the Functional Independence Measure (FIM) to reflect the cost of resources for supervising cognitively impaired individuals was also deemed beneficial. Shorter and less cumbersome instruments for clinical and research applications are needed, with measurement instruments adapted for cross-cultural use. Translating instruments into other languages is an obvious step in that regard. The instruments then could be validated in these cultures and modified, if necessary. Study findings might show that different norms exist for different cultures.[4]

MEASUREMENT OF QUALITY OF LIFE AND HEALTH STATUS

There is an urgent need to consolidate information regarding quality of life measures and to clarify the concept of quality of life and its principal components. There is a need to review, integrate, and consolidate the vast literature on quality of life as it applies to the field of medical rehabilitation and to develop a classification system for quality of life and health outcomes.[4] Special attention needs to be directed to components that generalize across disabling conditions, as well as to components that are relevant to particular disabling conditions.

THERAPEUTIC EFFICACY OF OUR TREATMENTS

In 1799, as George Washington, the Father of his country lay dying, some of the greatest physicians in

North America were gathered around his bedside. After great debate at the highest level of medical ethics and science, the physicians decided to bleed their patient. When he did not recover any strength, once more they bled him, and still once more. It was the considered opinion that he needed high colonic irrigation; so he had one or two of those on that same day. Finally the patient himself, mustering what strength remained, asked his concerned physicians to forbear; "No more, gentlemen," he said and soon after, in spite of the best efforts of his doctors, he died. Fresh debate ensued over whether the doctors had been remiss in their duties in not trying out further attempts to "save the President's life."[5]

Similar stories abound in the history of medicine. And yet, ironically, the high regard for the physician in the Middle Ages and Renaissance was far beyond the regard now given doctors in modern times. Even though much of what physicians did for many centuries now is known to be absolutely contrary to physiology and scientific management, they were credited—and I think correctly credited—with many cures and substantial improvement because of their activities.

How can this be? Much of what they did was inert by scientific standards; yet it worked! In my opinion, it worked better than much of what we do today except for the very specific target-oriented therapies such as antibiotics for specific bacteria, vaccination against specific viral and bacterial infections, replacement therapy for hormonal deficiencies, and various other specific replacement therapies. We must be suspicious of some surgery, quite clearly reserving judgment on about half of the surgery done in North America—not just the "improper" surgery, as it might be called. We should include for the time being the accepted and well-regarded surgery done routinely and semiautomatically for many conditions. My guess is that 50 percent of all the therapy done worldwide by physicians, surgeons, and therapists of all kinds may be either useless or harmful to the patient. The trouble is we cannot tell which 50 percent!

Perhaps even that guess is too conservative when one includes many things—both hackneyed and fringe—that a few rehabilitation professionals do that verge close to malpractice, even by the standards of today. I might give as examples the excessive use of complex diagnostic and treatment procedures that are invasive, much of the surgery of the spinal column, and our medieval modes of electrical stimulation and of bone setting. Quite correctly, our defense for much of the treatment procedures used today is that they are the best state of the art. This of course is also the argument for what goes on in television, advertising, politics, and so on. Such tolerance is unacceptable. A *better* state of the art is what we must seek to achieve. We must eliminate the bad and the mediocre.

THE POWERFUL BUT MYSTERIOUS PLACEBO

Rehabilitation—including oral and injected drug therapies; occupational, physical, speech, and sex therapies; counseling; and surgery—does not stand alone in its use of, reliance on, and unknowing dependence on, the very ancient art of placebo. Make no mistake. I greatly admire the effect achieved by placebos when they are administered with naive trust on the part of the administrator and patient. I condemn placebos used deliberately as deception either because of laziness or frustration. However, such therapy may occasionally be necessary (e.g., as a diagnostic test). My tolerance is for the placebo responses resulting from what will eventually be shown to be an inert substance or nonspecific method.

Intensive research to determine the specific effects of everything we do remains a top priority because, although I greatly advocate and admire the nonspecific effects of placebo treatment, science and plain honesty cannot be ignored. They demand that we learn as much about specific effects as possible while also learning more about the powerful tool of the nonspecific response.

Some would say that having a naive or ignorant or suggestible subject is important for the success of a nonspecific treatment or advice. In an editorial, *The Lancet*[6] described a remarkable experiment among a class of medical students asked to cooperate in a study of sedatives and stimulants. Participants were to take one of two capsules, half of which were blue and half were pink. Actually all of them were inert placebos. The medical students were more susceptible to placebo effect than other people. They became sedated on the blue capsules and elated on the pink capsules. What is more striking, there were marked changes in blood pressure in at least 65 percent of the students. That is, an actual morphologic or physiologic change occurred.

PLACEBO EFFECT OF MACHINES

Many rehabilitation professionals may feel smug because they use techniques and machines rather than drugs. They should know about the placebo effect of machines, too. In 1968, Schwitzgebel and Traugott[7] reported experiments with normal subjects who were attached by arm electrodes to electronic machines. It was implied that their performance on special tasks would be improved when the current was on and would decrease when it was off. In all cases, however, no current was ever turned on, and the hypothesis was borne out. When the subjects thought the current was on, their performance increased markedly. No doubt, in a rehabilitation setting the surroundings, equipment, and assured way in which clinicians handle the equipment have a strong influence on the patient.

There is no question that approaches other than chemotherapy have strong nonspecific influences. Byerly[8] pointed out that placebos seemed to work like magic incantations. Both require an object of concentration, and virtually anything can function as an object. Further, the improvement need not be simply of a subjective nature. Byerly cites a rheumatoid arthritis study in which placebos achieved the same level of effectiveness as aspirin in objective improvement in the swelling of the joints. Physical agents other than ingested chemicals may have the same powerful placebo response, as difficult as it is for people in rehabilitation to accept.

In a research study on the treatment of back problems, my colleagues and I[9] found that the electronic gear of the recording devices (inserted electrodes, electromyographic equipment, various electronic devices, and a computer) raised the placebo response in almost 200 patients with back problems from the 30 percent (or so) for sugar pills to about 50 percent. The superiority under these circumstances of a treatment with diazepam (Valium) for painful spasms of the back becomes hard to interpret; in another double-blind study using impressive recording apparatus, we found that diazepam suc-

ceeds at only about the 60 percent level.[10] Is the special effect of diazepam only 10 percent? I cannot give a final answer. But clinicians who do various complex things to patients, with and without machines, should be aware that physical and psychosocial procedures must surely have a strong placebo effect that is urgently in need of clarification.

THE THERAPIST IS VITAL

Despite everything said here, the therapist—whether a physical therapist, occupational therapist, psychotherapist, or physician—is vital. A human being surrounded by the mystique of a profession has the strongest influence. If that clinician is knowledgeable about the procedures and confident, and above all, comes in close contact with the patient, success of almost any treatment occurs in 30 to 50 percent of patients. A clinician who touches and manipulates the patient greatly enhances the effectiveness regardless of whether the current fad is carried out correctly or incorrectly. Hence, many patients will recover from disabilities of the musculoskeletal system by having an "improper" manipulation or traction rather than the "proper" manipulation advocated by some charismatic healer. It doesn't seem to matter whether transcutaneous electrical nerve stimulation or acupuncture is done absolutely "correctly." Many patients will achieve substantial success or cure. The important element seems to be a close contact between the patient and the therapist. This is *at least* as important as the specific effect of the treatment. But rabbits are not as lucky! Galiano and Leung[11] showed that acupuncture procedures do not produce significant changes of pain tolerance in rabbits. Probably the same is true of very young children who respond poorly to acupuncture treatments and to transcutaneous electrical nerve stimulation.

TREATMENTS AS OPPOSED TO TRAINING

What about the serious ailments caused by objective lesions of the central nervous system and the musculoskeletal system? It is beyond question that therapists in their clinical practice do many training procedures that are highly effective, for example, gait training of amputees, stroke patients, and cerebral palsy patients. But this is not really "therapy"; it is reeducation of the capabilities of patients who actually are doing the therapy themselves with only the assistance of a trained person. It is education or reeducation, not therapy in the classic medical model. When physiotherapists are engaged in this type of occupation, of course, there still is some overlay of nonspecific effect, but the main effect is one of learning.

In contrast is the complex of modalities in which the clinician does something *to* the patient, (e.g., various types of heat and cold treatment, manipulation, massage, various types of noninvasive internal deep therapies such as ultrasound and radiant energies in general, vibration, and electrical stimulation). These are *treatments* as opposed to *training*, and it is here where the nonspecific factor becomes an overwhelmingly important feature of the relationship between clinician and patient. Here is where the personality flows from the one to the other and enhances the specific effect of the treatment.

What specific effects do these various therapeutic conditions have that exceed the nonspecific effect? These areas require intensive exploration by the several rehabilitation professions.

Placebos have always been with us and always will. They certainly are an important factor in both Eastern and Western medicine. Anything can act as a placebo, whether chemical, electrical, mechanical, radiant, verbal and transmitted, or internal thought and faith.

THE MEDICAL USES OF HOPE

Buchholz[12] reported a dialogue he heard at a national meeting of the American Society of Clinical Oncology. One oncologist sadly complained that his results with exactly the same dosage and protocol for a set of experimental drugs were strikingly poorer than those of the colleague he was addressing. Both were using etoposide, cisplatin, vincristine sulfate, and hydroxyurea to treat metastatic lung cancer: he was getting a respectable 22 percent response rate, but the other oncologist got a 74 percent response rate.

The latter's explanation—too lengthy to report here—contrasted the style of the two physicians in their equally honest presentations of all factors, both positive and negative. There was one crucial difference—a powerful though subtle recruitment of motivation and hope by the more successful program. For example, the first physician had been calling the set of drugs by the eponym "EPOH," but the second physician chose the eponym "HOPE." Although not minimizing side effects and the current failure rates, the second physician emphasized to his patients the possibility of good outcomes and his pledge never to abandon them. Then he would faithfully help them through the entire possible scenario from realistic goal-setting switches (as needed) until even, together, they were preparing for death "that is comfortable and as meaningful as possible."

CONCLUSION

Let us not simply pour scorn upon the "placebo." Health professionals must learn what it is and how to use it wisely, humbly, and graciously in helping patients restore themselves to good health. Ultimately it is the patient, who, with the help of nature, recovers. It is the clinician's duty to learn to apply those elements of behavioral medicine that accelerate the recovery of those who suffer disturbances of the neuromusculoskeletal system of the body. This is a high calling that the rehabilitation team must not fail.

REFERENCES

1. American Physical Therapy Association's Task Force on Standards for Measurement in Physical Therapy: Standards for tests and measurements in physical therapy practice. Phys Ther 71:589, 1991
2. Johnston MV, Keith RA, Hinderer SR: Measurement standards for interdisciplinary medical rehabilitation. Arch Phys Med Rehabil 73:S3, 1992
3. Basmajian JV (ed): Physical Rehabilitation Outcome Measures. Canadian Physiotherapy Association, Toronto, 1994
4. Fuhrer MJ: Conference report: an agenda for medical rehabilitation outcomes research. Am J Phys Med Rehabil 74:243, 1995
5. Basmajian JV: I.O.U.: Adventures of a Medical Scientist. J&D Books, Hamilton, Ontario, 1993
6. Editorial: Drug or placebo? Lancet 2:122, 1972

7. Schwitzgebel RK, Traugott M: Initial note on the placebo effect of machines. Behav Sci 13:267, 1968

8. Byerly H: Explaining and exploring placebo effects. Perspect Biol Med 19:423, 1976

9. Basmajian JV: Effects of cyclobenzeprine HCl on skeletal muscle spasm in the lumbar region and back: two double-blind controlled clinical studies. Arch Phys Med Rehabil 60:59–63, 1978

10. Basmajian JV: Reflex cervical muscle spasm: treatment by diazepam, phenobarbital or placebo. Arch Phys Med Rehabil 64:121, 1983

11. Galiano C, Leung CY: Has acupuncture an analgesic effect on the rabbit? Pain 4:265, 1978

12. Buchholz WM: The medical use of hope. West J Med 148:69, 1988

Index

Page numbers followed by f *indicate figures; those followed by* t *indicate tables.*

Acetaminophen
  for acute low back pain, 69, 72
  for osteoarthritis, 210–211
Acupuncture
  for arthritis, 216
  for chronic pain, 103
  for low back pain
    acute, 78–79
    chronic, 103
Acute low back pain
  initial evaluation of, 90
  management protocol for neurologic
    signs or symptoms still evident
    after 4 weeks and, 91
  meta-analyses of treatment for, 102–103
  nonsurgical treatment of, 68–86
    acupuncture in, 78–79
    back school in, 77, 80
    bed rest in, 68–69, 77, 84t–85t
    biofeedback in, 80–81
    corsets and orthoses in, 79–80
    epidural injections in, 81–82
    exercise in, 75–77, 84t–85t
    facet injections in, 82
    manipulation in, 74–75, 76–77,
      84t–85t
    muscle relaxants in, 70–72
    narcotic analgesics in, 72–73, 76–77
    non-narcotic analgesics and nons-
      teroidal anti-inflammatory drugs
      in, 68–70, 84t–85t
    oral steroids in, 73
    physical modalities in, 76–77
    red flags and, 86, 86t
    traction in, 73–74
    transcutaneous electrical nerve stim-
      ulation in, 77–78
    trigger point and local injections in,
      83
  pathway of, 89
  phone triage of, 92
  physical modalities for, 103, 104
S-Adenosylmethionine, for fibromyalgia,
  191

β-Adrenergic blockers. *See* β-Blockers;
  specific drugs
Adrenocorticotropic hormone (ACTH), for
  myotonia, 194
Aerobic exercise
  for arthritis, 214
  for lower extremity amputees, 164–165
  for muscle diseases, 183
Agency for Health Care Policy and
  Research, "Clinical Practice Guideline No. 16: Poststroke Rehabilitation" of, 5. *See also* Stroke rehabilitation
β₂-Agonists, for chronic airflow limitation,
  125
Airflow limitation, pulmonary rehabilitation for. *See* Pulmonary rehabilitation
Alprazolam, for fibromyalgia, 191
Amantadine, for behavioral problems following traumatic brain injury, 47
Ambulation, in spinal cord injury, functional electrical stimulation to
  facilitate, 26–27
American Congress of Rehabilitation Medicine, 41
21-Aminosteroids, for acute spinal cord
  injury, 23
Amitriptyline
  for behavioral problems following trau-
    matic brain injury, 47
  for chronic pain, 100, 106, 112, 114
    in low back, 106
  for fibromyalgia, 106–107, 190–191
  for headaches, 108
  for myotonia, 194
Amnesia, following traumatic brain injury,
  45
Amoxicillin, following lower extremity
  amputation, 157, 158t
Amputations, lower extremity. *See* Lower
  extremity amputations
Amytal, for spasticity following spinal
  cord injury, 28

Analgesics. *See also specific drugs and*
    drug types
  non-narcotic
    for acute low back pain, 69–70, 72
    for chronic back pain,
      106
    for muscle spasm, 190
Anesthetics. *See* Local anesthetics
Ankle-foot systems, 166–167
  for muscle diseases, 184, 185
Anterior rhizotomy, for spasticity following spinal cord injury, 32
Antiarrhythmics, for myotonia, 193–194
Antibiotics. *See also specific drugs*
  for asymptomatic bacteriuria, 26
  for chronic airflow limitation, 126
  following lower extremity amputation,
    157–158, 158t
  for rheumatoid arthritis, 209
  for urinary tract infection prophylaxis,
    25–26
Anticholinergics, for chronic airflow limitation, 125
Anticonvulsants. *See also specific drugs*
  for behavioral problems following trau-
    matic brain injury, 47
  for chronic pain, 114
  for post-traumatic seizures, 46–47
  prophylactic, 46
Antidepressants. *See also specific drugs*
    and drug types
  for chronic pain, 100, 102, 105–106,
    111–112, 113, 114
    with depression, 108–109
  for fibromyalgia, 106–107, 190–191, 192
  for headaches, 108
  for phantom limb pain, 160–161
Anti-inflammatory agents. *See also specific*
    drugs and drug types
  for fibromyalgia, 191, 192
Antimalarials, for rheumatoid arthritis,
  207–208, 208t
Antioxidants, for rheumatoid arthritis,
  209

229

Anxiety
   in chronic airflow limitation, 122
      psychosocial interventions for,
         133–134
   exercise training and, 144
Anxiolytics, for fibromyalgia, 191, 192
Arachidonic acid metabolite modifiers, for
   rheumatoid arthritis, 209
Arachnoid scar tissue, low back pain and,
   59
Arteparon, for osteoarthritis, 212
Arthritis, 203–217. *See also* Osteoarthritis
   (OA); Rheumatoid arthritis (RA)
   nonpharmacologic management of,
      213–217
      acupuncture for, 216
      dietary, 216–217
      electrical stimulation for, 216
      exercise for, 214–215
      heat and cold for, 215–216
      hydrotherapy for, 215
      laser therapy for, 216
      rest for, 213
      splints, casts, and orthoses for,
         213–214
   research on, 203–205, 204t
   of spine, low back pain and, 60
Aspirin
   for fibromyalgia, 191
   for rheumatoid arthritis, 206, 206t
Assessment. *See also* Health status
      assessment
   Chedoke-McMaster Stroke Assessment
      for, 8, 12
   initial, in stroke rehabilitation, 10
   of psychosocial adjustment, 122
Auditory feedback, for acute low back
   pain, 80
Auranofin, for rheumatoid arthritis, 208t
Aurothioglucose, for rheumatoid arthritis,
   208
Aurothiomalate, for rheumatoid arthritis,
   208, 208t
Autogenic therapy, for chronic pain,
   101–102
Azapropazone, for osteoarthritis, 211
Azathioprine
   for Duchenne muscular dystrophy, 192
   for inclusion body myositis, 195
   for inflammatory myopathies, 195
   for rheumatoid arthritis, 208t, 208–209

Back pain. *See* Acute low back pain;
      Chronic low back pain; Low back
      pain
Back school
   for acute low back pain, 77, 80, 103

for chronic low back pain, 100
Baclofen (Lioresal)
   for acute low back pain, 71
   for spasticity
      following spinal cord injury, 28, 29t,
         30, 32
      following traumatic brain injury,
         47
Bacteruria, asymptomatic, treatment of, in
   spinal cord injury, 26
Beck Depression Inventory, 122
Becker's muscular dystrophy (BMD),
   strengthening exercise in, 181
Bed rest, for acute low back pain, 68–69,
   77, 103, 104
Behavioral interventions. *See* Multimodal
   pain programs; Unimodal chronic
   pain therapies; *specific interven-*
   tions
Behavioral problems, following traumatic
   brain injury, treatment of, 47
Benzodiazepines
   for behavioral problems following trau-
      matic brain injury, 47
   for chronic airflow limitation, 126
Beta-blockers. *See* β-Blockers; *specific*
   drugs
Biofeedback
   for acute low back pain, 80–81
   for chronic pain, 101–102
Biologic response modifiers, for rheumatoid arthritis, 209
Bladder, neurogenic. *See* Spinal cord
   injury (SCI), neurogenic bladder
   management for
Bladder retraining, in spinal cord injury,
   25
Bladder stones, in spinal cord injury, 24
β-Blockers. *See also specific drugs*
   for behavioral problems following trau-
      matic brain injury, 47
   for chronic pain, 114
   for headaches, 108
   for phantom limb pain, 160
Blood pressure, exercise training and,
   143–144
Boston Interhospital Amputation Study,
   154
Bracing. *See* Orthotics
Brain injury. *See* Traumatic brain injury
   (TBI) rehabilitation
Breathing retraining and control, for
   chronic airflow limitation,
   132–133
Bronchodilators, for chronic airflow limitation, 125–126
Brudzinski/Kernig test, in low back pain,
   62

Bupivacaine, epidural block using, for
   phantom limb pain, 159
Bursitis, low back pain and, 61

Calcitonin, for phantom limb pain, 159
Calcium, for muscle cramps, 190
Calcium channel blockers. *See also spe-*
   cific drugs
   for chronic pain, 114
   for Duchenne muscular dystrophy, 193
   for headaches, 108
   for myotonia, 194
Cancer, in dermatomyositis, 172
Capsaicin
   for chronic pain, 114
   for residual limb pain following lower
      extremity amputation, 159
Carbamazepine
   for behavioral problems following trau-
      matic brain injury, 47
   for chronic pain, 112
      with depression, 109
   for phantom limb pain, 160
   for post-traumatic seizures, 46–47
Carbocaine, trigger point and local injections of, for acute low back pain,
   83
Carbon monoxide, diffusing capacity for,
   120
Cardiac rehabilitation, 141–148
   rationale for physical training and,
      141–145
      external and internal workloads and,
         141
      glucose intolerance and, 144
      heart rate and oxygen uptake and,
         141–142, 142f
      hypertension and, 143–144
      left ventricular function and, 143
      myocardial perfusion and, 143
      peripheral adaptations and, 142–143
      potential improvements and, 145
      psychological effects and, 144–145
      serum lipids and, 143
   secondary prevention by, 145–147
      meta-analysis of, 145–146
      questions concerning, 146–147, 147t
Carisoprodol (Soma)
   for acute low back pain, 70
   for muscle cramps, 190
   for muscle spasm, 188–189, 190
Cartilage catabolism inhibitors, for
   rheumatoid arthritis, 209
Cartrofen, for osteoarthritis, 212
Case series, without controls, 3
Casts
   for arthritis, 213–214

plaster, following lower extremity amputations, 153–156, 156t
Catecholamines, plasma, exercise training and, 144
Catheterization
  indwelling catheters for, in spinal cord injury, 24–25
  intermittent, in spinal cord injury, 24
Cauda equina injuries, bullet removal in, 21
Cefoxitin, following lower extremity amputation, 158t
Cefuroxime, following lower extremity amputation, 158t
Charcot-Marie-Tooth disease, 177–178
Chedoke-McMaster Stroke Assessment, 8, 12
Chedoke-McMaster Stroke Team clinical decision-making paradigm, 5
Chiropractic manipulation, for low back pain
  acute, 74
  chronic, 104–105
Chlorambucil
  for inflammatory myopathies, 195
  for rheumatoid arthritis, 208
Chlorimipramine
  for fibromyalgia, 191
  for phantom limb pain, 160–161
Chlormezanone, for fibromyalgia, 191
Chlorpromazine
  for fibromyalgia, 191
  for phantom limb pain, 161
Chlorzoxazone, for muscle spasm, 188, 189
Cholesterol, exercise training and, 143
Chronic airflow limitation (CAL), pulmonary rehabilitation for. See Pulmonary rehabilitation
Chronic low back pain, 58
  acupuncture for, 103
  biofeedback training for, 101–102
  chiropractic manipulation for, 104–105
  exercise for, 103, 104
  intensiveness of treatment for, 104
  manipulation for, 104–105
  multimodal pain programs for, 95–96
  patient education for, 103
  pharmacologic therapy for, 106
    epidural injections, 103
Chronic obstruction pulmonary disease (COPD), pulmonary rehabilitation for. See Pulmonary rehabilitation
Chronic pain, 93–114
  algorithm for management of, 111–113, 112f
  in back. See Chronic low back pain

behavioral interventions for, 93. See also Multimodal pain programs; Unimodal chronic pain therapies
  meta-analyses of, 101–103
  with depression, pharmacologic treatment of, 108–109
  headaches and. See Headaches
  medical treatment of, 103–107, 114
    manipulation, 104–105
    pharmacologic. See Pharmacologic therapy, for chronic pain
    physical therapy, 103–104, 114
  prevention of, 98
Chronic Respiratory Disease Questionnaire (CRDQ), 121
Ciprofloxacin, for urinary tract infection prophylaxis, 25, 26
Claudication, spinal, 59
Client-centered practice, evidence-based practice versus, 5–7
  levels of evidence and, 6–7
Clinical data set, for stroke rehabilitation, 8–9
  contents of, 9, 9t
"Clinical Practice Guideline No. 16: Poststroke Rehabilitation," 5. See also Stroke rehabilitation
Clonazepam, for behavioral problems following traumatic brain injury, 47
Clonidine
  for muscle cramps, 190
  for spasticity following spinal cord injury, 29t, 31
Codeine, for acute low back pain, 72
Codetron, for arthritis, 216
Cognitive-behavioral therapy, for chronic pain, 100
Cognitive remediation. See Traumatic brain injury (TBI) rehabilitation, cognitive remediation in
Cognitive therapy, for chronic pain, 101–102
Cohort comparisons
  contemporaneous, 3
  historical, 3
Cold therapy, for arthritis, 216
Coma, 44
  early treatment for, 44, 45–46
  sensory stimulation for, 44
Community-based rehabilitation, for traumatic brain injury, 49–50
Community Integration Questionnaire, 43
Community reintegration, poststroke, 14
Compensation, prognosis of chronic pain and, 98
Compressed air, for chronic airflow limitation, 126–127

Computed tomography scans, in low back pain, 63
Computer aided design (CAD), of prosthetic sockets, 167–168
Conditioning exercise programs, for lower extremity amputees, 163–164
Contoured adducted trochanteric controlled alignment method (CAT-CAM) sockets, 165–166
Contractures, in Duchenne muscular dystrophy, 176
  exercise for, 180–181
  orthotics to prevent or correct, 183–184
Controlled environment treatment (CET), for residual limb following lower extremity amputation, 157
Controlled studies. See also Randomized controlled trials (RCTs)
  need for, 224
Coronary artery disease (CAD), cardiac rehabilitation and. See Cardiac rehabilitation
Cor pulmonale, oxygen therapy for, 126
Corsets, for acute low back pain, 79–80
Corticosteroids. See also specific drugs
  for chronic airflow limitation, 126
  epidural injections of, for acute low back pain, 81–82
  facet injections of, for acute low back pain, 82
  intra-articular, for osteoarthritis, 212
  for rheumatoid arthritis, 209
Cortisone, facet injections of, for acute low back pain, 82
Cram test, in low back pain, 62
Creatine kinase (CK), muscle injury and, 172
Cross-domain issues, 224
CT scans, in low back pain, 63
Cybex isokinetic exerciser, for muscle diseases, 181, 182f
Cyclobenzaprine (Flexeril)
  for acute low back pain, 69–70, 71
  for chronic pain, 114
  for fibromyalgia, 106–107, 191
  for muscle spasm, 188, 189–190
Cyclophosphamide
  for inflammatory myopathies, 195
  for rheumatoid arthritis, 208

Dantrolene (Dantrium)
  for acute low back pain, 71
  for Duchenne muscular dystrophy, 193
  hepatic injury caused by, 31
  for spasticity

Dantrolene (Dantrium) *(Continued)*
  following spinal cord injury, 29t,
    30–31, 32
  following traumatic brain injury, 47
Decompressive surgery, for spinal cord
    injury. *See* Spinal cord injury
    (SCI), surgical treatment of
Delflazacort, for Duchenne muscular dys-
    trophy, 193
Depression
  in chronic airflow limitation, 122
    psychosocial interventions for, 133
  exercise training and, 144
  pain with, pharmacologic therapy for,
    108–109
Dermatomyositis, 171–172
  malignancies coexisting with, 172
  prednisone for, 194
  rest for, 172
Design issues, 224
Desipramine, for chronic pain, 112
  with depression, 109
Detoxification, for headaches, 107–108
Detrusor hyperreflexia, in spinal cord
    injury, 25
Dexamethasone, for acute low back pain,
    73
Dextrose, trigger point and local injec-
    tions of, for acute low back pain,
    83
Diabetic polyneuropathy, 178
Diathermy
  for acute low back pain, 75, 76–77
Diazepam
  for acute low back pain, 70
  for myotonia, 194
  for spasticity
    following spinal cord injury, 28, 29t,
      32
    following traumatic brain injury, 47
Diclofenac
  for acute low back pain, 69, 77
  for osteoarthritis, 211
  for rheumatoid arthritis, 206t
Dietary manipulation, for arthritis,
    216–217
Diffusing capacity for carbon monoxide
    (DCO), 120
Diflunisal
  for acute low back pain, 69–70, 72,
    76–77
  for rheumatoid arthritis, 206t
Dihydroergotamine, for headaches, 107,
    114
Diphenylhydantoin (Phenytoin)
  for myotonia, 193–194
  for post-traumatic seizures, 46
Disability

in chronic airflow limitation, measure-
    ment of, 120, 121f, 123
  definition of, 119
    World Health Organization, 7
  measurement of, 224
  severity of, pulmonary rehabilitation
    and, 134, 135f
  in traumatic brain injury, 43
Disc degeneration, low back pain and, 61
Disc extrusion, low back pain and, 59
Discharge planning, in stroke rehabilita-
    tion, 13–14
Disc herniation, low back pain and, 59
Discography, in low back pain, 64
Discriminant measures, of health status, 7
Disease modifying antirheumatic drugs
    (DMARDs), for rheumatoid arthri-
    tis, 207–209, 208t, 210
Disopyramide, for myotonia, 193, 194
Distal myopathy, hereditary, strengthen-
    ing exercise for, 182
Distance walked (WD), 120
Dorsal column stimulation, for phantom
    limb pain, 161–162
Dorsal root entry zone lesions, postampu-
    tation pain and, 162
Dothiepin, for fibromyalgia, 191
Doxepin
  for chronic pain, 112
    in back, 106
  for depression, in chronic airflow limi-
    tation, 134
Dry powder inhalers, for chronic airflow
    limitation, 125
Duchenne muscular dystrophy (DMD),
    172–173, 173f–176f, 175–176
  exercise in
    flexibility, 180–181
    strengthening, 181, 182f
  orthotics for, to prevent or correct
    deformities, 183–184
  pharmacologic therapy for, 192–193

Elastic crepe bandages, for swelling of
    residual limb following lower
    extremity amputation, 162–163
Elastic shrinker socks, for swelling of
    residual limb following lower
    extremity amputation, 162
Electrical stimulation. *See also* Functional
    electrical stimulation (FES); Tran-
    scutaneous electrical nerve stimu-
    lation (TENS)
  for arthritis, 216
  for muscle diseases, 181–182
Electromyographic feedback
  for acute low back pain, 80–81

for headaches, 101
Electromyography, in low back pain, 64
Employment
  following traumatic brain injury, 50–51
  prognosis of chronic pain and, 98
Energy conservation, for chronic airflow
    limitation, 133
Epidural injections
  for low back pain
    acute, 81–82
    chronic, 103
  for phantom limb pain, 159
Epidural scar tissue, low back pain and,
    59
Epidural venography, in low back pain, 63
Error
  false-negative, levels of evidence and,
    2
  false-positive, levels of evidence and, 2
Ethylchloride spray, for acute low back
    pain, 83
Etidronate disodium, for heterotopic ossi-
    fication, following traumatic brain
    injury, 47
Etodolac, for rheumatoid arthritis, 206t
Evaluation. *See* Assessment; Health status
    assessment
Evidence
  levels of, 1–4
    "Clinical Practice Guideline No. 16:
      Poststroke Rehabilitation" and,
      6–7
    grading of recommendations and,
      3–4, 4t
    nonexperimental, overestimation of
      treatment efficacy by, 1
Evidence-based practice, client-centered
    practice versus, 5–7
  levels of evidence and, 6–7
Exercise. *See also specific specific types of
    exercise*
  for arthritis, 214–215
  in cardiac rehabilitation. *See* Cardiac
    rehabilitation
  for chronic airflow limitation. *See* Pul-
    monary rehabilitation, exercise in
  for chronic pain, 103, 114
    in back, 103, 104
  for low back pain
    acute, 75–77, 103, 104
    chronic, 103, 104
  in lower extremity amputees, 163–165
  for muscle diseases. *See* Muscle dis-
    eases
Expanded disability status scale (EDSS),
    180
Expectorants, for chronic airflow limita-
    tion, 126

Extension exercises, for acute low back pain, 75–77

Facet injections
  for acute pain, in low back, 82
  for chronic pain, 103
Facet syndromes, low back pain and, 61
Facioscapulohumeral (FSH) dystrophy, 172, 176–177, 177f
  orthotics for, 184
Failed back, 59
False-negative error, levels of evidence and, 2
False-positive error, levels of evidence and, 2
Faradic stimulation, for arthritis, 216
Fenoprofen, for rheumatoid arthritis, 206t
Fibromyalgia (fibrositis)
  low back pain and, 60
  pharmacologic therapy for, 106–107, 190–192
Financial compensation, prognosis of chronic pain and, 98
Fish oil, for arthritis, 216
Flexeril. See Cyclobenzaprine (Flexeril)
Flex Foot, 166–167
Flexibility exercise, for muscle diseases, 180–181
Flucloxacillin, following lower extremity amputation, 157, 158t
Flunarizine, for Duchenne muscular dystrophy, 193
Fluoxetine, for fibromyalgia, 191
Flurbiprofen, for rheumatoid arthritis, 206t
Forced expiratory volume in 1 second (FEV$_1$), 120
Foreign body removal, in spinal cord injury, 21
Functional approach, to cognitive remediation, 48
Functional electrical stimulation (FES), for spinal cord injury, 26–27
  lower extremity stimulation using, 26–27
  upper extremity stimulation using, 27
Functional Independence Measure (FIM), 43

Gait
  In Duchenne muscular dystrophy, 175
  in poliomyelitis, 178
  in polyneuropathies, 178
Gamma globulin, intravenous, for inflammatory myopathies, 195
Gangliosides, for acute spinal cord injury, 22–23

Gender differences
  in chronic pain treatment outcomes, 99
  in complications following spinal cord injury, 25
Glucocorticoids, for osteoarthritis, 210
Glucose intolerance, exercise training and, 144
Glycerine, trigger point and local injections of, for acute low back pain, 83
GM$_1$-ganglioside, for acute spinal cord injury, 22–23
Goal setting
  for pulmonary rehabilitation, 134
  for stroke rehabilitation, 12, 12t
Gower's sign, In Duchenne muscular dystrophy, 172, 173f–175f
Ground reaction force (GRF), ankle-foot systems and, 166

Handicap
  in chronic airflow limitation, measurement of, 120–122, 123
  definition of, 119
    World Health Organization, 7
  measurement of, 224
  as motivating factor, 7
  severity of, pulmonary rehabilitation and, 134, 136f
  in traumatic brain injury, 43
Headaches
  chronic, 107–108
    detoxification for, 107–108
    physical therapies for, 108
    prophylaxis of, 108
    psychological treatment of, 108
    treatment of, 114
  migraine
    relaxation therapy for, 100–101
    treatment of, 102
  tension
    biofeedback for, 101
    relaxation therapy for, 101
    treatment of, 100
Head injury. See Traumatic brain injury (TBI) rehabilitation
Head Injury Interdisciplinary Special Interest Group (HI SIG), 41
Health status assessment, 7–8
  discriminant measures for, 7
  evaluative measures for, 8
  future directions for, 224
  prediction of risk-adjusted outcomes using, 8
  predictive measures for, 7–8
  standardized measures for, 8
Heart disease. See Cardiac rehabilitation

Heart rate, oxygen uptake and, 141–142, 142f
Heat therapy, for arthritis, 215–216
Heel-cord shortening, In Duchenne muscular dystrophy, 175
Hepatotoxicity, of dantrolene sodium, 31
Heterocyclic antidepressants, for chronic pain, 106
Heterotopic ossification, following traumatic brain injury, treatment of, 47
High-density lipoprotein (HDL) cholesterol, exercise training and, 143
History taking, in low back pain, 62
Home-based rehabilitation, for traumatic brain injury, 49–50
Hoover test, in low back pain, 62
Hope, medical uses of, 227
Hospital-based rehabilitation, for traumatic brain injury, limitations of, 49–50
Hospitalization
  length of stay and, for spinal cord injury, 20
  reduction in, pulmonary rehabilitation and, 134–135
Hot packs, for arthritis, 216
Hyaluranon, for osteoarthritis, 212
Hyaluronic acid, for osteoarthritis, 212
Hydrocodone, for acute low back pain, 72
Hydrocortisone, for headaches, 107, 114
Hydrotherapy, for arthritis, 215
Hydroxychloroquine, for rheumatoid arthritis, 208–209
5-Hydroxy-L-tryptophan, for fibromyalgia, 191
Hypertension, exercise training and, 143–144
Hypnosis, for chronic pain, 101–102

Ibuprofen
  for fibromyalgia, 191
  for heterotopic ossification following traumatic brain injury, 47
  for osteoarthritis, 211
  for rheumatoid arthritis, 206, 206t
Ice packs, for arthritis, 216
Iliac crest pain syndrome, local injections for, 83
Ilioconduit, in spinal cord-injured men, 25
Imagery, for headaches, 101
Imaging, in low back pain, 63–64
Imipramine
  for fibromyalgia, 191
  for myotonia, 194
Immediate postoperative prosthetic fitting (IPOP), 153–154, 155, 157t

Immunomodulators, for rheumatoid arthritis, 209
Immunosuppressants. *See also specific drugs*
    for inclusion body myositis, 195
    for inflammatory myopathies, 195
    for rheumatoid arthritis, 209
Impairment
    definition of, 119
        World Health Organization, 7
    determination of nature and severity of, in stroke rehabilitation, 11
    severity of, pulmonary rehabilitation and, 134
    in traumatic brain injury, 43
Inclusion body myositis, pharmacologic therapy for, 195
Indomethacin
    for heterotopic ossification following traumatic brain injury, 47
    for osteoarthritis, 211–212
    for rheumatoid arthritis, 206, 206t
Indwelling catheters, in spinal cord injury, 24–25
Infection, following lower extremity amputation, treatment of, 157–158, 158t
Inflammatory myopathies, orthotics for, 184–185
Infrared therapy
    for acute low back pain, 77
    for arthritis, 216
Inotropic drugs, for chronic airflow limitation, 126
Intermittent catheterization, in spinal cord injury, 24
International Classification of Impairment, Disability and Handicap (ICIDH), 7
Intra-articular therapy, for osteoarthritis, 212
Intrathecal treatment, for spasticity following spinal cord injury, 32
Intravenous gamma globulin, for inflammatory myopathies, 195
Isokinetic exerciser, for muscle diseases, 181, 182f
Isometric exercise
    for acute low back pain, 75
    for lower extremity amputees, 165

Ketoprofen
    for osteoarthritis, 211
    for rheumatoid arthritis, 206t
Ketorolac, for rheumatoid arthritis, 206t
Kidney stones, in spinal cord injury, 24
Knee-ankle-foot orthoses, for muscle diseases, 184–185

Kyphoscoliosis, In Duchenne muscular dystrophy, 176

Laser therapy, for arthritis, 216
Left ventricular function, following exercise training, 143
Leucine, for Duchenne muscular dystrophy, 193
Leucovorin, for inclusion body myositis, 195
Levels of evidence, 1–4
    "Clinical Practice Guideline No. 16: Poststroke Rehabilitation" and, 6–7
    grading of recommendations and, 3–4, 4t
Lidocaine, trigger point and local injections of, for acute low back pain, 83
Lignocaine, trigger point and local injections of, for acute low back pain, 83
Lioresal. *See* Baclofen (Lioresal)
Lipids, serum, exercise training and, 143
Lithium
    for chronic pain, 112
        with depression, 109
    for fibromyalgia, 191
    for myotonia, 194
Liver, hepatotoxicity of dantrolene sodium and, 31
Local anesthetics
    epidural injections of
        for acute low back pain, 81–82
        for phantom limb pain, 159
    facet injections of
        for acute low back pain, 82
        for chronic pain, 103
    local injections of, for acute low back pain, 83
    trigger point injections of, for acute low back pain, 83
Lorazepam, for behavioral problems following traumatic brain injury, 47
Lordosis, In Duchenne muscular dystrophy, 173, 175, 175f–176f
Low back pain, 55–92
    acute. *See* Acute low back pain
    causes of, 59–61
        arachnoid and epidural scar, 59
        bursitis, 61
        degenerative, 60
        disc degeneration, 61
        disc herniation and/or extrusion, 59
        facet syndromes, 61
        piriformis syndrome, 61
        rheumatologic, 59–60

        sacroiliac joint syndrome, 61
        segmental instability, 61
        spinal stenosis, 60
        spondylolysis and spondylolisthesis, 60–61
    chronic. *See* Chronic low back pain
    clinical syndromes and, 56–57, 57f, 57t, 58–59
        acute lumbago, 58
        chronic back pain, 58
        failed back, 59
        recurrent mechanical back pain, 58
        sciatica, 58
        spinal claudication, 59
    clinicopathologic taxonomy of, 56–58
        clinical syndromes and, 56–57, 57f, 57t
        heuristic diagnosis and, 57–58, 58t
        hypothetical conditions and, 58
    diagnostic methods for, 61–64
        electromyography, 64
        history taking, 62
        imaging, 63–64
        physical examination, 62
    literature search on, 55–56, 56t
    manipulation for, 104–105
    physical modalities for, 103–104
    structural diagnoses for, 56–57, 57f, 57t
Low-density lipoprotein (LDL) cholesterol, exercise training and, 143
Lower extremities
    amputation of. *See* Lower extremity amputations
    functional electrical stimulation of, in spinal cord injury, 26–27
Lower extremity amputations, 153–168
    above-knee, open versus locked knee prostheses for, 165
    controlled environment treatment for, 157
    exercise following, 163–165
    phantom limb pain following, 159–162, 163t
        β-adrenergic blockade for, 160
        algorithm for treatment of, 164f
        antidepressants for, 160–161
        calcitonin for, 159
        carbamazepine for, 160
        dorsal column stimulation for, 161–162
        dorsal root entry zone lesions and, 162
        epidural block for, 159
        mexiletine for, 159–160
        peripheral stimulation for, 161
        relaxation training for, 162
    pneumatic sleeve for, 157, 157t
    prosthetic ankle and foot, 166–167

prosthetic sockets for
  computer aided design and manufacture of, 167–168
  contoured adducted trochanteric controlled alignment method, 165–166
  normal shape/normal alignment, 165
  quadrilateral versus CAT-CAM, 165–166
  residual limb healing following antibiotics and, 157–158, 158t
    nutritional status and, 158
  residual limb pain following, 158–159
  residual limb volume reduction and, 162–163
  rigid plaster cast versus soft dressing and weight-bearing for, 153–156, 156t
  weight-bearing and, timing of, 156
Lumbago, acute, 58
Lumbar corsets, for acute low back pain, 79–80
Lung function. See also Pulmonary rehabilitation
  impairment of, measurement of, 120

Machines
  Cybex isokinetic exerciser, for muscle diseases, 181, 182f
  microdyne, for arthritis, 216
  placebo effect of, 226
  Tru Trac apparatus, for acute low back pain, 73–74
McKenzie extension exercises, for acute low back pain, 75–76
Magnesium choline salicylate, for rheumatoid arthritis, 206t
Magnetic resonance imaging (MRI), in low back pain, 63
Malignancies, in dermatomyositis, 172
Malnutrition
  in chronic airflow limitation, 131–132
  residual limb healing following lower extremity amputation and, 158
Management plan, for stroke rehabilitation, 12–13, 13t
Manipulation
  for acute pain, in low back, 74–75, 76–77, 103
  for chronic pain, 102, 114
  in low back, 104–105
Maprotiline, for fibromyalgia, 191
Marcaine, facet injections of, for acute low back pain, 82
Massage, for acute low back pain, 77, 104
Maximum exercise capacity (Wmax), 120

Mazindol, for Duchenne muscular dystrophy, 193
Meclofenamate sodium, for rheumatoid arthritis, 206t
Memory loss, following traumatic brain injury, 45
Metabolic exercise, for muscle diseases, 183
Metaxalone, for muscle spasm, 187
Metered-dose inhalers, for chronic airflow limitation, 125
Methenamine, for urinary tract infection prophylaxis, 25, 26
Methocarbamol, for muscle spasm, 187–188
Methotrexate
  for inclusion body myositis, 195
  for inflammatory myopathies, 195
  for rheumatoid arthritis, 208t, 208–209
Methylprednisolone
  for acute spinal cord injury, 22, 23
  epidural injections of, for acute low back pain, 81
  facet injections of, for acute low back pain, 82
  for rheumatoid arthritis, 209
Methylxanthines, for chronic airflow limitation, 125
Methysergide, for Duchenne muscular dystrophy, 193
Meticillin, following lower extremity amputation, 158t
Metoprolol
  for headaches, 108
  for phantom limb pain, 160
Mexiletine
  for myotonia, 193, 194
  for phantom limb pain, 159–160
Microdyne machines, for arthritis, 216
Migraine headaches
  relaxation therapy for, 100–101
  treatment of, 102
Milgram test, in low back pain, 62
Minnesota Multiphasic Personality Inventory (MMPI), employability following traumatic brain injury measured by, 51
Mobilization
  for chronic pain, 114
  early, in stroke rehabilitation, 10
Molded body jackets, for Duchenne muscular dystrophy, 184
Monitoring, of progress in stroke rehabilitation, 13
Monoamine oxidase inhibitors (MAOIs). See also specific drugs
  for chronic pain, 106, 113

with depression, 109
for headaches, 108
Morphine
  derivatives of, for acute low back pain, 72
  epidural block using, for phantom limb pain, 159
  for spasticity following spinal cord injury, 32
Motivation
  degree of handicap and, 7
  for pulmonary rehabilitation, 134
MRI, in low back pain, 63
Mucolytics, for chronic airflow limitation, 126
Multidisciplinary team care
  in chronic airflow limitation, 123–124
  in stroke rehabilitation, 10
  in traumatic brain injury. See Traumatic brain injury (TBI) rehabilitation
Multimodal pain programs, 93–99, 113f, 113–114
  for chronic pain, 101–102
  long-term outcome with, 96–97
  pain prevention and, 98
  prognostic factors and, 97–98
  randomized controlled trials and
    chronic low back pain diagnosis and, 95–96
    mixed chronic pain diagnoses and, 94–95
  trials using untreated control groups and, 93–94
Multiple sclerosis, 179–180
  exercise in, flexibility, 181
  orthotics for, 184
  strengthening exercise for, 182
Muscle cramps, pharmacologic therapy for, 190
Muscle diseases, 171–195. See also specific diseases
  exercise for, 180–183
    in acute anterior poliomyelitis, 178–179, 179f, 180f
    aerobic or metabolic training, 183
    flexibility, 180–181
    strengthening, 181–183
  inflammatory versus hereditary, 171–177
    muscular dystrophies and, 172t, 172–177
    polymyositis and, 171–172
  multiple sclerosis, 179–180
  neurogenic, 177–179
    acute anterior poliomyelitis, 178–189
    peripheral neuropathy, 177–178
  orthotics for, 183–185

Muscle diseases *(Continued)*
  to prevent or correct deformities,
    183–184
  for weakness, 184–185
  pharmacologic therapy for, 187–195
    for Duchenne muscular dystrophy,
      192–193
    for fibromyalgia, 190–192
    for inclusion body myositis, 195
    for inflammatory myopathies,
      194–195
    for muscle cramp, 190
    for muscle spasm, 187–190, 189f
    for myotonia, 193–194
Muscle relaxants
  for acute pain, in low back, 70–72
  for chronic pain, 114
  for muscle spasm, 187–190, 189f
Muscle spasm, muscle relaxants for,
  187–190, 189f
Muscular dystrophies, 172, 172t. *See also*
  Duchenne muscular dystrophy
    (DMD)
  Becker's, strengthening exercise in, 181
  facioscapulohumeral, 172, 176–177,
    177f
  orthotics for, 184
Myelography, in low back pain, 63
Myelotomy, for spasticity following spinal
  cord injury, 33
Myocardial perfusion, following exercise
  training, 143
Myolastan (Tetrazepam), for acute low
  back pain, 71–72
Myopathy, inflammatory. *See also specific
  disorders*
  pharmacologic therapy for, 194–195
Myositis, inclusion body, pharmacologic
  therapy for, 195
Myotonia, pharmacologic therapy for,
  193–194

Nabumetone, for rheumatoid arthritis,
  206t
Naffziger test, in low back pain, 62
Naproxen
  for osteoarthritis, 211
  for rheumatoid arthritis, 206t
Narcotic agents. *See also specific drugs*
  for acute low back pain, 72–73, 76–77
  for chronic airflow limitation, 126
  epidural injections of
    for acute low back pain, 81–82
    for phantom limb pain, 159
  for osteoarthritis, 211
National Acute Spinal Cord Injury Studies
  (NASCIS), 22, 23

Neurectomy, for spasticity following
  spinal cord injury, 33
Neurogenic bladder management. *See*
  Spinal cord injury (SCI), neuro-
    genic bladder management for
Neurogenic muscle weakness, 177–179
  in acute anterior poliomyelitis, 178–179
  in peripheral neuropathy, 177–178
Neurological function, surgery to
    improve, in spinal cord injury. *See*
    Spinal cord injury (SCI), surgical
    treatment of
Neuromuscular atrophy, 177–178
Neuropathies
  acquired, 178
  inherited, 177–178
Neuroprobes, for arthritis, 216
Nifedipine
  for Duchenne muscular dystrophy, 193
  for myotonia, 194
Nocturnal Oxygen Therapy Trial, 126
Nonexperimental evidence, overestima-
    tion of treatment efficacy by, 1
Nonsteroidal anti-inflammatory drugs
    (NSAIDs)
  for acute low back pain, 69, 70, 103
  for fibromyalgia, 191, 192
  for heterotopic ossification following
    traumatic brain injury, 47
  for osteoarthritis, 210–211, 210–212
  for rheumatoid arthritis, 206t, 206–207,
    209
Norflex. *See* Orphenadrine (Norflex)
Normal shape/normal alignment sockets
    (NSNA), 165
Nortriptyline, for phantom limb pain,
    160–161
Nutrition
  in arthritis, 216–217
  in chronic airflow limitation, 131–132
  measurement of nutritional impairment
    and, 122
  residual limb healing following lower
    extremity amputation and, 158

Obesity, in chronic airflow limitation, 131
Operant conditioning, for chronic pain,
    101–102
Opioids. *See* Narcotic agents; *specific spe-
    cific drugs*
Orgotein, for osteoarthritis, 212
Oropharyngeal drug deposition, for
    chronic airflow limitation, 125
Orphenadrine (Norflex)
  for acute low back pain, 70–71
  for muscle cramps, 190
  for muscle spasm, 189

Orthotics
  for acute low back pain, 79–80
  for arthritis, 213–214
  for muscle diseases
    to prevent or correct deformities,
      183–184
    for weakness, 184–185
Ossification, heterotopic, following trau-
    matic brain injury, treatment of, 47
Osteoarthritis (OA), 203. *See also* Arthritis
  pharmacologic therapy for, 210–212
  prognosis of, 212
  research on, 203–205, 204t
Osteochondritis, vertebral, 60
Osteochondrosis, low back pain and, 60
Osteopathic manipulation, for acute low
    back pain, 74, 77
Outcomes
  criteria for, in traumatic brain injury, 41
  measures of, 223, 224
    in stroke rehabilitation, 14
    of traumatic brain injury rehabilita-
      tion, 46
  of multimodal pain programs, gender
    differences in, 99
  risk-adjusted, predicting, 8
    in stroke rehabilitation, 11–12
  values and, 223
Oxaprozin, for rheumatoid arthritis, 206t
Oxygen therapy, for chronic airflow limi-
    tation, 126–127
  with exercise, 126–127
Oxygen uptake, heart rate and, 141–142,
    142f

Pain
  acute. *See also* Acute low back pain
    algorithm for management of,
      109–110
  algorithms for management of, 109–114
    acute pain and, 109–110
    persistent pain and, 111–113, 112f
    subacute pain and, 110, 111f
  in back. *See* Acute low back pain;
      Chronic low back pain; Low back
      pain
  chronic. *See* Chronic low back pain;
      Chronic pain; Multimodal pain
      programs; Unimodal chronic pain
      therapies
  phantom limb. *See* Lower extremity
      amputations, phantom limb pain
      following
  in residual limb following lower
      extremity amputation, 158–159
  subacute, algorithm for management
      of, 110, 111f

Panic disorders, in chronic airflow limitation, 122
  psychosocial interventions for, 133–134
Paracetamol, for acute low back pain, 69, 103
Paraplegia. *See also* Spinal cord injury (SCI)
  thoracic, incomplete, surgical decompression in, 20–21
Patient education
  for chronic low back pain, 103
  in pulmonary rehabilitation, 132
Pelvic traction, for acute low back pain, 73–74
Penicillamine
  for Duchenne muscular dystrophy, 192
  for rheumatoid arthritis, 208, 208t
Penicillin, following lower extremity amputation, 158t
Peripheral muscle function, measurement of, 122
Peripheral muscle training, for chronic airflow limitation, 127–128
Peripheral neuropathies, orthotics for, 185
Peripheral stimulation, for phantom limb pain, 161
Peroneal atrophy, 177–178
Persistent pain. *See* Chronic low back pain; Chronic pain; Multimodal pain programs; Unimodal chronic pain therapies
Personality, type A, 144–145
Phantom limb pain. *See* Lower extremity amputations, phantom limb pain following
Pharmacologic therapy. *See also specific drugs and drug types*
  for acute low back pain. *See* Acute low back pain, nonsurgical treatment of
  for acute spinal cord injury, 22–23
  for behavioral problems following traumatic brain injury, 47
  for chronic airflow limitation. *See* Pulmonary rehabilitation, pharmacologic therapy in
  for chronic pain, 102, 105–109, 111–113, 114
    analgesics for, 106–107
    antidepressants for, 105–106
    in back, 106
    with depression, 108–109
    in fibromyalgia, 106–107
    in headache, 107–108
    in low back, 103, 106
  for heterotopic ossification following traumatic brain injury, 47

  for muscle diseases. *See* Muscle diseases, pharmacologic therapy for
  for osteoarthritis, 210–212
  for post-traumatic seizures, 46–47
  for spasticity
    following spinal cord injury, 27–32, 29t
    following traumatic brain injury, 47
Phenothiazines, for fibromyalgia, 191, 192
Phenylbutazone, for rheumatoid arthritis, 206t
Phenytoin (diphenylhydantoin)
  for myotonia, 193–194, 194
  for post-traumatic seizures, 46
Physical examination, in low back pain, 62
Physical modalities. *See also specific modalities*
  for acute pain, in low back, 76–77
  for arthritis, 215–216
  for chronic pain, 103–104, 114
  for headaches, 108
Piriformis syndrome, low back pain and, 61
Piroxicam
  for acute low back pain, 69
  for rheumatoid arthritis, 206t
Pizotyline, for headaches, 108
Placebo effect, 225–226
  of machines, 226
Plain radiographs, in low back pain, 63
Plaster casts, following lower extremity amputations, 153–156, 156t
Pneumatic sleeve, for residual limb following lower extremity amputation, 157, 157t
Poliomyelitis
  anterior, acute, 178–179
    post-polio syndrome and, 178
    weight training and exercise effects in, 178–179, 179f, 180f
  orthotics for, 184
Polymyalgia rheumatica, low back pain and, 60
Polymyositis, 171–172
  prednisone for, 194
  rest for, 172
Polyneuropathies
  acquired, 178
  inherited, 177–178
Popeye arm, in facioscapulohumeral dystrophy, 177, 177f
Post-polio syndrome, 178
Post-traumatic amnesia (PTA), 45
Predictive measures, of health status, 7–8
Prednisone
  for Duchenne muscular dystrophy, 192, 193

  for fibromyalgia, 191
  for inclusion body myositis, 195
  for inflammatory myopathies, 195
  for myotonia, 193, 194
  for polymyositis/dermatomyositis, 194
  for rheumatoid arthritis, 209
Primer on the Rheumatic Diseases, 171
Procaine, epidural injections of, for acute low back pain, 81
Procaine amide, for myotonia, 193, 194
Process approach, to cognitive remediation, 47
Prolonged unresponsiveness, sensory stimulation for, 44
Propoxyphene, for osteoarthritis, 211
Propranolol
  for chronic pain, 102
  for headaches, 108
  for phantom limb pain, 160
Prostheses, for lower extremity amputees. *See* Lower extremity amputations
Psychological factors. *See also* Anxiety; Depression
  exercise training and, 144–145
  prognosis of chronic pain and, 98
Psychological therapy
  for chronic airflow limitation, 133–134
  for chronic pain, 99–102, 113
    with depression, 109
  for headaches, 101, 108
  supportive, for chronic pain, 100, 113
Psychosocial adjustment, measurement of, 122
Psychosocial Adjustment to Illness Scale (PAIS-SR), 122
Pulmonary rehabilitation, 119–136
  breathing retraining and control in, 132–133
  definitions in, 119–120
  energy conservation in, 133
  exercise in, 127–130
    combined rehabilitation and ventilatory muscle training and, 130
    general exercise training and, 127
    with oxygen therapy, 126–127
    specific peripheral muscle training and, 127–128
    strength training and, 128–129
    ventilatory muscle training and, 129–130
  general education in, 132
  improvement in hospitalizations, cost, and survival due to, 134–135
  literature review and, 122–123
  measurements in, 120–122
    of disability, 120, 121f
    of handicap, 120–122
    of lung function impairment, 120

Pulmonary rehabilitation (Continued)
    of nutritional impairment, 122
    of peripheral muscle function, 122
    of psychosocial adjustment prob-
        lems, 122
    of respiratory muscle function, 122
    of respiratory ventricular dysfunc-
        tion, 122
    motivation and goal setting for, 134
    multidisciplinary, 123–124
    nutrition and, 131–132
    pharmacologic therapy in, 125–127
        bronchodilators in, 125–126
        oxygen in, 126–127
        steroids in, 126
    psychosocial interventions in, 133–134
    severity of impairment, disability, and
        handicap and, 134, 135f, 136f
    ventilatory muscle rest in, 130–131
Pursed-lip breathing, for chronic airflow
    limitation, 132

Quadrilateral sockets, 165
Quadriplegia. See also Spinal cord injury
        (SCI)
    complete, functional recovery in, 19–20
Quality of life, measurement of, 224
Quick Reference Guide for Clinicians, 8
Quinine
    for muscle cramps, 190
    for myotonia, 193

Radiographs, plain, in low back pain, 63
Randomized controlled trials (RCTs)
    with high false-positive and/or high
        false-negative errors, 2
    with low false-positive and/or low
        false-negative errors, 2
    for multimodal pain programs, 94–96
        chronic low back pain diagnosis
            and, 95–96
        mixed chronic pain diagnoses and,
            94–95
    subgroup analyses in, 2–3
    for traumatic brain injury rehabilitation,
        42
Recommendations, grading of, 3–4, 4t
Rehabilitation, definition of, 119
REHABT, 47
Relaxation training
    for chronic pain, 100–102
    for phantom limb pain, 162
Respiratory muscle function, measure-
    ment of, 122
Respiratory rehabilitation. See Pulmonary
    rehabilitation

Respiratory stimulants, for chronic airflow
    limitation, 126
Respiratory tract
    involvement in Duchenne muscular
        dystrophy, 176
    ventricular dysfunction of, measure-
        ment of, 122
Rest
    for acute low back pain, 68–69, 77,
        103, 104
    for arthritis, 213
    for polymyositis/dermatomyositis,
        172
Rheumatoid arthritis (RA), 203. See also
        Arthritis
    dietary manipulation for, 216
    low back pain and, 60
    pharmacologic therapy for, 205–209
        corticosteroids in, 209
        disease modifying antirheumatic
            drugs in, 207–209, 208t
        nonsteroidal anti-inflammatory drugs
            in, 206t, 206–207
        pyramidal approach to, 205f,
            205–206, 209
    prognosis of, 209–210
    research on, 203–205, 204t
Rheumatologic disease. See also specific
        disorders
    low back pain and, 59–60
Rhizotomy, anterior, for spasticity follow-
        ing spinal cord injury, 32
Right ventricular dysfunction, measure-
        ment of, 122
Risk-adjusted outcomes, predicting, 8
    in stroke rehabilitation, 11–12
Rumalon, for osteoarthritis, 212

SACH foot, 167
Sacroiliac joint syndrome, low back pain
        and, 61
Sacroiliitis, low back pain and, 59
St. George's Respiratory Questionnaire,
        121
Salicylate, for rheumatoid arthritis, 207
Salsalate, for rheumatoid arthritis, 206t
Scar tissue, arachnoid and epidural, low
        back pain and, 59
Scheuermann's disease, low back pain
        and, 60
Sciatica, 58
Scoliosis, in Duchenne muscular dystro-
        phy, spinal orthotics for, 184
Seattle Foot, 166–167
Sedatives, for fibromyalgia, 191, 192
Segmental instability, low back pain and,
        61

Seizures, following traumatic brain injury,
        treatment of, 46–47
Selective serotonin reuptake inhibitors
        (SSRIs)
    for chronic pain, 106, 112
        with depression, 109
    for headaches, 108
Selenium, for myotonia, 194
Sensory stimulation, for coma and vegeta-
        tive state, 44
Sensory Stimulation Assessment Measure
        (SSAM), 44
Septra (sulfamethoxazole), for urinary
        tract infection prophylaxis, 25, 26
Serum lipids, exercise training and, 143
Settings, for traumatic brain injury rehabil-
        itation, 42
Shuttle walking test, 120
Sickness Impact Profile, 120–121
Single-case experimental designs, for
        traumatic brain injury rehabilita-
        tion, 42
Skeletal hyperostosis, idiopathic, diffuse,
        low back pain and, 60
Sockets, prosthetic. See Lower extremity
        amputations
Sodium valproate
    for behavioral problems following trau-
        matic brain injury, 47
    for post-traumatic seizures, 46–47
Soft dressings, following lower extremity
        amputations, 153–156, 156t
Soma. See Carisoprodol (Soma)
Somatic amplification, in low back pain,
        clinical tests for, 62
Somatoform disorders, chronic pain in,
        treatment of, 100
Spacer devices, for chronic airflow limita-
        tion, 125
Spasticity
    following spinal cord injury. See Spinal
        cord injury (SCI), spasticity in
    following traumatic brain injury, treat-
        ment of, 47
Spinal claudication, 59
    spinal stenosis as cause of, 60
Spinal cord injury (SCI), 19–34
    functional electrical stimulation for,
        26–27
        lower extremity, 26–27
        upper extremity, 27
    neurogenic bladder management for,
        23–26
        asymptomatic bacteriuria treatment
            and, 26
        bladder emptying and, 23–25
        urinary tract infection prophylaxis
            and, 25–26

pattern of recovery following, 19–20
pharmacologic treatment during acute phase, 22–23
sequence of events during acute phase of, 22
spasticity in, treatment of, 27–34
  intrathecal, 32
  pharmacologic, 27–32, 29t
  spinal cord stimulation for, 33–34
  surgical, 32–33
surgical intervention for, 19–22
  decompression to improve neurological outcome, 19–21
  for foreign body removal, 21
  for spasticity, 32–33
  timing of, 21–22
surgical treatment of, for neurogenic bladder, 23
Spinal cord stimulation (SCS), for spasticity, 33–34
Spinal manipulation. See Manipulation
Spinal orthoses, for Duchenne muscular dystrophy, 184
Spinal stenosis, low back pain and, 60
Splints, for arthritis, 213–214
Spondylolisthesis, low back pain and, 61
Spondylolysis, low back pain and, 60–61
Spondylosis deformans, low back pain and, 60
Standardized measures, 8
Standing, in spinal cord injury, functional electrical stimulation to facilitate, 26–27
Standing devices, for Duchenne muscular dystrophy, 183–184
Steroids. See also Corticosteroids; specific steroids
  for chronic airflow limitation, 126
  for Duchenne muscular dystrophy, 192, 193
  epidural injections of
    for acute low back pain, 81–82
    for chronic low back pain, 103
  facet injections of
    for acute low back pain, 82
    for chronic pain, 103
  for fibromyalgia, 191
  for inclusion body myositis, 195
  for myotonia, 193, 194
  oral, for acute low back pain, 73
  trigger point and local injections of, for acute low back pain, 83
Stimulants, respiratory, for chronic airflow limitation, 126
Stooptest, in low back pain, 62
Straight leg raising test, for sciatica, 58
Strategy issues, 224

Strengthening exercise
  for chronic airflow limitation, 128–129
  for muscle diseases, 181–183
    active strengthening exercises, 182
    decision making regarding, 182–183
    electrical stimulation and, 181–182
    isokinetic exerciser for, 181, 182f
Stress-coping training, for headaches, 100–101
Stroke rehabilitation, 5–14
  in acute setting, 9
  client-based versus evidence-based practice and, 5–7
    levels of evidence and, 6–7
  clinical data set for, 8–9
    contents of, 9, 9t
  clinical decision-making steps in, 10–14, 11f
    determination of nature and severity of problems, 11
    discharge planning and outcome evaluation, 13–14
    initial data gathering, 10
    management plan development and selection of specific interventions, 12–13, 13t
    prediction of risk-adjusted outcomes, 11–12
    reintegration into community, 14
    treatment goal development, 12, 12t
    treatment provision and monitoring, 13
    treatment target specification, 13
  health status assessment and. See Health status assessment
  setting for, choice of, 10
  World Health Organization classification and, 7
Subgroup analysis, 2–3
Sulfamethoxazole (Septra), for urinary tract infection prophylaxis, 25, 26
Sulfasalazine, for rheumatoid arthritis, 208t, 208–209
Sulindac, for rheumatoid arthritis, 206t
Supported employment, for traumatic brain injury patients, 51
Supportive therapy, for chronic pain, 100, 113
Surgical treatment
  for back pain, failed back and, 59
  for heterotopic ossification following traumatic brain injury, 47
  for spinal cord injury. See Spinal cord injury (SCI), surgical treatment of
Survival, increased, pulmonary rehabilitation and, 135

Swelling, of residual limb following lower extremity amputation, 162
Sympathomimetics, for chronic airflow limitation, 125

Taurine
  for muscle cramps, 190
  for myotonia, 194
Team, multidisciplinary. See Multidisciplinary team care
TENS/Codetron treatments, for acute low back pain, 78
Tension headaches. See Headaches, tension
Tetrazepam (myolastan), for acute low back pain, 71–72
Theophylline, for chronic airflow limitation, 125–126
Therapies. See Treatment entries; specific treatments
Therapist, vital role played by, 226
Thermal biofeedback, for chronic pain, 102
Thermography, in low back pain, 64
Thermotherapy, for acute low back pain, 104
Thoracolumbosacral orthoses, for Duchenne muscular dystrophy, 184
Tirilazad, for acute spinal cord injury, 23
Tizanidine, for spasticity following spinal cord injury, 29t, 31, 32
Tocainide, for myotonia, 193
Toe-walking, In Duchenne muscular dystrophy, 175
Tolmetin, for rheumatoid arthritis, 206t
Traction, for acute low back pain, 3–74
Training, treatments versus, 226–227
Transcutaneous electrical nerve stimulation (TENS)
  for acute pain, in low back, 77–78
  for arthritis, 216
  for chronic pain, 101–102
  for phantom limb pain, 161
Traumatic brain injury (TBI) rehabilitation, 41–51
  acute phase of, 45
  behavioral problems and, 47
  cognitive remediation in, 47–49
    functional approach to, 48
    process approach to, 47
    questions concerning, 48–49
    research on, 47–48
  coma and vegetative state and, 44
    early treatment of, 44
    sensory stimulation for, 44

Traumatic brain injury (TBI) rehabilitation *(Continued)*
  community-based, 49–50
  experimental design for, 42–43
  heterogeneity of client problems in, 42
  heterotopic ossification and, 47
  literature review of, 43
  multiple environments and disciplines in treatment of, 42
  outcome criteria for, controversy regarding, 41
  recovery and
    biologic constraints limiting, 42
    natural, duration of, 42
  research in clinical decision making in, 43
  return to work and, 50–51
  seizures and, 46–47
  spasticity and, 47
  traditional multidisciplinary programs for, 45–46
    basic questions concerning, 45
    complex factors in, 46
    early rehabilitation and, 45–46
    intensity of intervention and, 46
    outcome measures for, 46
Trazodone, for chronic pain, 112
  with depression, 109
Treatment. *See also specific treatments*
  efficacy of, 224–225
    overestimation by nonexperimental evidence, 1
    training versus, 226–227
Treatment goals
  for pulmonary rehabilitation, 134
  for stroke rehabilitation, 12, 12t
Treatment targets, for stroke rehabilitation, 13
Triamcinolone, epidural injections of, for acute low back pain, 81
Triaprofenic acid, for fibromyalgia, 191
Tricyclic antidepressants (TCAs). *See also specific drugs*
  for chronic pain, 100, 105–106, 111–112, 114
    with depression, 109
  for depression, in chronic airflow limitation, 134

for fibromyalgia, 106–107, 190–191
  for headaches, 108
  for myotonia, 194
  for phantom limb pain, 160–161
Trigger point injections, for acute low back pain, 83
Tru Trac apparatus, for acute low back pain, 73–74
Type A personality disorder, 144–145

Ultrasound
  for acute low back pain, 76–77
  for arthritis, 216
Uniform Data Set for Medical Rehabilitation (UDS$_{MR}$), 8–9
Unimodal chronic pain therapies, 99–101
  biofeedback training, 101
  relaxation, 100–101
Unresponsiveness, prolonged, sensory stimulation for, 44
Upper extremities
  functional electrical stimulation of, in spinal cord injury, 27
  Popeye arm, in facioscapulohumeral dystrophy, 177, 177f
Urinary tract infections (UTIs), in spinal cord injury, 25–26
  prophylaxis of, 25–26
  treatment of, 26

Valproic acid. *See also* Sodium valproate
  for behavioral problems following traumatic brain injury, 47
  for post-traumatic seizures, 46–47
Values, outcomes and, 223
Vegetative state, 44
  early treatment for, 44
  sensory stimulation for, 44
Venlafaxine, for chronic pain, with depression, 109
Venography, epidural, in low back pain, 63
Ventilatory muscle rest, for chronic airflow limitation, 130–131
Ventilatory muscles
  impairment of, nutrition and, 131

training of, for chronic airflow limitation, 129–130
Verapamil
  for muscle cramps, 190
  for myotonia, 194
Vertebral osteochondritis, low back pain and, 60
Vibratory stimulation, for phantom limb pain, 161
Viscosupplementation, for osteoarthritis, 212
Vitamin E
  for Duchenne muscular dystrophy, 192–193
  for muscle cramps, 190
  for myotonia, 194
Vocational rehabilitation, following traumatic brain injury, 50–51

Wax baths, for arthritis, 216
Weakness, muscular, 177–179
  in acute anterior poliomyelitis, 178–179
  in peripheral neuropathy, 177–178
Weight-bearing, following lower extremity amputations, timing of, 153–156, 156t
Weight-lifting belts, for acute low back pain, 79
Weight loss, in chronic airflow limitation, 131–132
Weight training, in acute anterior poliomyelitis, 178–179, 179f, 180f
Work
  prognosis of chronic pain and, 98
  return to, following traumatic brain injury, 50–51
World Health Organization (WHO), International Classification of Impairment, Disability and Handicap of, 7, 119
Wound infection, following lower extremity amputation, treatment of, 157–158, 158t

Zopiclone, for fibromyalgia, 191